T0073680

Advance Praise for *When Brains Meet Buildings*

"For couple of decades there has been an attraction between neuroscience and architecture. However, the real interactions between the two disciplines have rarely been presented or discussed. Due to the internal complexities of architecture and its dialogical relation with life, the largely preconscious and embodied intuitions of the creative mind tend to escape scientific definition. Michael Arbib's exceptionally wide scientific background, combined with his deep interest in the arts and architecture, makes him well equipped to cross this gap. His current book is a devoted study of the neural basis of architecture and the applicability of this knowledge in the design of buildings, especially intelligent buildings, which are deliberately conceived as extensions of our neural capacities."

—JUHANI PALLASMAA, Architect HonSAFA, HonFAIA, IntFRIBA,
Academician, International Academy of Architecture,
Professor emeritus, Aalto University, Helsinki

"This book is one of the most valuable contributions, from a neuroscientific perspective, of the interplay between the architectural environment and human beings."

—DAVIDE RUZZON, Architect,
Director and Founder of *Neuroscience Applied to
Architectural Design,* NAAD Postgraduate Course,
at the University Iuav Venice and POLI Design Milan

When Brains Meet Buildings

*A Conversation Between Neuroscience
and Architecture*

MICHAEL A. ARBIB

UNIVERSITY OF CALIFORNIA AT SAN DIEGO, LA JOLLA

UNIVERSITY OF SOUTHERN CALIFORNIA

ACADEMY OF NEUROSCIENCE FOR ARCHITECTURE

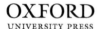

OXFORD
UNIVERSITY PRESS

Oxford University Press is a department of the University of Oxford. It furthers
the University's objective of excellence in research, scholarship, and education
by publishing worldwide. Oxford is a registered trade mark of Oxford University
Press in the UK and certain other countries.

Published in the United States of America by Oxford University Press
198 Madison Avenue, New York, NY 10016, United States of America.

Library of Congress Cataloging-in-Publication Data
Names: Arbib, Michael A., author.
Title: When brains meet buildings : a conversation between neuroscience
and architecture / Michael A. Arbib.
Description: New York, NY : Oxford University Press, [2021] |
Includes bibliographical references and index.
Identifiers: LCCN 2021015055 (print) | LCCN 2021015056 (ebook) |
ISBN 9780190060954 (hardback) | ISBN 9780190060978 (epub) |
ISBN 9780190060985 (online)
Subjects: MESH: Brain—physiology | Mental Processes—physiology |
Architecture | Cognitive Neuroscience | Environment | Adaptation, Physiological
Classification: LCC QP356 (print) | LCC QP356 (ebook) |
NLM WL 337 | DDC 612.8/2—dc23
LC record available at https://lccn.loc.gov/2021015055
LC ebook record available at https://lccn.loc.gov/2021015056

DOI: 10.1093/med/9780190060954.001.0001

Production of this book was supported in part
by a grantfrom the Driehaus Foundation

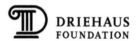

To Prue and Ben
for their imagination
and their flair for design

CONTENTS

We humans evolved to live on the savannah, but most of us today live within a built environment, whether rural or urban. In recent years, there has been an upsurge of interest in how we are affected by the built environment, on various scales from rooms to buildings to villages and all the way up to the hustle and bustle of the largest cities.

The title *When Brains Meet Buildings* signals that understanding "how the brain works" is a major motivation for this book and that buildings provide a key locus in which the entwining of the social and the physical offers fresh challenges for cog/neuroscience. This includes learning through neuroscience in its strict sense of the study of brains, and learning through psychology and cognitive science, studies of the mind without a necessary concern for "how the brain does it." The broad conception of architecture here relates buildings both to the rooms they contain and to the larger environments of which they are part, and embraces "ordinary" buildings as well as "famous" buildings. In each case, the interaction between the aesthetics and the utility of buildings provides a crucial aspect of our conversation.

The book provides a broad conversation between architecture and neuroscience—an A↔N conversation—that is designed to offer new insights to architects and neuroscientists in the practice of their craft, but also to offer new ways for each of us, even with no professional involvement, to think about how we experience buildings and develop intuitions about how they might serve us better. At the price of a small amount of repetition, each chapter begins with an extended synopsis of its various themes.

The built environment makes physically manifest the results of historical trends and individual creativity in ways that directly affect individual experience and behavior. The book shows how understanding our brains can enrich our understanding of the ways we act and interact in a complex world, and how our experience of the built environment helps shape who we are—and yet can be shaped by us in turn. Our focus on how people experience the built environment generally suggests many issues that must be taken into account by the architect. We thus consider, too, how the brains and minds of architects operate, with particular concern for the interaction of memory and imagination, pursuing the idea that each of these is a form of *mental construction* that, in the case of architecture, is constrained by the idea that the design must eventually reach a form that can guide the *physical construction* of buildings.

I come to this effort with decades spent exploring how brains—both human and nonhuman, natural and artificial—can mediate the linkage of perception with ongoing behavior within a variety of environments. A particular challenge has been to develop *schema theory* as a cognitive-level bridge between the phenomena of everyday experience and the detailed processes within neural circuitry. But I augment my personal research on neuroscience with what I have learned from conversations, conferences, and reading of the literature in neuroscience broadly construed to include, as noted previously, cognitive science, psychology, and the scientific analysis of social interactions. Much of my own work has focused on understanding the brain mechanisms that link vision and action in diverse species, developing *action-oriented perception* as a unifying theme. Further work on spatial navigation, memory, and imagination laid the basis for exploring what it is about the biological and cultural evolution of humans that allows us to master the gift of language. My work on "How the brain got language" is an example of that part of neuroscience that concerns social interaction, and thus offered one entry point for a concern with the importance of neuroscience for understanding architecture as a social practice. I argue that the language-ready brain is also an architecture-ready brain.

Neuroscience embraces a vast array of subtopics. Thus, the way *I* think is different from the way many other neuroscientists think. Still, the exposure to my general way of thinking may help prepare architects to conduct discussions with other neuroscientists who have the focused expertise relevant to a specific challenge in evidence-based design. For example, an expert on the auditory system who might help with an acoustics problem would be unable to help address memory problems relevant to design of a home for Alzheimer's patients. Architects go broad; scientists go deep (though of course they will be aware of many findings from outside their own lab).

As for the architecture end of the conversation, I not only have enjoyed the experience of visiting and thinking about buildings and rural areas and cities around the world, but also have been privileged to get to know many architects with whom I have had a range of conversations that inform the views of architecture offered in this book. I have learned much from other architects as well, whether directly, or through their writings, or through experience of their buildings.

The aim of the A↔N conversation here is to engage architects to learn more about the impact of their buildings on the minds, brains, and bodies of others, as well as to gain insight into the mental and neural processes that underlie their own design processes, while also engaging neuroscientists in exploring how their highly focused studies in the laboratory, the clinic, or at the computer might relate to life in the built environment, in all its messy complexity. Moreover, because I must explain architecture to neuroscientists and neuroscience to architects, I hope that the exposition will attract nonspecialists who would like to listen in on the conversation because, like most of us, they share a fascination with both the brains within them and the buildings around them.

There are many styles of conversation: The witty epigrammatic style of the classic Parisian salons, where one listens to others only for the opportunity to deliver a *bon mot* whose brilliance will be appreciated by all; the exchange of gossip; or the simple companionship of sharing together memories of, say, a recent football match. However, this book's conversation is intended to be one in which each partner in the conversation wishes to discuss a topic of mutual interest, both sharing what they know and learning from the other. Architects and neuroscientists think about the world in very different ways, and I hope to exemplify the excitement and challenge of learning much that is new because of these differences. This book aims to catalyze further conversations by enriching the shared vocabulary of all concerned, with diverse examples linking particular buildings to the scientific principles that illuminate them and can be illuminated by them in turn.

In addition to the two primary themes of the neuroscience (broadly conceived) of the *experience* and *design* of architecture, the book develops two further themes.

The first, which is touched on primarily in a single chapter, is *neuromorphic architecture*, which seeks to understand how lessons we get from neuroethology—the study of brain mechanisms underlying the behavior of animals—might be extended to a "neuroscience" of smart buildings that have both sensors and effectors that allow them to interact both with the users of the building and with the physical environment.

A deeper theme that permeates the whole conversation is the *EvoDevoSocio* view of how brains evolved so that humans can shape and be shaped by the built environment. Humans are seen as both embodied brains and embrained bodies developing in a milieu that is both physical and social. The *Evo* stresses the biological evolution that gave us the genes that underlie the development of human brains and bodies. The *Devo* reminds us that the genes in themselves do not specify exactly how we will develop—this development depends crucially on both our physical and social environment. For the former, consider the effects of malnutrition or disease in impairing what might be considered normal growth; for the latter, consider the very real difference in the brains of those who have developed in a language-rich environment from those who have not. Finally, the *Socio* reminds us that we are not only shaped by our environment but that we can shape it ourselves as we change the culture by constructing new aspects of the physical and social environments.

This is not a "how-to" book on experimental or evidence-based architecture. It does not provide a manual on how to assess brain activity of people experiencing or designing buildings, though it does consider a few examples. Nor does it provide a blueprint for incorporating neuroscience data into the architectural design process, though I review some key papers that have initiated collaborations in this area. Rather, a primary goal of this A↔N conversation is to deepen the architect's understanding of the human beings whose life her building should be designed to enrich and to appreciate what goes on "in the head" and beyond the body in the users of buildings.

[An aside on pronouns. I use "I" for myself, the author; I use "you" to address you, the reader; and I use "we" in two ways: when talking about general human experience, and when I am hopeful that you now share, or will soon share, certain ideas presented in the book. For third-person singular pronouns, I use the gendered version for gendered individuals, and almost always use "they" otherwise.]

To give some sense of the conversation that is to come, here is a sampling of the architecture discussed in this book, along with the neuroscience concepts that they are used to introduce:

Peter Zumthor's Therme at Vals introduces the *action–perception cycle* of the users of buildings, as well as *affordances* for action and the *multimodality of perception*, but also gets us thinking about the relation between the *physical construction* of the building and the *mental construction* involved in its design.

Lina Bo Bardi's São Paulo Art Museum introduces the notions of *wayfinding* and *cognitive maps*, but also gets us to consider the extent to which architects engage with *scripts* for how people will behave in buildings of a certain type and yet can defy those scripts in innovative ways.

Discussion of the Parthenon and various works by Le Corbusier illustrates the challenge of integrating "engineering aesthetics" and "architectural aesthetics" as a variation on the form–function theme. It also leads into discussion of the ways in which a particular style of architecture can be considered a language, and ways in which it should not.

A temple garden in Kyoto and a stroll in Edinburgh help introduce the notion of *atmosphere*, and extend the notion of *affordances* as perceptual cues for action from the realm of practical action to the realm of mood and emotion. Discussion of the Todai-Ji temple in Nara and Notre-Dame de Paris then leads us into a brain imaging study that seeks to probe the underpinnings of contemplative architecture.

Libraries in Stockholm, Berlin, Los Angeles, and Seattle are used to further our discussion of wayfinding and cognitive maps, but also to introduce the role of *symbolism in architecture*—leading us to assess the relation between such symbolism and the use of symbols in conveying meaning through language. Later, I not only place language in an evolutionary framework but also do so in ways that relate language to manual skills in general and to drawing and model-making in particular.

The interactive space Ada, developed for the 2002 Swiss Expo in Lausanne, was designed to interact with visitors in a manner driven in some sense by its "emotions." This leads into the discussion of neuromorphic architecture, of "brains" for buildings, more generally.

WOHA's Kampung Admiralty in Singapore emphasizes the role that buildings can play in creating a *sense of community*, exemplifies *biophilia* by bringing nature into the urban environment, and views architecture as creating *systems of systems*.

Finally, detailed case studies of Jørn Utzon's design of the Sydney Opera House and Frank Gehry's design of the Guggenheim Museum Bilbao set the stage for linking spatial navigation, visual perception, action, memory, and imagination as the basis for charting the beginnings of a new cognitive neuroscience of design.

Since a number of these buildings are famous, let me stress that the book uses cog/neuroscience to enrich our understanding of the built environment in general. However, the advantage of famous buildings is that they are often well documented, and readers are more likely to know something about them that can enrich their understanding of the related part of the A↔N conversation. In any case, you are invited to assess how well the insights I offer do apply to buildings with which you are familiar.

The conversation between neuroscience and architecture is in its early days. To the extent that there are books at the architecture–neuroscience interface, they have been written primarily by architects for architects and the architecturally inclined, but I offer a riff on a famous speech by John Fitzgerald Kennedy: Ask not only what neuroscience can do for architecture, but also what architecture can do for neuroscience. The challenge is this: Certainly, a number of architects are now interested in how knowledge of the brain's function may contribute to design thinking, but fewer neuroscientists are assessing the challenges that arise from looking at architecture. At the annual meeting of the Society for Neuroscience, there are about 15,000 talks and posters for the 20,000 to 30,000 attendees each year, but (almost) none of them specifically address the neuroscience of the built environment, even though a good number do address processes in the brain that are relevant to our enterprise. This book aims to help architects deepen their understanding of what cog/neuroscience has to offer, and to help neuroscientists understand ways in which architecture may entice them to move beyond the laboratory.

If, as I hope will be the case, I succeed in my aims, then there will be a double payoff—not only raising the level of interaction between architecture and neuroscience but also providing an accessible introduction to the interplay of brains and buildings for *anyone* who thinks about buildings and is intrigued by ongoing attempts to unravel the brain's mysteries.

Michael A. Arbib

La Jolla, 2020

ACKNOWLEDGMENTS

I write as a neuroscientist for whom architecture is a lifelong interest that has only recently become a major professional focus. If I appear knowledgeable about architecture, it is thanks in great part to the many architects who have discussed their subject with me and offered much friendly criticism of my ideas, all of it constructive.

Among all I owe to my parents, let me mention here the gift of worldwide travel, the gift of a Bayko building set, and my father's development as a master builder after founding Australian Steel Prefabrications. My wife, Prue, shares my love of architecture, and has a great sense of design that she has passed on to our architect son, Ben.

The professional link from my neuroscience career to architecture was triggered by the work of two computational neuroscientists, Rodney Douglas and Paul Verschure, who led the team that created an "intelligent space," Ada, that interacted with visitors at the Swiss Expo in Lausanne in 2002. This led me in 2003 and 2004 to have my students at the University of Southern California conduct projects on "intelligent rooms" whose intelligence was based in part on brain operating principles. Thus, "brains for buildings" provided my rather off-center entry point into the linkage of architecture and neuroscience, and thence to the invitation from Eduardo Macagno to become a Board member of the Academy of Neuroscience for Architecture (ANFA, www.anfarch.org). Eduardo's successor as ANFA President, Alison Whitelaw, nominated me to Sarah Robinson to give a talk at Taliesin West, where I shared the platform with Juhani Pallasmaa, the Finnish architect and architectural scholar. Discussions with Juhani have been crucial in my development as an A↔N conversationalist. This marked the beginning of many friendships and intense and informative discussions with architects, not only Sarah and Juhani but also Harry Mallgrave, Bob Condia, Barbara Lamprecht, Mark Hewitt, Bob Hart, Pedro Borges de Araújo, Julio Bermudez, Edwin Chan, Richard Leplastrier—and many more, including my son, Ben Arbib. A number of my ideas were developed while teaching at NewSchool of Architecture and Design in San Diego (with help on "talking to architecture students" from Tatiana Berger) and at the University of California at San Diego. Special thanks go to Mitra Kanaani, who took on the onerous task of helping me reshape the text to better engage the interest of architects, with further input from Bob Condia and Bob Hart. Meanwhile, Eduardo Macagno, Tom Albright, David Kirsh, and Colin Ellard are among the cog/neuroscientists contributing vigorously to this conversation. Since I have learned from so many people whose books and papers I have read, or whose conversations have enriched my understanding of architecture, I apologize in advance to all whose names I have omitted here.

My research in recent years on the evolution of the language-ready brain and on the linkage of neuroscience to architecture has been supported in part by the National Science Foundation (NSF) under Grant No. BCS-1343544 "INSPIRE Track 1: Action, Vision and Language, and Their Brain Mechanisms in Evolutionary Relationship" (Michael A. Arbib, Principal Investigator). My thanks to Betty Tuller for her work in building an environment at NSF that made such support possible.

Finally, my thanks to the Driehaus Foundation for their support in defraying costs for editing of this volume and for its production, with the aim of making the book accessible and affordable for a wider audience.

Brains in bodies in the — social, built, and natural — environment

1.1. Linking physical and mental construction
1.2. Framing the A↔N conversation
1.3. How brains meet buildings
1.4. The many levels of the brain
1.5. A key debate: Is neuroscience relevant to architecture?

Brains meet buildings: Our concern with brains extends to how each brain enlivens a body in interaction with the social and physical environment. Our concern with buildings is centered on how people act and interact within and around buildings. Buildings reshape the environment and reshape people in turn, and this informs our insights into the neuroscience of architectural design. This chapter provides a foundation for our A↔N conversation between architecture and neuroscience, introducing key ideas from neuroscience, an appropriate perspective on architecture, and the possibilities these offer for the conversation.

The grounding tenet is that buildings are not just to be looked at; they are also to be used and experienced, and that experience engages a cycle of action and perception. The actions may include praxis (practical actions directly affecting the environment) and contemplative actions (whether for emotional satisfaction or to better understand the current situation). A tour of Peter Zumthor's Therme at Vals plunges us into the A↔N conversation by linking the success of that work to ways the actions of users fuse with the multimodal nature of their experience, and the interplay of the interior with the surroundings.

As we experience the world, our goals and motivation change. This affects how we act and, through directing our attention, changes the way we perceive the world. And so the action–perception cycle continues. But, of course, the way we act depends on who we are, and this depends on our memories, both conscious and unconscious, as well as our current needs and social interactions. Thus, not only are action and perception and emotion intertwined, but so are remembering and imagination. As we imagine different ways to proceed in a given situation, so does our behavior depend on our memories but in turn may change our skills and the facts and events we remember.

Quotes from Zumthor introduce and bring together two themes that will run through the book: the notion of *construction* and the relation between *memory and imagination*. Certainly, architectural design leads to the *physical construction* of buildings—but we will also explore the idea that much of what our brains achieve can be seen as a form of *mental construction*. Whether it engages the construction of our understanding of the world around us or our construction of plans of action or the neuroscientist's design of an experiment or the architect's design of a building, such mental construction exploits diverse memories to ground those feats of imagination that can yield new ideas and understandings.

It is common to speak of form and function in architecture, and we analyze what Louis Sullivan meant by his observation that "form ever follows function." However, we will more often talk of aesthetics and utility, though there is no hard and fast line between them. A building may be beautiful or affect our feelings in other ways and yet be hard to use; a building may be functional and yet offer little appeal to the senses beyond providing cues for necessary actions. Given the needs and the budget in the program for a new building, it may be impossible to achieve maximal utility or maximal aesthetic impact; rather, a tradeoff between the two must be found.

Often, the neural details are less important to the architect than making contact with the personal analysis of experience and behavior. We may thus distinguish the strict sense of neuroscience (in which the focus is on the structure and function of brain regions and their neural activity) from the broad sense—call it cognitive science or psychology—which analyzes action, perception, learning and memory, emotion, and more, without necessarily seeking their neural underpinnings. The hybrid term *cog/neuroscience* may be used to span this spectrum of approaches. I leave it to the reader to infer when I use "neuroscience" in this broad sense, and when it is limited to studies in which the structure and function of the brain are explicitly involved.

With this understanding of the N, the chapter will sketch the four themes of the A↔N conversation as developed in this book:

- *The neuroscience of the experience of architecture*: What goes on in the brain of a person—a brain in a body in the social, built, and natural environment—experiencing a building, interacting with and within it? Interesting questions here focus on how different groups of people may have different types of brains that affect how they experience their environment, and the related notion of lifespan architecture.
- *The neuroscience of the design of architecture*: What goes on in the brain of the architect—a brain in a body in the social, built, and natural environment—designing a building?
- *Neuromorphic architecture*: The notion that neuroscience might influence the design of "brains" for buildings considered as dynamic, interactive, and adaptive systems.
- *The EvoDevoSocio framework*: We are formed not only by our genetic inheritance shaped by biological evolution but also by the physical and social milieux, shaped by cultural evolution, in which we develop. Architecture has a special role to play in structuring the physical

environment, thus closing the loop between the actions of architects and the users of the buildings they design.

One terminological concern: we typically reserve the term *architect* for someone who designs buildings and the term *client* for someone who engages and/or pays for the design and subsequent construction. But what of those who live in a house, or work in a factory, or study in a school or library, or worship in a sacred space, or simply shop in a store or get some cash at a bank? I have settled on the term *user* and note that a building may be designed with many different types of user in mind.

With this, we can turn to the first brief overview of narrow-sense neuroscience—many further details will be discussed later as their relevance emerges to our developing conversation. A crucial issue will be the back and forth between the structure and function of each brain. These can be studied at many different levels, ranging from the whole person in interaction with the social and physical environment down to the minute details of the molecular biology and genetics of the mechanisms within the neurons and the *synapses* that connect them. It is worth pausing to contrast how our perceptions, emotions, and actions may often be summarized in a few words per second with the astonishing fact that there are about 10 billion neurons in each human brain and maybe thousands times as many synapses connecting them. No amount of *direct introspection* can let us monitor the different parts of our brains, let alone the activity of the neural circuits within them. In short, we must understand that much of what our brains do is *subconscious*. An intriguing challenge for our conversation, then, is to appreciate the ways in which conscious and subconscious influences are linked, and the way in which much of what our bodies do proceeds with little or no conscious intervention.

An important challenge for cog/neuroscience is to develop a bridge between the levels of psychological and cognitive analysis and the understanding of how these are made possible by the dynamic interactions of myriad neurons in diverse circuits and interacting regions of the brain. The bridge that I offer is a version of what is called *schema theory*, and we will see in later chapters that schemas may be analyzed purely at a psychological or cognitive level, or in terms of their neural implementation, or in terms of overall patterns of thought and behavior shared by a community.

My feeling is that most of the *cooperation* between architects and neuroscientists will proceed via highly focused studies in psychology or cognitive science—but that the key lessons of these disciplines will be continuously enriched by neuroscience research. My aim is to create a framework for a *conversation* that enables the architect and neuroscientist to better understand each other's work as the means for defining new challenges that draw on their initially disparate resources. We will briefly examine some of the ways in which brain and behavior can be measured, and some focused studies at the architecture/neuroscience interface will be discussed in later chapters.

This book does, I believe, demonstrate conclusively that the conversation between architecture and neuroscience not only is of general interest but also can yield specific insights relevant to the practice of both architects and neuroscientists. Some architects have expressed the fear that the conversation between architecture and neuroscience will strip the architect of any creativity. However, this book will show that deeper understanding of what goes on in our heads as we experience buildings can enrich their design.

Nonetheless, some skepticism remains, and the chapter concludes by offering some general arguments before we proceed to the convincing examples that occupy chapter after chapter. We will examine the interdependence of science and art and then offer a philosophical framework, *two-way reduction*, linking the phenomenology of the first-person experience of architecture at least in part with the detailed workings of the brain. As readers of the popular neurology writings of Oliver Sacks well know, damage to the brain can yield many unexpected changes in the behavior and experience of the world. Such human case studies, combined with much that we learn from both human brain imaging studies and detailed studies of the neural networks of animals, demonstrate that our first-person being-in-the-world rides atop a vast diversity of neural processes.

Thus, neuroscience can "dissect" phenomenology by showing how first-person experiences arise from melding diverse subconscious processes. This raises the intriguing possibility that neuroscience can extend the effectiveness of architectural design by showing how different aspects of a building may affect human experience in subtle ways that are simply not apparent to self-reflection.

That is the spirit of this A↔N conversation: there is neither the claim that architecture offers all the problems that are of interest to neuroscientists nor the claim that neuroscientists can solve all the problems faced by architects. Rather, there are two main claims: that the conversation may be of interest in a nonprofessional sense of general enrichment, and that each partner in the conversation may learn something of use to them, without in any way exhausting all the concerns that they must address themselves.

1.1. LINKING PHYSICAL AND MENTAL CONSTRUCTION

Action and multimodal perception are intertwined

Consider one of the masterpieces of the Swiss Architect Peter Zumthor, the thermal baths at Vals in Switzerland (Zumthor, 2011; Figure 1.1). The chosen material (gneiss from local quarries) and the design of the exterior blend with the Swiss alpine landscape. The landscape is brought into the building in some places by framing it. Grass sod on some of the roofs harmonizes with the landscape. But all this is complementary to the rooms that give access to different thermal pools. These offer multisensory experiences that vary as you move through the spaces. As you enter a room, there is the visual impact, and then you immerse yourself, feeling the temperature of the water on your skin, and the water's resistance to and support of your movements. At least one of the rooms has flowers floating in the water, bringing in the sense of smell. There is one doorway that requires pushing aside a heavy leather curtain, adding a new tactile

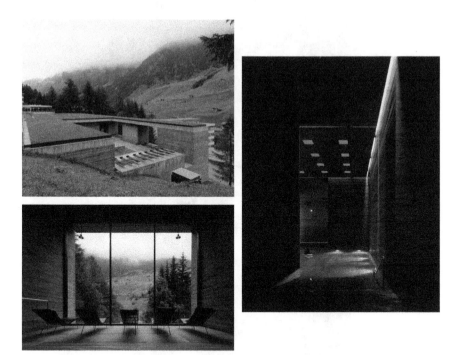

Figure 1.1 A montage of views of Peter Zumthor's Therme at Vals, Switzerland. It is built from gneiss, a stone quarried from the region. The views indicate the way the building has been designed both to fit into the alpine landscape and to frame it from certain vantage points. Within the building, different rooms frame their pools in different ways, and the users' experiences involve many senses as they move into, through, and out of the pools, and from one space to another. (All photos © Fujimoto Kazunori, with permission.)

element beyond that of walking, immersing, and floating, to highlight the transition from one thermal experience to another.[1]

Despite the use of photos here, one should not think of a building merely as a source of visual experience but must take multisensory experience into account, as powerfully argued by the Finnish architect and scholar Juhani Pallasmaa in his book, *The Eyes of the Skin* (Pallasmaa, 2012; Figure 1.2). He stressed the importance of touch and

1. I speak here based on my architect son Ben Arbib's experience. Unfortunately, I have not been to Vals myself.

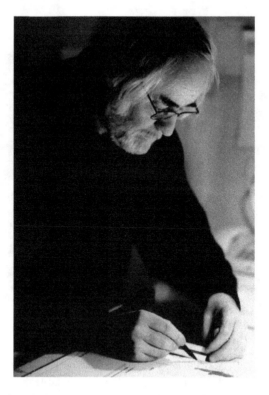

Figure 1.2 Finnish architect Juhani Pallasmaa. (Photo © Knut Thyberg, with permission.)

other senses; I stress *the linkage of action and multisensory perception*—not just vision and touch but also audition and even, in come cases (consider restaurants, for example), smell and taste. In everyday experience, we can reach into a pocket and confidently select an object by hapsis (the sense of touch) alone. We might even choose one key from a keyring before it leaves the pocket, and then combine sight and touch to insert the key into its lock, after which hapsis and audition work together to confirm that we have successfully locked or unlocked a door. When we eat food, sight, mouth feel, smell, and taste combine to determine our experience and modify the actions of hands, lips, tongue, jaws, and swallowing.

Let's use the term *action-oriented perception* to stress that much (though not all) of our experience intertwines action and perception. A sound or a touch that is meaningful at one stage is irrelevant at another, unless it is so discordant that it sets off an alarm that triggers a new course of action. In the same way, each building can support functional and aesthetic aspects of a host of behaviors, each engaging a dynamic range of actions and perceptions.

The architect must think through the diverse multisensory experiences and behavior of different users of a building. For example, in designing a restaurant, noise levels and the control of aromas complement visual experience, and the public area must integrate the experience of servers and diners. This area must also have a smooth interface with the staff area, where meals are prepared and dispatched, and thus where many ancillary tasks must be performed.

Architects know this, and I do not presume to offer them a practical guide for any type of building. Rather, my aim is to help the reader better understand what goes on in our minds and brains and bodies as we experience architecture, or as the architect designs a building with potential future experiences in mind. The aim is threefold:

- To enrich architectural design through a deeper understanding of action-oriented perception and its many ramifications;
- To enrich the experience of all of us as we venture in and around buildings by linking this specific experience to a better understanding of our selves; and
- To invite neuroscientists to consider architecture as a new domain for "translational science" beyond the laboratory.

One more crucial point: the environment, whether built or natural, may at times be a setting for the lone individual to act or to contemplate their surroundings, but it will often provide a stage on which the human drama unfolds as we interact with those around us. We are socially enculturated beings. Given this, let's focus directly on the chapter's title, "Brains in bodies in the—social, built, and natural—environment," and clarify how this book's concern with the brain comports with a somewhat different emphasis that has gained some traction with architects.

Considering form and function

Back to Peter Zumthor. In his essay, "A Way of Looking at Things," from his book, *Thinking Architecture* (Zumthor, 2012), Zumthor says,

> Unlike the sculptor, I have to start with functional and technical requirements.

As an architect, he must consider how the building is to be used and expected to perform. At the Therme, it is not enough to make it easy for people to experience the different springs and move from one to another; one must worry about a shower room and a changing room and mundane issues like the utilities. But as the photos made clear, such considerations constrain the design of the final building only lightly. The placement of the springs and the movement of people within and between them, while respecting the beauty of the landscape, provides the essential program that the building is to satisfy.

For the architect, the *program*, or project brief, provides the initial specifications that provide the setting for the design process—very different from the computer scientist's sense of the *program* as the detailed coding of specific instructions that together meet the specifications. However, the architect's sense is somewhat closer to the earlier notion of the program for a play or concert that gives a high-level view of what is to be performed.

We adapt Louis Sullivan's slogan "form follows function" by suggesting that there is a dynamic interaction of considerations of form and function as design proceeds. A clearer understanding of this comes from its source, Sullivan's essay, "The Tall Office Building Artistically Considered" (Sullivan, 1896).[2] The major part of Sullivan's article

2. I had not read "The Tall Office Building Artistically Considered" until Robert Lamb Hart read an earlier draft of this chapter and suggested that were I to do so, I would see that "form follows function" is probably as good a conceptual scheme for studying architecture as any, provided both are defined in broad overlapping terms.

distinguishes three functions of the tall office building: that of the ground floor, that of the repeated floors of office space, and that of the "attic," which contains a range of machinery to complete the work of that in the basement. Whereas some would argue for the tripartite division of the form of the tall office building on the basis of the three parts of a tree (roots, trunk, branches) or a Greek column, Sullivan argued that such ideas are mistaken—the tripartite *form* of the building follows from its tripartite *function*. It is only after he has argued this case that he then makes the *observation*:

> Whether it be the sweeping eagle in his flight or the open apple-blossom, the toiling work-horse, the blithe swan, the branching oak, the winding stream at its base, the drifting clouds, over all the coursing sun, *form ever follows function*, and this is the law. Where function does not change form does not change. . . . Shall we, then, daily violate this law in our art? Are we so decadent, so imbecile, so utterly weak of eyesight, that we cannot perceive this truth so simple, so very simple? [My italics.]

However, this does not imply that forms are defined down to their details by their functions, any more than an oak should resemble a willow. Indeed, earlier in his essay, Sullivan asserts:

> [The loftiness] of the tall office building . . . is to the artist-nature its thrilling aspect. . . . It must be tall, every inch of it tall. The force and power of altitude must be in it, the glory and pride of exaltation must be in it. It must be every inch a proud and soaring thing, rising in sheer exultation that from bottom to top it is a unit without a single dissenting line . . .

Three buildings shown in his essay demonstrate how little the *generalities* of function-following-form limit the architect's imagination (Figure 1.3).

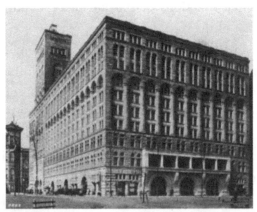

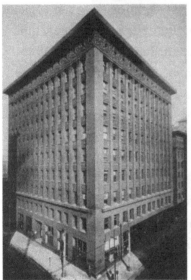

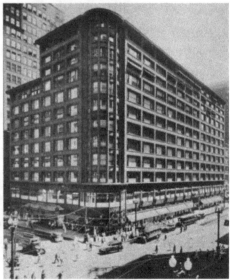

Figure 1.3 Three figures from Sullivan's essay, "The Tall Office Building Artistically Considered," in which he made the observation "form follows function" somewhat differently from how it is understood today. (*Top*) Auditorium Building, from the East, Chicago (Chicago Architectural Photograph Co.). (*Bottom left*) Wainwright Building, St. Louis (Keystone View Co.). (*Bottom right*) Carson Pirie Scott Store, Chicago (Chicago Architectural Photograph Co.).Public domain. All three reproduced from Sullivan, L. H. [1896]. The tall office building artistically considered. *Lippincott's Magazine*, 57[March], 403–409.)

In this book, we will focus our notion of "function" in architecture down from Sullivan's lofty tripart division to consider the range of actions that a building offers its users, from the practical to the contemplative. In this spirit, we may echo the dictum of another great organic American architect, Louis Kahn: "Architecture is the thoughtful making of spaces. It is the creating of spaces that evoke a feeling of appropriate use." The point for us is that each space may have a plurality of uses, so that its overall form must achieve balance between a variety of more localized forms, some of which may be fashioned to serve multiple functions. In this, we may be channeling the concerns of Sullivan's former partner Dankmar Adler that

> architectural form evolves from the complex web of functions, materials, and techniques available to the designer and builder . . . [while] environment, which Adler took to include the technical and *sociocultural milieu* of a project, plays an important role in the dialogues, negotiations, and compromises that ultimately inform building design. [My italics.] (Leslie, 2010, p. 83)

In the end, Zumthor's Therme is a success for the way it blends with the landscape, it is considered beautiful by many of its visitors,[3] and it works well as a place to experience the different springs. The key issue here is what has been dubbed *performativity* (Kanaani, 2019). In the final building, the various functions must be performed well (by some criteria) for the client and the relevant users. This notion of performativity can then be extended to embrace the aesthetic experience afforded by the final form of the building. Simply listing functions and saying "perform them well" will not of itself dictate the form of the building, but a successful design may involve initially disparate ideas, whether for achieving various functions or for the form of different parts of a building, and these will affect each other as design proceeds.

---

3. Beautiful to whom? "Beauty" is a loaded term in architecture. Judgment of beauty varies so much from one person to another that some architects avoid the term, while others use it in idiosyncratic ways. I will have more to say about this in §3.1.

The action–perception cycle is a learning cycle too

Our visit to Zumthor's thermal baths at Vals in Switzerland stressed how perceptual experience was shaped by ongoing behavior. To tease out the general implications of these ideas, we will repeatedly assess *action-oriented perception* (Arbib, 1972) in the context of the *action–perception cycle* (Neisser, 1976). We will explore the action–perception cycles of users within and around a building as we analyze the *experience* of architecture, and architects must imagine what typical such cycles might be when they *design* a building.

Before our guided tour of Figure 1.4, let me briefly introduce the key concept of a *schema*. For many writers, the "schema" captures the overall structure of a particular situation, and an architect may talk of the overall "scheme" of a building. In my own work, however, a finer scale has proved crucial. If I walk into a room, how do I come to master the "overall situation"? It is only because I can recognize certain key objects and their disposition. Entering one of the rooms at the Therme, I would make sense of it because I can see the pool, the steps, the handrail, the walls, the exit to the next room, and more—and the relations between them. My brain has different *perceptual schemas* for recognizing these objects and, crucially, the ability to recognize properties of the various "instances" of these objects and the relations between them. Such perception can not only affect my contemplation of the scene but also provide the details necessary for action. This involves activating various *motor schemas* for actions like "move toward handrail," "grasp handrail," "descend the steps into the pool," and so on. In particular, as I look around, and start to move, the details that I attend to will change, and so too will the actions available to me at that moment.

Figure 1.4 shows two cycles that link "the world": the knowledge of the person (or animal or other agent), and the actions that the person takes, acting back on the world. The inner cycle stresses "perceptual" actions— such as eye movements, or sniffing for odors, or active touch—that serve perceptual exploration. The outer cycle stresses actions that change both our relation to the external environment and our knowledge of that environment (which, in humans and thanks to language and other media, can

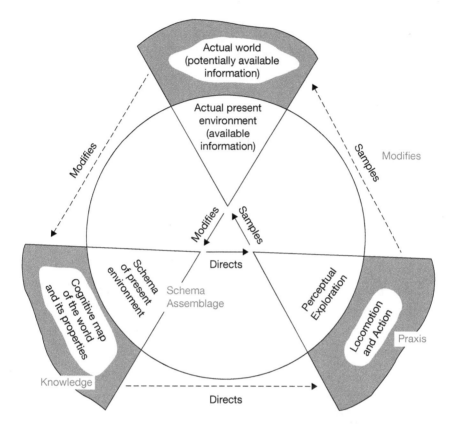

Figure 1.4 The action–perception cycle, adapted from Neisser (1976). Where Neisser speaks of *schema of present environment*, I will use *schema **assemblage** of present environment*; and where Neisser speaks of the *cognitive map of the world and its properties*, I will speak of ***knowledge*** *of the world and its properties*. I use *praxis* as an umbrella term that includes locomotion and those actions that have a direct effect in changing the physical world; it thus *modifies* rather than *samples* the "actual world." An extension of this figure could include communicative actions that change the mental states of others who might then change the physical state of the world. (Adapted by the author from Neisser, U. [1976]. *Cognition and reality: Principles and implications of cognitive psychology*. San Francisco: W. H. Freeman.)

extend far beyond our own immediate experiences). Let's consider the three triangles of figure in turn:

Top: Out there is the "actual" world, but at any time there is only a small part of it, the "available information," that we could possibly

sample, owing to our spatial relationships with the external world, the type of brain and sensors we possess, and our previous experience. Different people may have very different impressions of the same passing scene.

Left: (Outer) At any time, we have built up what Neisser calls a "cognitive map," but he uses the term in a different sense from that we use when talking about wayfinding, so let's understand this as *knowledge (or long-term memory [LTM]) of the world.* This knowledge may be tacit or explicit. **(Inner)** Here Neisser talks of the schema of the present environment, but I will talk of the *schema assemblage for the present environment*, stressing that our perception of the environment may take in many different actions and objects. Our behavior depends in part on this working memory (WM) of our current relation with what is around us as defined by this schema assemblage. Input from the top triangle may modify both our knowledge of the world and our sense of the current environment. Different people may have very different impressions of the same passing scene, both because their current aims may differ and because their experience (encoded as schemas) allows them to be responsive to different features of the environment.

Right: The division here is between *two types of action*, but each is guided by our knowledge of the world in general and our understanding of the current environment. "Inner" actions include eye movements, moving to change our viewpoint, or running our hand over an object, each intended to extend our sampling of the world around us. "Outer" actions allow us to change the world, not just sample it, even in as simple an act as cutting a slice of bread. These include "practical" actions, *praxis.* In later chapters I will extend this to consider communicative actions and contemplative actions, and the roles of emotions. The world itself is continually changing without need of our intervention, and that world includes other people so that action includes social interaction, which may involve conversations that can change both our knowledge and our current views.

Our current "schema assemblage" includes not only perceptions of the external world and plans for overt action but also fleeting thoughts and ideas for future behavior, as well as our current emotional state and motivation—and these in turn change with our perception of the environment and affect our ongoing action and social interaction.

The action–perception cycle is a learning cycle too. As we act and perceive, we may come to remember certain episodes and also to learn new facts, while developing new skills and honing others. In other words, the stock of schemas and the relations between them are dynamic. Our thoughts combine with subconscious neural processes not only to change our understanding of the world but also to allow us to plan how we will act, with some appreciation of the near-term or long-term consequences.

In this book, I emphasize human experience and behavior in and around buildings but also include the planning and construction of buildings as willful interventions to change parts of the external world on a long-term basis. This reminds us that the action–perception cycle also runs in "contemplation mode" or "planning mode," where our ideas develop through the dynamics of our mental processes without necessarily yielding immediate overt action. If we are in an art gallery, contemplation (with attendant eye movements) may serve to enrich our appreciation of that which is contemplated, but it may also serve to enrich our store of related schemas to prepare us should we choose to act in relation to some aspects of the gallery at some later time, as in noting where the exits are, or returning to an artwork admired earlier only in passing.

Construction, memory, and imagination

The experience of architects as users of buildings provides a core for their expertise as designers of buildings. I return to Zumthor several times in this section to establish this interaction:

Construction is the art of making a meaningful whole out of many parts. . . .

I feel respect for the art of joining, the ability of craftsmen and engineers . . . the knowledge of how to make things. . . . (Zumthor, 2012, p. 11)

Zumthor is in part expressing here his early experience as a cabinet-maker. It is not enough to sketch a beautiful shape; the architect must (eventually) think through the building (process) of the building (the end result). Of course, joining is just one approach to construction. We may contrast *additive processes* (joining pieces together) with *subtractive processes* (as in sculpting—e.g., separating pieces from a block of marble to "reveal" the final form) as classic alternatives. Other processes form new shapes (whether bending wood or steel, molding plastic, or pouring concrete on novel wooden forms). Technology changes the mix, too, as we go from wooden structures to brick structures to the rise of steel girders that allow the construction of skyscrapers, and on to work, such as Frank Gehry's, where a computer is necessary to calculate with swirling curvatures (so distinct from the constant curvature of a cylinder or sphere) to exploit novel forms of assembly based on individually shaped components.

Unlike the sculptor's, the architect's work stops short of the actual process of *physical* construction. Nonetheless, the design must spell out how basic forms are to be produced and assembled in ways achievable with the construction technology chosen for the building. In this way, the design process is itself a form of construction, but it is a process of *mental* construction, the development of ideas memorialized in preliminary sketches and models. Some of these are rough, some detailed; some offer general ideas, and some focus on small parts of the building.

Indeed, the quest to understand "construction" as a very general process will be a recurring theme in this book. We will chart its importance in visual perception and in memory as a basis for understanding its importance in imagination. It applies to any of us in *planning* our future behavior, constructing a plan as an assemblage of possible actions. And it even applies to language.

In designing a building, the architect must envisage a range of possible action–perception cycles for future users of the building. In looking at an object or a building, we can recognize *what it is*, but we can also recognize *what actions it makes possible.* Following J. J. Gibson (Gibson, 1979), we use the term *affordances* for perceptual cues for the actions that an object makes possible. In turn, these affordances depend on our own *effectivities* in the sense of the actions of which we are capable—a rock face might afford climbing for some people, but not for most of us. Thus, the designers must understand the effectivities, the capabilities, of potential users of the building while providing the means to carry out certain actions within the building, along with appropriate affordances to alert users and possibly guide them in their chosen actions.

I am being careful to distinguish an affordance from the action it affords, but the distinction is a subtle one. Consider a door handle. Its visual appearance will provide the affordance for reaching out to grasp it. However, when it is grasped, tactile feedback may be the primary cue for successful operation, and success requires attention to ensuring that the grasp does not slip, that the handle can be turned with little exertion, and that the grasp will remain firm as the door is opened. Since the latter stages play little role in the major steps of architectural design, the relevant affordances will be little discussed in what follows. But here is the crucial distinction: the architect provides the affordances; the user executes the actions. (More on affordances and effectivities in Chapter 2.)

Of course, the architect is not omniscient, and indeed may (whether intentionally or not) offer users opportunities to discover unplanned affordances as they build up routines for an often-visited building, such as a home, an office, or a school, or explore a seldom-visited building. A space may succeed because it evokes a sense of play. And, at least in the home, each of us may continue the work of the architect as we add furniture, and move it, and perhaps even remodel the building, to better adapt the building to our behaviors, even as we adapt our behaviors to the building. In some sense, then, *the action–perception cycle applies to the building in its response to us, even as it applies to our behavior in and around it*—an idea from which I extrapolate in Chapter 7, where I consider what it might mean for buildings to have "brains."

Zumthor further notes that the designer must meet

> the challenge of developing a whole out of innumerable details, out of various functions and forms, materials and dimensions.
> Details . . . lead to an understanding of the whole of which they are an intrinsic part. (Zumthor, 2012, p.15)

In visual perception, one seeks to make sense of an observed scene. One can quickly recognize its gist and then (and these processes are often subconscious) go back and forth between rectifying one's overall impression and filling in the details.[4] What is perceived is greatly dependent on the attention, motivation, and *prior experience* of the observer.

The artist or architect in some sense *reverses* or *inverts* the process, creating a painting or building that will direct our attention and support our experience in certain ways—although, of course, our own experience may differ from those they intended. Though design thus proceeds, in some sense, in the opposite direction to perception, much the same processes hold in developing a design. The whole may be imagined first as a frame for developing details, but as the design develops, as the interaction of various functions and forms and the choice of materials and dimensions proceeds, these details may lead to a new understanding, and even reshaping, of the whole of which they are part. The designer does not fully know what the building will be before working on the details. Only when the

---

4. More generally, the gist is the essential point of any matter. However, in this book I will focus on the visual gist of a scene or episode—usually with an emphasis on the first impression of its overall nature that may or may not be verified as one attends to further details. I haven't thought in any detail about gist for other sensory modalities, but one could certainly get an auditory first impression of, for example, a railway station interior versus a lively party versus a city street. Since it lacks spatial structure for humans, olfaction would provide less detailed cues, while touch will generally require tactile exploration to gather details in spatial relationship to each other before any overall impression begins to emerge. Of course, in real life, any and all modalities can contribute to one's understanding of a situation, both its gist in the general sense [*sic*] and its details. In Chapter 4 we will explore the notion of "atmosphere" of a building, and we may note its parallels with gist in my restricted sense.

whole and its parts are in balance can the design specify how the physical construction of the building is to proceed. The details may be purely practical—some are required to make the wall stable, others to ensure a doorway is wide enough—but other detailing may be aesthetic.

Another crucial challenge comes from Zumthor's reflection on the relation between memory and imagination:

> When I think about architecture, images come into my mind. . . .
> When I design a building, I frequently find myself sinking into old, half-forgotten memories. . . . Yet, at the same time, I know that all is new and that there is no direct reference to a former work of architecture. (Zumthor, 2012, pp.7-8)

Of course, not all images that come to an architect's mind are new, and architects may make direct references to earlier buildings, even posting drawings and photographs of their own and others' buildings as reference points. With the advent of computer-aided design, some architects have assembled digital catalogs of favored details. But the key point remains: What is crucial in imagination is not accuracy of recall but rather to somehow extract something new from the combined effect of multiple recalled images.

Often, when we use the terms *image* or *imagination*, we refer to visual images. However, our quick look at the thermal baths in Vals reminds us that *the architect's images may be multisensory, with vision, hearing, and other senses combining with action.* Imagine the feel of a door handle as you turn it, the quiet thud as the door closes.

It's not that the designer thinks, "I have to build a doorway, so let me pull out doorway 173 from memory and plug it in here." And yet, remembering that doorway and considering it in the context of the planned-for building may suggest features that become candidates for inclusion in the new design—or dire warnings of mistakes to be avoided. We are in the realm of mental construction that may at first proceed with limited constraint from consideration of the physical construction that must in due course be specified. Each memory of a particular episode in our lives—like each perception of a visual scene—is itself a construct, so that fragments of different memories can provide elements for constructing something new. For the architect, the current design challenge is creating new "site-specific" ideas to enter into the mix. In the case of the Therme, this would include the topography and appearance of the valley, the specific qualities of gneiss, and the thermal properties of each pool and the spatial relations between them. Certain items become "islands of reliability," configurations that, although they may be changed later, are stable enough for now to provide ideas around which the next stage of design can be organized.

The actual building, when constructed, will be relatively static (doors and windows open and close, lifts and escalators may move people between floors), though we will consider more dynamic architectures in Chapter 7. During design, though, the building is strangely amorphous and dynamic as the architect's imagination flows *outward* from the actions and perceptions of the imagined users and *inward* from the morphing forms of the building—at places precise, at others vague—that will contain those users and provide their affordances and shape their experiences.

In summary, the architects' role is not limited to the measurable details that are needed for construction plans. They do not construct the physical building, but *must (though to varying degrees at different stages) keep construction in mind* in both senses of this expression—the physical process of constructing the building, and the mental process of developing the design. The latter notion of "construction as a general capability of the brain, exemplified in many modes," will be a recurring theme of this book.

1.2. FRAMING THE A↔N CONVERSATION

I seek to further a conversation between architect and neuroscientist that explores both the design and experience of architecture—so the time has come to explore key findings about the workings of brains. As the book proceeds, we will add further findings as we show their relevance to our conversation. But first a warning. Neuroscience embraces a vast array of subtopics. Thus, the way *I* think is different from the way many other neuroscientists think. Still, the exposure to my general way of thinking may help prepare architects to conduct more focused discussion with neuroscientists who have the expertise relevant to a specific challenge in evidence-based design. For example, an expert on the auditory system who might help with an acoustics problem would be unable to help address memory problems relevant to design of a home for Alzheimer's patients. Architects go broad; scientists go deep (though of course they will be aware of many findings from outside their own labs).

Cog/neuroscience considered

This chapter introduces a delicate balancing act, seeking to tell architects more about brains without turning off the neuroscientists, and seeking to tell neuroscientists more about "how an architect thinks about the design and experience of buildings" without turning off the architects—and to do so in a way that may appeal to a broader public beyond these professions.

Actually, it is more delicate than this. For the last decade, I have been active in the Academy of Neuroscience for Architecture (ANFA), whose website (www.anfarch.org) states its mission to be "to promote and advance knowledge that links neuroscience research to a growing understanding of human responses to the built environment." However, at ANFA's biennial conferences, most of the architects want to talk about "the brain" at the level of "how people perceive feel, remember, act, and so forth," rather than in terms of neural circuitry, and few neuroscientists take part. Thus, my balancing act is complicated by the fact that many architects or general readers may tend to skip details of neuroscience that may nonetheless be crucial to the A↔N conversation. My solution in later chapters is the following: any text that gets into those details will come in two parts: a discussion of the general implications of the material, followed by a "skippable" presentation of those details set off by double lines. Nonetheless, I do hope that many readers will at least skim those details. My concern that this material might put off some non-neuroscientists brought to mind a book review by Peter Medawar (July 16, 1981),[5] in which he commented on the excessive use of mathematical formulas, and added:

> I asked a distinguished anatomist friend, Professor S., what he did when in the course of reading a paper he came across mathematical formulas he did not fully understand. "*I hum them,*" he said. . . . [My italics.]

As for mathematics, so for the details of neuroscience. I have done my best to strip out many details inessential to our conversation. Nonetheless, for details that remain, I suggest you follow the practice of Professor S., and *hum the detailed neuroscience* wherever it appears daunting, then return to the material as desired when reading later chapters. To hum is human, to understand is divine.

Neuroscience can be pursued with specific medical aims in mind, including the treatment of neurological disorders. But in this book we align with those who study the brain to better understand human experience and behavior, linking neuroscience with a broader perspective on *cognitive science* and *artificial intelligence* (AI), in which cognitive processes are explored without insisting on neural correlates. We can explore action, perception, memory, social interaction, and language in terms of interacting systems "in the head," whether or not we can yet relate these systems to specific regions of the brain, let alone the details of activity in neural circuitry. For different challenges, and at different stages of scientific progress, different levels of detail, from "purely cognitive" to "neurally

---

5. A nice challenge for neuroscience! How could my concern about explaining neuroscience to architects bring to mind an article read almost 40 years earlier, linking (at least) the name of the author, the name of the journal, and the phrase "hum the mathematics"? These provided sufficient cues to go online to download the article and retrieve the quotes, finding that I had recalled some further details but not others. How did the remembered details get linked and stored in memory? What associations led to their recall? In this case, the memory had come to mind a few times in the intervening decades. In other cases, a vivid memory full of the hustle and bustle of lived experience can resurface even though it has never sprung to mind before. Questions like this can spice the A↔N conversation even if the potential answers offer no immediate "plug-in" for the design of buildings.

detailed," will be appropriate. In what follows, then, I will often use "cognitive science" for the science of human experience and behavior that includes psychology but ignores the structure or function of the brain, while reserving "neuroscience" for the science of brains and neurons. I will often use the hybrid term *cog/neuroscience* to replace "neuroscience" in the loose sense employed by ANFA.

The brain has specialized and interacting subsystems, and a constant challenge is to understand how they work together to make us who we are. But what is "the" brain? Usually, we will refer to the structure and function of the human brain, but one may need to be more specific about which type of human brain, as when contrasting the needs of a child going to kindergarten and a person suffering from Alzheimer's disease. Moreover, I will talk about what is going on "in the head" of the user or architect of a building whenever I want to explore what has been achieved, or remains to be achieved, in cognitive science and neuroscience—without in any way denying the importance of the body, the linkage of the nervous system with receptors and effectors, and the fact that mental activity and neural activity involve the dynamic balance between "inside" and "outside" within the ongoing action–perception cycle.

However, *we cannot understand the human brain if we study only the human brain.* This may seem paradoxical—but in many cases our insights into the human brain are reached only through comparative studies of humans with other creatures. For example, we might use brain imaging to assess the relative activity of different regions of the brain as humans perform different tasks, but only in animals can we probe the underlying details of neural circuitry. For example, we have learned much about human brain mechanisms supporting wayfinding by studying the rat's neural circuitry supporting spatial navigation. Of course, there is a catch—nonhumans not only have different bodies from ours, they also have different brains. Nonetheless, hypotheses on how we and they may have evolved from shared but distant ancestors may let us relate, for example, the brain mechanisms linking eye and hand in monkeys and humans—and even yield insight into distinctively human brain mechanisms. Chapter 8 assesses how biological evolution yields a human brain with diverse capabilities, but with much of what is distinctively human, including language, emerging only through cultural evolution. To take just one example of interest to architects, cities are relatively recent human inventions, and much of what we may take for granted in possible life-styles follows on from this basic invention. Anyway, we end this paragraph with a counterpoint:

- we cannot understand the human brain if we study only the human brain; and yet,
- we cannot fully understand the human brain if we study only the brains of nonhumans, ignoring the relationships between the human brain and body and the diverse social and physical environments that shape them.

We seek to understand *functions* like perception, thought, memory, emotion, the control of action, and more in terms of the interaction of diverse processes. For example, vision include processes for depth perception, motion perception, object recognition, and the passing of parameters to action controllers. Such analysis of high-level functions in terms of interacting processes will be of value whether or not we have yet succeeded in showing how these processes are instantiated in the *structures* of the brain. As we seek to break these immense questions into manageable subparts, we will find that some of the questions we pose can indeed be answered by linkage to known brain processes. In general, however, we must take a two-step approach: Having come up with an answer to the question, "What cognitive processes could underlie this aspect of the experience or design of architecture?" we can then ask, "And how might the brain carry out these processes?" In some cases, an answer to these questions will be available; in other cases, the questions will pose challenges that can be answered only by new research on the brain. Having said this, it should be stressed that an answer to the first question will often suffice to advance our understanding, whether or not the relevant findings in neuroscience are currently available.

From social cooperation to consciousness

In many (but not all cases), A↔N conversations—architecture for neuro-science, neuroscience for architecture –will involve two stages:

Architecture ↔ Cognitive Science ↔ Neuroscience

When architects seek to collaborate on studies of human behavior and experience in buildings, they usually do so at the level of cognitive science and psychology, leaving it to the cognitive scientist to interact with neu-roscientists to determine which neuroscience findings can be "brought back" to extend understanding at the cognitive level. Indeed, there is a field, cognitive neuroscience, that supports the latter bridge, but the bridge of Architecture ↔ Cognitive Science is still in its early stages and will grow in tandem with novel approaches to environmental psychol-ogy. Indeed, our concern for the human mind in its interaction with the environment—a mixture of the natural, the social, and the built—can only be fully addressed by understanding something of our bodily physiology, and something of the environment's ecology, and how both biological and cultural evolution operate at the population level. (Figures 1.5 and 1.6 offer an architectural example and a Venn diagram to illustrate these ideas).

A crucial "philosophical" point: when I talk about my own behavior, I will often say "I decided to do X"; yet when I wear my neuroscience hat, I might ascribe my choice to a decision mechanism embedded in spe-cific regions of the brain. Many people feel uncomfortable with the lat-ter formulation, but this is just another instance of our ability to describe the same situation at different levels of explanation, just as we might talk about the sun rising and setting, or explain this phenomenon in terms of the Earth's rotation around its axis.

We have billions of neurons and cannot keep track of their detailed activity. Thus, when we "make decisions," this may rest more on myriad subconscious neural operations than on those of which we are conscious or put into words. For example, in choosing the main course for dinner at a restaurant, you may consciously decide against the chicken because

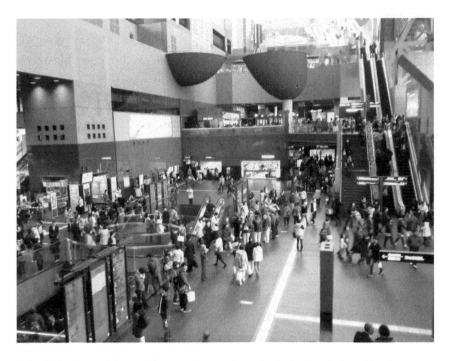

Figure 1.5 A partial view of the extension to Kyoto Train Station designed by the architect Hiroshi Hara and completed in 1997. Here, many people are interacting with other people or with the built environment, but at each moment their behavior is shaped by their current goals (getting to a train, trying to find the ticket office, looking for a place to eat, meeting a colleague) and by their previous experience (how to ride an escalator, knowledge of Japanese, and so much more). (Author's photo.)

you had chicken for lunch, yet be unable to articulate why you eventually chose the salmon rather than the halibut beyond saying, "I just felt like it." Thus, when we review mental processes involved in the experience and design of architecture, much will, similarly, be subconscious. But if the subconscious can achieve so much (and please do not confuse the term "subconscious" as used here with the "unconscious" of Freudian analysis), then what role does consciousness serve? There are many thousands of books about consciousness, but rather than try to review them, I will just offer one account (Arbib & Hesse, 1986) that seems consistent with my Chapter 8 account of evolution of the language-ready brain.

Human consciousness as we normally experience it is a mental experience, but rooted in properties of the brain. Our brains can support forms

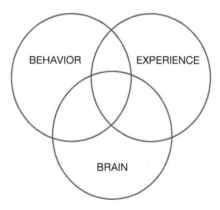

Figure 1.6 But what is going on in the head of each person at Kyoto Station, and how does the building shape their behavior? This Venn diagram leaves implicit the human body and the structure of the environment, but homes in on behavior, experience, and brain. Behavior is constituted by embodied interaction with the environment. Experience can focus on the current moment but may also become part of the memories that can shape further experience. If we focus solely on the relation between behavior and experience, we are in the realm of psychology or cognitive science. If we study their linkage with the structure and function of brains, then we are in the realm of neuroscience in the strict sense. Our attempts to engage in the A↔N conversation may be further enriched by insights from ecology, sociology, and more. And, of course, we all can be enriched by an appreciation of literature and the arts.

of "animal awareness" that may enrich human consciousness in ways that seem qualitatively different from conscious reflection. What makes human consciousness so different is that it includes the possibility of communicating something of our thoughts to others: consider the Latin *con* + *scio*, to know together.

Primate communication serves coordination of the members of a social group. There is a real continuity from controlling one's own body, to using tools, to "using" another member of one's group to complete some action. However, processes that coordinate a group member need not involve consciousness. Hesse and I argue that the ability to form a "précis"—a gesturable representation—of intended future actions evolved in protohumans as a way of coordinating more complex behaviors between different members of a group (Arbib & Hesse, 1986). Our further point is that this *communication plexus*—comprising the circuits involved in generating this representation—enriches the "information environment" for the rest of the brain, providing further evolutionary possibilities.

The basis for this was the observation from 19th-century British neurologist John Hughlings Jackson (Critchley & Critchley, 1998) that the evolution of a new brain system provides an environment for the further evolution of older systems. This led us to hypothesize that a new process of evolution begins whereby the précis comes to serve not only as a basis for coordination between the members of a group but also as a resource for planning and coordination within the brain itself. Our thesis is that it is the extension of this co-evolved system that imparts a specifically human dimension to consciousness.

Since subconscious activity can often proceed successfully without this highest level coordination, consciousness may sometimes be active, if active at all, as a monitor rather than as a director of action. In other cases, this précis plays the crucial role in determining our future course of action as, for example, we consciously compare verbally expressible alternatives. In particular, much of our ongoing experience and behavior—and much of that within the built environment—involve the interaction of consciously accessible and subconscious processes, and depend on the subconscious accumulation of details that shapes our schemas. Turning to design, our study of Gehry's use of sketching in Chapter 9 will reveal an interesting interaction: Drawing the sketch may be a semiautomatic process, with the motion of the pen across paper reflecting subconscious feelings about the form of the building; however, after the sketch exists, it can be consciously reviewed by Gehry and his colleagues as the basis for new ideas for extending the ongoing process of design.

Architecture considered

"Architecture" refers both to the process whereby buildings are designed and to the buildings that emerge from that design process. While our focus will be more on rooms and buildings, the concepts developed here can be extended from a single room to diverse buildings embedded in landscape or cityscape. Thus, the book offers no hard and fast distinction between urbanism, architecture, and interior design, just as we have blurred the line between cognitive science and neuroscience (and will, indeed, bring evolutionary, environmental, and cultural issues into this scientific arena).[6]

In this book (starting with the Therme at Vals), most of the buildings I discuss will be famous—with the advantage that their familiarity for some of you (directly, or through videos or reading) will enrich your engagement with my discussion. Yet much of the brain responds similarly for buildings whatever their merits—indeed, what seems meritorious to one person will be a failure to another—and so we will often use *architecture* as shorthand for *the design and experience of rooms, buildings, and larger ensembles*, whether or not they succeed functionally or aesthetically.

It is only within this broader setting that we can succeed in understanding how the built environment helps shape us as human beings and seek to assess what this might mean for a "better" architecture informed by the findings of cog/neuroscience. (Assessing what "better" might mean will be a recurring challenge.) Nonetheless, it still makes sense to take note of architecture in its aspirational sense. For example, Will Miller (whose father was instrumental in making Columbus, Indiana, a mecca for great architects) made an interesting distinction between building, sculpture, and architecture[7]:

If it's space that physically encloses a human activity and functions at a reasonable level but has no capacity to elicit from you a desire to go further, think spiritually, worry about your fellow man, then it's just a building.

---

6. *Neuroscience for Cities* (Camargo, Artus, & Spiers, 2018) assesses how buildings fit into the larger environment and its impact on the people who use it.

7. "Columbus, Ind.: A Midwestern Mecca of Architecture," an interview by Susan Stamberg on NPR, July 31, 2012, https://www.npr.org/2012/08/04/157675872/columbus-ind-a-midwestern-mecca-of-architecture.

If it's an enormously elaborate, beautiful, moving space that you can inhabit but it was designed as a symphony hall and you can't hear the orchestra in the back, then it's large-scale sculpture.

Architecture to me is that fantastic combination of the two where it enhances and encloses human activity, but it actually inspires you to do better.

The challenge of combining the two will continue to pose great challenges to architects—and to the A↔N conversation. I will return to this in §3.1.

1.3. HOW BRAINS MEET BUILDINGS

In the laboratory, the neurophysiologist must maintain a narrow focus, seeking, for example, to assess how different features of visual stimuli are encoded in different parts of the monkey brain, or how activity of cells in a rat's hippocampus varies depending on the place where the rat is in a maze, or how the activity of human brains, as studied by brain imaging, varies between two different but precisely delimited tasks. However, the experience of architecture is not that of responding to a well-designed stimulus. And we do not just "appreciate" a building—we "use" it, whether to learn, or to play, or to worship, or to work . . . and for each of these, the form of the building must be conformable to our bodies and wants, needs, and expectations, which may include social interaction as well as solitary pursuits. A major challenge of this book, then, is to weave a diversity of focused findings and theories about specific aspects of brain function into a convincing overall tapestry that offers new patterns for our thinking about architecture.

We next consider our two main, interconnected, themes of the *neuroscience of the experience of architecture* and the *neuroscience of the design process*, followed by a brief introduction to *neuromorphic architecture*, before turning to a fourth theme that permeates the book, the *EvoDevoSocio framework integrating evolution, development, and society.*

Neuroscience of the experience of architecture

An important precursor for the current A↔N conversation was provided by the book *Survival Through Design* (Neutra, 1954) by Richard Neutra, who was born in Vienna but spent the majority of his career in Southern California, where he came to be considered among the most important modernist architects. His book sought to integrate his extensive reading in both biology and psychology with his views on the importance of architecture for human survival in an increasingly incoherent world. Barbara Lamprecht offers a perspective on Neutra's architecture as a whole in *Neutra: Complete Works* (Lamprecht, 2010) that includes an essay on "Biorealism: Bodily Substrate of the Mental Life," focusing most closely on the themes of the book.

Turning more specifically to neuroscience, John Eberhard—Founding President of ANFA—set forth his manifesto in the book *Brain Landscape: The Coexistence of Neuroscience and Architecture* (Eberhard, 2008a). His guiding vision, and the main concern of ANFA, was with the *neuroscience of the experience of architecture.* The notion here is that by understanding the neuroscience of how different types of people experience and behave within different types of buildings, architects will support better design of each building to afford appropriate experiences to users other than themselves, such as a young child or a factory worker. Eberhard argued that architecture will benefit from increased understanding of how the brain reacts to and is influenced by different environments and advocated the establishment (yet unrealized) of *a neuroscience database on human responses to architecture,* as a basis for enhancing the quality of life through reduction of stress, increased cognition, prolonged productivity, and enhanced spiritual and emotional response.

A crucial observation was that buildings where people spend much time can *influence the fundamental structure of the brain* and thus affect people's thoughts and behaviors (both conscious and subconscious). For example, Eberhard posited that neuroscience will change architects' understanding of how classroom design affects the cognitive processes of children, how the design of hospital rooms could affect the recovery rate of patients, how working environments affect workers' productivity, and how sacred spaces instill a sense of awe in those who worship there. Contrast building an elementary school for children who are learning so much about their environments (Eberhard, 2008b) and a retirement home for patients with Alzheimer's disease whose memories of a lifetime are rapidly disappearing (Zeisel, 2006). The architects' own experience of many buildings informs their understanding of how users will experience each new building they design, but that is not enough when a particular typology of building demands an understanding of the embodied experience and behavior of very different people who will use it.

However, Eberhard seems too concerned with building a database of "narrow sense" neuroscience, whereas the insights that may best inform the activity of the architect will usually come from psychology and cognitive science. Nonetheless, the neuroscience remains pertinent for those who wish to seek a richer understanding. For the architect this understanding may be a form of mental enrichment rather than being "plugged in" to design, but for the cognitive scientist it may (but may not) be essential to uncovering phenomena that would otherwise have remained invisible. To take an example from John Zeisel's book, *Inquiry by Design: Environment/ Behavior/Neuroscience in Architecture, Interiors, Landscape, and Planning* (Zeisel, 2006), we know that Alzheimer's disease starts with disruption of the hippocampus, a brain region whose role in episodic memory we will meet later. For the architect, this location within the brain may be irrelevant; the progression of memory loss and consequent disorientation and loss of personal connection may set guidelines for the design of housing for people suffering such loss—and further understanding of the progressive symptoms can inform the caregivers who attend to these people as their inner world appears to disintegrate. Complementing all this, neuroscientists are currently engaged in an ongoing search to understand the underlying changes in the brain in the desperate hope of discovering how the progress of the disease may be stopped or, at least, slowed down and the patient's condition ameliorated. Understanding such research, at least at a general level, may deepen architects' understanding of the human beings whose life their buildings should be designed to enrich.

Neuroscience of the design of architecture

Understanding how people experience buildings informs our understanding of what goes on in the brain of an architect, and we gained some preliminary insight into the *neuroscience of the design process* in discussing Zumthor's comments. Design must anticipate, in some sense, the experience of the people who will use the building. Most architects begin design by investigating client needs, and then transform this shared understanding into a novel building. Different architects bring diverse skills and experiences to their designs. Thus, when we consider the work of a particular architect, we make no claim that the way they design is in any sense "canonical." Rather, the aim is to reflect on their work as the basis for extracting underlying cognitive processes that are deployed in varying combinations by all designers.

Two complementary challenges are involved in Eberhard's concerns. One is to understand the way the brain changes through a typical lifespan, understanding the changes in action, perception, learning, and memory and the underlying brain mechanisms that come with different "stages" of life. This is augmented by understanding the capabilities of special populations, including an assessment of whether and where shortfalls in some capacities may be offset to some extent by increased capacity in others. The other challenge is to assess how experience of buildings of different types can be improved by design that is informed by an understanding of these diverse capabilities.

Building on this, Eduardo Macagno, a developmental neurobiologist and former ANFA President, speaks of *lifespan architecture*—thinking through how a building might be designed so that it can be readily updated over time. Consider, for example, a house that in turn might accommodate a newlywed couple, the same couple with young children, the couple with teenagers, the couple leading a vigorous life in their (not always) empty nest, and then the couple facing the rigors of the last few years of life. This is a crucial case of what Stewart Brand (1995) considers in his book, *How Buildings Learn*—not considering (as we may increasingly do in future) how the building itself forms an adaptive system, but rather how humans may restructure it over time to meet different needs. All this poses intrigu-ing challenges for both cog/neuroscience and architecture.

The challenges of lifespan architecture will receive little attention in this book. John Zeisel's book is an excellent place to start for those wishing practical guidance in pursuing this alternate path. Here, my aim will be to help develop the shared knowledge that can increase the bandwidth of the A↔N conversation in assessing the experience of architecture, while also encouraging nonprofessionals to join in. I will pay particular attention to the role of the hand in experience and design, to locomotion as a basic human activity in support of other actions, enriched by some discussion of aesthetics and atmosphere. Throughout the book, we will see the way in which understanding the diversity of experience of architecture provides strong lessons for the architect, but our especial focus on design will come with the case studies of Chapter 9, and the extraction from them of gen-eral insights that will guide our steps toward a cognitive neuroscience of architectural design in Chapter 10.

Neuromorphic architecture—buildings with "brains"

Since every building with a thermostat is already an interactive one, and since many people are now welcoming voice-activated digital assistants into their homes, it is timely to explore whether neuroscience will contrib-ute to the further factoring of interactivity into architecture. What I call *neuromorphic architecture* focuses not on what happens to the brain of someone experiencing or designing a building, but rather on what it might mean for a building to have a "brain." Chapter 7 will introduce the interac-tive space Ada, a perceiving, acting, and adapting entity, interacting with the people inside the space. It had a "brain" based in part on artificial neu-ral networks, had "emotions," and in some sense wanted to play with "her" visitors. Ada may be considered to be an "inside-out" robot. There is no implication that a building with a "brain" (and the scare quotes are crucial) has anything close to human autonomy or consciousness—neuromorphic architecture seeks neurobiological inspiration from the bodies and brains of diverse animals. Neuromorphic architecture integrates the "neural space," encompassing not only the "brain" (computational infrastructure) of the building but also its sensors and effectors, with the "physical space" of the actual building. I suggest that, in future, design of the neural and physical spaces will develop in tandem to yield new ideas for the physical design of buildings.

The EvoDevoSocio perspective

Christopher Egan, a San Antonio architect, now deceased, talked about emotion and behavior in the architectural setting[8]:

> Architecture moves us. It can comfort us or intimidate us; it can enlighten us or mystify us; it can bring joy, or tear at our hearts. Architecture moves us by touching three layers of memory. Through primal space it can touch our deepest emotional core; evoking shadow memories of the womb, the cave, the forest, and light. It can recall memories of culture, or our place in the historical world. Personal memories add overlays of subjective meanings, as buildings are associated with events in our lives.

I have some trouble with "evoking shadow memories of the womb, the cave, the forest, and the light." I doubt that we have memories of the womb, but I can accept that our subjectivity is in part genetically based. Most people find watching a fire intriguing, and are scared by snakes and spiders. They enjoy a beautiful sunset and a walk in the countryside, so there does seem to be some innate substrate for our aesthetic experience, perhaps the residue of biological adaptation to the weather, to the uses and dangers of fire, and to the challenges of hunting, foraging, and avoiding predators.

8. Cited by John Eberhard (2008a) in *Brain Landscape: The Coexistence of Neuroscience and Architecture*, p. 89.

Just as the growth of the body may be stunted by malnutrition and disease, so may it be enhanced by good nutrition and healthy exercise—but these environmental effects depend on our genetic makeup, which is itself the result of the biological evolution of the species and the happenstances of our parentage. In this spirit, we adopt the *EvoDevoSocio perspective* of brains in bodies of agents in social and physical interaction with the world around them, a perspective enriched by the view that biological evolution defines developmental systems that can both shape and be shaped by cultural evolution, the dynamic emergence of patterns of social interaction. Such an approach seeks to illuminate how biological evolution yielded brains and bodies (Evo) that could develop (Devo) in a setting that already had some form of culture (Socio) so that children could master their local culture with the help of caregivers to support their development as active members of that culture.

Moreover, our biological heritage emerged from landscape and the need for shelter and refuge. Buildings can evoke some of that, but we have been transformed by 200 millennia or more of cultural evolution, and especially the vast transformations of the past few centuries and even the past few decades. Perhaps it is not so much that architecture explicitly recalls ancestral memories as that the culture in which we grow up shapes our development in ways that in turn shape our expectations and our desires. A recurrent theme, one that moves to center stage in Chapter 8, is thus to replace nebulous terms like "ancestral memory" with ideas gathered from the EvoDevoSocio analysis—evolutionary, developmental, and social— that situates our individual development within the framework set by biological and cultural evolution.

Back to neuroscience. Many laboratory studies are based on limited manipulation of a few variables in the isolated subject: Put a human in the scanner and see how the brain responds during a limited set of tasks; put an animal in a small enclosure and correlate neuron activity with well-controlled changes in the animal's behavior. However, humans (like most other creatures) evolved as social beings. In this book, we will explore the relevance of neuroscience to understanding how people interact in the physical and social environment they inhabit. This environment may be referred to as the "ecological niche" of a human group—but, crucially, humans are constantly changing that niche, and so we speak of *niche construction* (Iriki & Sakura, 2008; Laland, Odling-Smee, & Feldman, 2000; Odling-Smee, Laland, & Feldman, 2003). Where, in the study of beavers, we might note how their damming of rivers physically constructs a new ecological niche, human niche construction is cognitive as well as physical. Although we will not make much explicit use of the term "niche construction" in what follows, it will be implicit as we think about different buildings and the extent to which a new niche makes them possible or is made possible by them—as in the way the development of elevators and innovations in construction created the niche in which Sullivan's tall buildings became possible.

Our capacity for experience and the skills we deploy depend on the cultural environment in which we develop. Here, the term "culture" has no implication of evaluating high or low cultures—it just refers to the fact that, for example, your adult behavior will reflect the language, politics, and morality of the group or larger society in which you were raised. Whether you conform or rebel, your experiences and behaviors are shaped by the reflection in your brain of your individual experience within a particular set of cultural or social milieux. But then, of course, the individual experiences of diverse people within a society will cohere in varying patterns to reshape that sociocultural framework over the years.

A word of caution: Evolution is a process of change—but with no guarantee of "progress." In *biological* evolution, random mutations may be correlated with an increased rate at which a population produces offspring, but this reproductive "fitness" may not necessarily result from the mutation but from an increased availability of food in the area in which the mutation occurs. In this case, "natural selection" may yield a change in the population that is detrimental in the long run, after the fluctuation has passed. In *cultural* evolution, some changes will be of benefit to many members of a population, some will cater to the tastes of an elite with little impact on others, and some will involve strengthening the power of one group only at the cost of the subjugation of others. Short-term gains may breed long-term disasters—the exploitation of fossil fuels had diverse benefits from increased personal mobility to ready availability of energy to diverse uses of petrochemicals, and yet has now led to the urgent challenges of global warming. Turning to architecture, then, there is no reason to regard the architectural innovations produced in a society as necessarily improving on that of preceding generations. Our challenge in what follows will be to deepen our understanding of architecture through a conversation that engages with neuroscience within a broader setting. This requires recognizing the current state of *biological* evolution in setting the biological basis for development of human individuals, while also recognizing that the social and physical environment in which they develop will be shaped by the *cultural* evolution of the family and the environment. The architect, in particular, is thus shaped by cultural evolution—but is also an agent for helping change it. Will those changes constitute "progress," and if so, in what sense and for whom?

1.4. THE MANY LEVELS OF THE BRAIN

Having seen the relevance of neuroscience in the broad sense to architecture, it is now time to at last introduce some details of the structure and functioning of various regions and neural circuitry of the human brain—noting again the importance of comparative study with other creatures in developing our knowledge in neuroscience. This section is pitched at such a level that most of it will be accessible to all readers (though there is no need to memorize the details).

When we analyze the brain, we divide the brain into different regions, but we are not in the realm of phrenology where a bulge in the skull signals an enlarged brain region devoted to some particular trait like "acquisitiveness." Rather, while each region has a particular role to play, our perception, action, and more each depend on the coordinated activity of diverse regions—*the brain is a system of systems.*

Structure and function in the brain

What do structure and function mean for neuroscience?

> *Structure*: In looking at the mammalian brain, we can delimit large
> regions such as cerebral cortex, hippocampus, and cerebellum, all
> the way down to individual neurons and even smaller components
> such as the synapses where one neuron influences another.
> *Function*: The functions we consider include vision and other forms
> of perception, emotion, locomotion and other forms of action,
> learning, and memory, as well as social interaction and aesthetic
> appreciation.

In neuroscience, we seek to understand how this diversity of structures supports this multiplicity of functions and their interaction, including the way in which many functions will rest on the coordinated activity of multiple brain regions.

Figure 1.7 presents a double hierarchy linking society and neurons, one functional (left = hand path) and the other structural (the forms that implement the functions; right-hand path). The aim here is to seek the mechanisms that enable the brain to function through its integration into a body whose sensors and effectors mediate the person's interactions within the physical and social environment, and how these interactions shape new memories that continually modify the individual self of each person even as the actions of diverse people change the environment.

When we explore the interactions of persons in a society and seek to understand the underlying processes from the perspective of cognitive science, we may employ *schemas* as our units of analysis (left-hand path). These are units of distributed computation that underlie our cognitive processes. As noted in our discussion of the action–perception cycle, we will consider various *perceptual and motor schemas* but also a range of related concepts. Explanation of some cognitive function in terms of interacting schemas may suffice when we work under the banner of cognitive science, the locus for what will most engage architects in their pragmatic pursuit

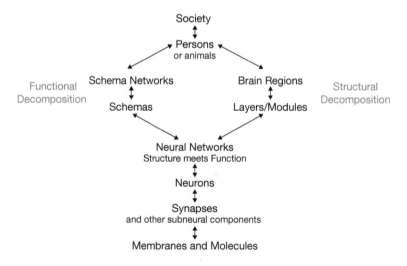

Figure 1.7 Two hierarchies for neuroscience. In either case we seek to understand people (or animals) interacting within the social and physical environment (to both of which the built environment contributes). The term "decomposition" here reflects a methodology that is the opposite of "composition"—seeking component processes whose composition explains a function; seeking substructures whose integration offers a finer grain analysis of some structure of the brain. In any particular instance, we may seek to understand some behavior or experience by breaking it down functionally into interacting processes that are here called "schemas"—and this functional analysis (left-hand path) may satisfy the cognitive scientist. The neuroscientist may start with a structural decomposition (right-hand path), and this may suffice for initial analysis of brain imaging data. However, such analyses may be refined by seeking to understand how the various functions are implemented by neural networks. For architecture, the descent down the hierarchy may stop at very simple analysis of "learning rules" that modify synapses to allow experience to change the performance of neural networks over time. For some neuroscientists—but not us, in this book—the descent continues downward to explore the biophysics, molecular biology, and genetics of synapses, neurons, and networks. (From Arbib, M. A. [2016]. From neuron to cognition: An opening perspective. In M. A. Arbib & J. J. Bonaiuto [Eds.], *From neuron to cognition via computational neuroscience* (pp. 1–71). Cambridge, MA: MIT Press.)

of the A↔N conversation. However, there will be relevant insights from gaining at least some entry into the neuroscientist's domain. Initial ideas about how interacting schemas serve some function of interest may prove wrong as we seek to match schemas to interacting brain regions (e.g., if we are looking only at brain imaging or lesion data) or to details of activity in neural circuits (if we can assess how animal data might relate to human circuitry).

The details of synapses at present seem relevant to our discussion of architecture only to the extent that they provide the loci of *synaptic plasticity*—as changes in synapses, the connections between neurons, mediate the changing function of neural circuits. The level of membranes and molecules may be crucial for understanding genetics and the effects of drugs on the brain but are not directly relevant (at least for now) to the A↔N conversation.

We use the term "gross anatomy" for the parcellation of the brain into distinguishable regions, as distinct from the "fine anatomy" at the level of single neurons and their connectivity. The left of Figure 1.8 gives a medial (middle) view as it might be revealed were we to slice the head in half, so that the midbrain structures may be clearly seen. The brains of mammals, and especially of humans, are distinguished from those of other species by the "explosion" of cerebral cortex that is new in evolutionary terms—*neocortex*. This comes in humans to dominate the rest of the brain, as is clear in the lateral (side) view of a human brain at right, where the outfoldings of neocortex completely hide the midbrain from view. The human cerebral cortex is a sheet only 50 to 100 neurons in depth, but it contains so many billions of neurons that it must fold, and fold again, to fit into the space within the skull. This great expansion of forebrain comes with evolution to greatly modify circuitry in the brainstem and spinal cord. Indeed, we cannot understand the human brain by focusing on the cerebral cortex alone—it only gains its power through interaction with diverse subcortical structures. The *cerebellum* is necessary to allow us to move gracefully; the *basal ganglia* is involved in action selection and reward; and the *hippocampus* is a key player (but not the only one) in spatial navigation and episodic memory.

While the *thalamus* is shown simply as a floating oval in Figure 1.8, it is divided into diverse structures (*nuclei*) that are richly connected with other brain regions. In particular, all sensory systems except olfaction send signals from the sensors to neurons in a dedicated nucleus of thalamus, and the neurons of this nucleus send these signals on to the primary

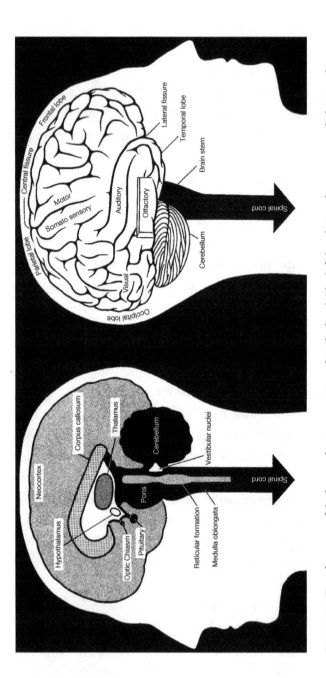

Figure 1.8 Two diagrams of the human brain as positioned in the head. The left-hand view diagrams a *medial* view, what we would see were we to slice down the middle of the head from the outside after removal of the skull. The *spinal cord* runs up through the vertebrae of the spine, receiving signals from the limbs and trunk, and contains the motoneurons that control limb and trunk muscles. The spinal cord leads into the *brainstem*, behind which is the outswelling of the *cerebellum*. Then, overshadowing all, is the great outfolding of the *neocortex* of the cerebral hemispheres. At left we can see the *midbrain* and other structures that are obscured by the neocortex at right. (From Arbib, M. A. [1972]. *The metaphorical brain: An introduction to cybernetics as artificial intelligence and brain theory*. New York, Wiley-Interscience.)

sensory cortex for that modality after some further processing. For example, messages from the retina go to a part of the thalamus called the *lateral geniculate nucleus*, and this projects in turn to primary visual cortex.

Here is a crucial fact: There are more fibers extending "down" to the retina from the lateral geniculate nucleus to the retina than there are going "up" from the retina. This introduces a key partnership that is very much part of the action–perception cycle: all perceptual processing integrates *bottom-up* processes moving up from the sensors with *top-down* processes that modulate activity in terms of current goals and hypotheses based on an immense stock of schemas in long-term memory encapsulating the diversity of an individual's experience.

The cerebral cortex is divided into four lobes whose names provide the basic terminology for locating diverse brain regions: the *frontal lobe* in the region of the forehead; the *temporal lobe*, which is to the sides in the region of the temples; the *parietal lobe*, which is at the top rear where the parietal bones form part of the skull; and the *occipital lobe*, from the Latin *occipitus*, meaning back of the head. A groove in the cortex may be called a *fissure* or a *sulcus*, and the upfolded tissue between two sulci is a *gyrus*. Pathways connecting regions in the two halves of the brain are called *commissures*. The largest is the *corpus callosum*, which connects the two cerebral hemispheres.

The motoneurons, which synapse upon the muscles of the body and limbs and thus control their contractions, are contained in the spinal cord, *not* the forebrain, but the circuitry for the control of eye movements is contained within the head. The brain also contain neurons that directly control a different kind of effector. The *pituitary gland* releases various subtle hormones that are broadcast through the bloodstream to control endocrine organs. This endocrine chemical messenger system is another "chain of command" in addition to the neural. We should complement this reminder of the variety of effector mechanisms by noting, similarly, that the sensory surface of the organism is *not* just the external surface. In fact, there are two sensory surfaces in addition to the external (*exteroceptive*) inputs from the body surface and such sense organs as the eyes, ears, and nose. There are *proprioceptive* fibers providing feedback information on movement and orientation from muscles, joints, tendons, otoliths, and the semicircular canals; and there are *interoceptive* fibers bringing signals from the glands and viscera.

Certain areas of cortex can be dubbed *sensory* because they primarily process information from one modality—this includes not only the area labeled *somatosensory* in Figure 1.8, which receives information relayed via the spinal cord from the body surface and joints and muscles of the limbs, but also the *visual, auditory,* and *olfactory* areas (the last shown in cutaway because it is not on the outer surface), which receive information from the distance receptors in the head. The *motor* cortex is a source of fibers that control muscular activity, some indirectly via multiple intervening areas, while others exercise direct control of those motor neurons engaged in fine control of the fingers. Phylogenetically, somatosensory and motor cortex form a tightly coupled system, and it is thus common to refer to the regions of frontal and parietal cortex adjoining the central fissure as *sensorimotor cortex.*

The rest of the cortex is called *association* cortex, but this is a misnomer that reflects an erroneous 19th-century view that the job of these areas was simply to "associate" the different sensory inputs to provide the proper instructions to be relayed by the motor cortex. The absolutely false idea that 90% of the brain is "unused" probably arose from a layman's misinterpretation of the fact that the exact functions of many of these "association areas" are only now being understood.

In the early years of the 20th century, the German neurologist Korbinian Brodmann (1905, 1909) noted that the neurons of all parts of cerebral cortex could be characterized as forming six layers, but that the density and depth of these layers varied from region to region. He used this to characterize the cerebral cortex at a finer level than the four lobes. He defined 52 regions, each with a distinctive cellular arrangement of its layers, and numbered them in a way that is not particularly clear. Figure 1.9 shows both a lateral (side) view and a medial view of cerebral cortex labeled with Brodmann areas. Only a few of these numbers will appear in later pages. There is no need to memorize them here, but they may come in handy if you decide to read the primary literature. Here are some examples:

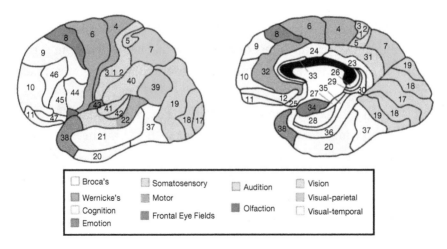

Figure 1.9 Lateral and medial views of the Brodmann areas of the human cerebral cortex, with color-coding of a basic view of their functionality. However, this labeling is only a first approximation to the finer subdivisions discovered through subsequent research. (From Arbib, M. A. [2012]. *How the brain got language: The mirror system hypothesis*. New York and Oxford: Oxford University Press.)

- Area 17 is the primary visual cortex, feeding into secondary visual cortex in areas 18 and 19.
- The input pathway for touch and body sense enters cortex at area 1, primary somatosensory cortex, and continues to areas 2 and 3.
- Area 4 is primary motor cortex with fibers sending signals down to various regions engaged in motor (muscle) control, some even projecting directly to motoneurons in the spinal cord that control finger movements.
- At a higher level, the perception and production of language involves many areas, including Wernicke's area (area 22) and Broca's area (areas 44 and 45).

However, behavior and cognition will involve the integrated competition and cooperation of multiple brain regions, and not just these. As already noted, the brain is a system of systems. As we learn more about the brain, we can refine the regions characterized by Brodmann and explore the pathways that connect them to support their coordinated activity.

All this, without even getting into the detail of neural networks, suggests something of the treasure house of knowledge that neuroscience may have to offer to our further quest to understand more fully the experience and design of buildings.

It is worth emphasizing how very different a brain is from a contemporary desktop computer. Only a small part of such a computer is engaged in actively following the instructions of a computer program, one or a few steps at a time. Vast reams of data are stored in a passive electronic memory, with a few items to be retrieved when needed in the ongoing serial computation, and to be updated as computations progress. But just because the brain looks like a bowl of porridge doesn't mean it's a serial computer. Each region of the brain is a vast network of millions or more neurons, each constantly active and exchanging signals and transforming those they receive. Memory and processing are intertwined—the same neurons are processing the signals they receive and changing in ways that will affect how they later perform. There is thus a dynamic memory in the current exchange of signals throughout the network, and a more enduring form of memory captured by longer term changes within the neurons— later we will pay attention to the learning mechanisms that affect the "strength" of the synapses whereby neurons affect each other.

In short, a brain is not a general-purpose computer to which we may simply download new software as needed. Rather, the brain's computation style is *cooperative computation*—it operates through vast, dynamic patterns of *competition and cooperation*, whether characterized at the level of schemas or of neurons, that must yield some sort of consensus in committing the organism to a course of action or other "decision."

Moreover, different brain regions, while changeable through protracted activity, involve different types of neurons and different patterns of neural connectivity, thus contributing to their unique contribution to the ongoing computations. Figure 1.10 is a photograph including Janós (John) Szentágothai, one of the neuroanatomists whose work we sample in Figure 1.11 to depict something of the diversity of neurons and their interconnections (showing a selected few of the neurons so that their shape

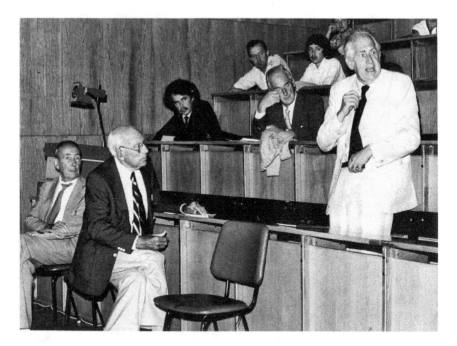

Figure 1.10 The great Hungarian neuroanatomists Janós (John) Szentágothai (1912–1994) speaking, with his usual vigor, at the conference in Pécs, Hungary, organized for his 70th birthday in 1982. Next to the very attentive Sir John Eccles (the Australian Nobel Laureate) is Richard Jung (Freiburg); next to John is the less attentive Donald MacKay (the Scottish cybernetician); and in the same row left is Hendrick Van der Loos (discoverer of "barrels" in rat somatosensory cortex). (The picture was taken by Mrs. Márta Soltész, photographer of the Anatomy Department at Pécs, and is used here with kind permission of Gyula Lázár and Miklós Réthelyi.)

and positioning can be sketched clearly) that distinguish one brain region from another.[9] These drawings give some sense of the beauty of another form of architecture, the neural architecture of the brain, but the insights to be gained from studying their details lie outside the scope of this book.

9. I coauthored two books with Szentágothai: Szentágothai and Arbib (1975), and Arbib, Érdi, and Szentágothai (1998). The latter, *Neural Organization: Structure, Function, and Dynamics*, was still in preparation when John died in 1994. Peter Érdi and I completed it thereafter, using the material he had prepared on *Structure*, integrating it with my material on *Function* and Peter's on *Dynamics*.

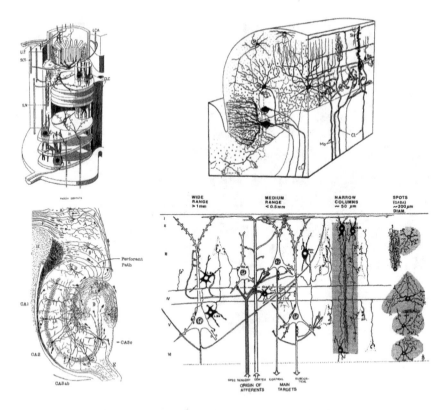

Figure 1.11 The diversity of neural architecture in the mammalian brain. (*Top left*) Spinal cord. (*Top right*) Cerebellum. (*Bottom left*) Hippocampus. (*Bottom right*) Cerebral cortex. The drawing of the cross section of rat hippocampus is by the great Spanish neuroanatomist Santiago Ramón y Cajal, the other three are by John Szentágothai. (From Arbib, M. A., Érdi, P., & Szentágothai, J. [1998]. *Neural organization: Structure, function, and dynamics.* Cambridge, MA: MIT Press.)

Measuring brain and behavior

Classic work in the 19th century on people with *aphasia* (defects in language behavior associated with brain damage) started with Broca's (1861, 1861/1960) description of a patient with a lesion in the *anterior* region (i.e., a region toward the front) marked B on the cortex in Figure 1.12, what is now called Broca's region. Broca's aphasia seemed essentially *motoric* in that the patient was able to comprehend speech but could speak only

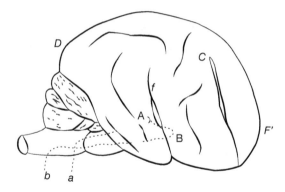

Figure 1.12 Wernicke's 1874 diagram showing the principal pathways for language suggested by his and Broca's data: (a to A) peripheral auditory pathway → sound center for words; (B to b) motor center for words → peripheral motor pathways for speech. Strangely, Wernicke shows what we now call Wernicke's area (A) and Broca's area (B) on the right (i.e., wrong) hemisphere: in most humans the key language mechanisms are located in the left hemisphere, though with some related mechanisms (such as speech prosody) on the right. Compare the locations as shown in our schematic of the Brodmann areas—BA 44 and 45 for Broca; BA 22 for Wernicke. (Adapted from Wernicke, C. [1874]. *Der aphasische symptomencomplex.* Breslau: Cohn and Weigert. The letters A and B are my changes from a and b, respectively. Public domain.)

with effort and then only "telegrammatically" in short utterances omitting most of the grammatical markers.

By contrast, Wernicke (1874) described a patient with a lesion in the *posterior* region (towards the rear), marked A on the cortex, now called Wernicke's region. Wernicke's aphasia seemed essentially *sensory*, in that the patient seemed not to comprehend speech (but was not deaf to auditory stimuli) and would speak a fluent but meaningless stream of syllables. It should also be added that later work established that for most people (even 90% of left-handers, whose dominant hand is controlled by the right motor cortex), it is the left hemisphere that is predominantly involved in language, with lesions of the right hemisphere causing few or no aphasic symptoms, but possibly affecting the prosody of speech.

A problem with assessing the effects of brain lesions is that the observation that damage to region R blocks function X does *not* guarantee that region R supports the key processing for function X—any more than the fact that a car's failure to move after the wheels are removed would imply that the wheels provide the car's motor. Naturally, neurologists combine data from studies of many different patients in the quest for more reliable inferences.

Such 19th-century (and much 20th-century) knowledge of the human brain derived from correlating behavioral and cognitive disorders with postmortem analysis of where the brain was damaged. This was supplemented by studies of the effects of surgery that removed parts of the brain and, later, by electrical stimulation of parts of the brain (Penfield & Rasmussen, 1950) during neurosurgery to help design cuts that would have minimal impact on language and cognition and the ability to care for oneself. In the past few decades, these insights have been dramatically expanded using brain imaging—in this book we focus on functional magnetic resonance imaging (fMRI)—which can be used even with participants with no medical problems to study the relative activity of parts of the brain when they carry out different tasks. We will explore one such study in detail in Chapter 4.

One drawback of fMRI is that the "blobs" of activity it records are enormous compared to the scale of individual neurons. Most functions depend on interactions between diverse brain regions. Thus, when I'm working as a neuroscientist (whether or not I am worrying about architecture), one of my big concerns is to understand what is really going on in the underlying neural interactions during various tasks, and why this yields certain types of fMRI images. I see fMRI data not just as phenomena of interest in themselves but as windows on the details of "how the brain works." However, the windows have fogged up, and to better make sense of what they reveal I will often seek to reconcile these views with what is known from more detailed studies of neural circuitry in animals.

Animal studies range from the genetics and molecular biology of basic cellular mechanisms including synaptic plasticity, via single-cell and multicell recordings of neural activity during specific tasks, all the way to observations of behavior in single animals and groups both in the lab and in the wild. The microelectrodes that make possible the recording of the activity of single neurons, or groups of single neurons, in awake behaving animals became available only in 1948. In Chapter 2, we will look at data from monkey neurophysiology relevant to the study of eye–hand coordination, while Chapter 3 will offer an interesting perspective on vision by contrasting neural circuitry in the frog and monkey. Chapter 5 will show how "mirror neurons" were discovered in the brains of macaque monkeys and how this in turn inspired the discovery of "mirror systems" in the human brain—and we will explore how mirror systems work with systems "beyond the mirror" to support imitation, empathy, and language in humans and even an action-oriented view of aesthetic experience. Our discussion of wayfinding in Chapter 6 will be enriched by reviewing neurophysiology of circuitry in the brains of rats exploring mazes.

But what of the challenges of measuring human response within the built environment, as distinct from, say, lying in an fMRI scanner and responding to photos of buildings? Eduardo Macagno (personal communication) stresses that just putting a headset on a subject to measure brainwaves does not mean that one can interpret the waveforms. Any experiment requires something like this methodology, *whether the methodology is linked to cognitive science, neuroscience, or statistical polling of a population*:

- Define a question of interest.
- Narrow it down to an answerable form.
- Select the best methodology to gather data, for example, using a questionnaire or physiological measurements.
- Design the experimental paradigm and controls.
- Do double-blind analysis of data to avoid bias in the interpretation.

Functional MRI offers good spatial resolution and poor temporal resolution of brain activity, but requires the subject to lie in a scanner with little or no movement. Electroencephalography (EEG), recording the summed electrical activity of vast populations of neurons as recorded through electrodes placed on the scalp, offers poor spatial resolution but excellent temporal resolution and has the advantage of portability (but I will say very little about EEG further in this book). Behavioral analysis can track overt movements, including eye movements, whether of the individual or group.[10] One may seek to study action in the built environment or evocation of certain emotions as a design goal. For the latter, pupil dilation and galvanic skin response may provide relevant data. Light, wearable devices make measuring responses to the real environment more practicable. Studies may employ virtual reality (VR), but one then needs to study at least some of the functions in the real environment to establish how well the two types of data may be correlated.

It is outside the scope of this book to provide a "how-to" manual for monitoring human brain and behavior within the A↔N framework. However, this brief note on some of the relevant methodologies may provide an entry point to the relevant literature. The reader will find several examples of such studies later in the book.

1.5. A KEY DEBATE: IS NEUROSCIENCE RELEVANT TO ARCHITECTURE?

Phenomenology is the study of structures of consciousness as experienced from the first-person point of view:

> The central structure of an experience is its intentionality, its being directed toward something, as it is an experience of or about some object. An experience is directed toward an object by virtue of its content or meaning (which represents the object) together with appropriate enabling conditions. . . . Phenomenology . . . came into its own in the early 20th century in the works of Husserl, Heidegger, Sartre, Merleau-Ponty and others. Phenomenological

---

10. An essay by Ann Sussman and Janice M. Ward in *Common Edge* argues that "Game-Changing Eye-Tracking Studies Reveal How We Actually See Architecture," https://commonedge.org/game-changing-eye-tracking-studies-reveal-how-we-actually-see-architecture/. Of course, they do not "reveal how we actually see" but do give us powerful insights into what we attend to. More on this in Chapter 3.

issues of intentionality, consciousness, qualia, and first-person perspective have been prominent in recent philosophy of mind. (Smith, 2018)

Each of us has a clear set of experiences of our body and how it moves in space, and architects develop a rich understanding of the experience of people in the built environment. For some architects, the linkage of this to cog/neuroscience is certainly *interesting*, but this leaves open its *relevance* to the practice of architecture. This book seeks to settle that debate, but here we consider some of the issues more explicitly.

The interdependence of science and art

One of the strongest proponents of the phenomenological stance in architecture has been Juhani Pallasmaa,

[who introduced] phenomenological aspects of kinesthetic and multisensory perception of the human body into architecture theory. He argues that hand-drawing is a vital spatial and haptic exercise in facilitating architectural design. Through this process, architecture can emerge as the very "material" existence of human embodied "immaterial" emotion, feelings and wisdom. Hence, for Pallasmaa, architecture can be seen as an artistic practice, which entails multisensory and embodied thought in order to establish the sense of being in the world. (Tamari, 2016, p. 91)

I have already stressed the importance of Pallasmaa's (2012) book, *The Eyes of the Skin*, but my current aim is to resolve the tension between the first-person phenomenology of Pallasmaa and the third-person emphasis of the neuroscientist seeking the neural basis of experience. To start this process of reconciliation, consider an excerpt from Pallasmaa's contribution to the concluding discussion in *Architecture and Atmosphere* (Tidwell, 2015):

The field of neuroscience is now somewhat gaining a grasp on the mental processes and phenomena that support the idea of emergent rather than finite understanding. And there has been increasing value placed on the idea that *consciousness may not be something that we contain in our brains* but something that is 'out there' in our relationship with the world. [My italics.] (Pallasmaa in Tidwell, 2015, p. 68)

But if we had no brain, we could not have a relationship with the external world in the sense Pallasmaa intends. A human body with an aardvark brain would not be human, and would not have a human consciousness. However, a human brain in a body that is incapable of almost all movement may yield a human with a human consciousness, as revealed in a case described to me by the Italian pediatric neurologist Giuseppe Cozzu (personal communication, 1999). He was approached at a conference by the caregiver for a boy who had only one movement, a quick inclination of the head that seemed to occur at random intervals, and who showed no apparent understanding of what was said to him. The caregiver told Cozzu that, nonetheless, she was sure that "there was someone in there" and asked him to examine the boy. He agreed to do so, but felt somewhat foolish as he gave instructions (in Italian) to the boy. "I am going to show you objects, and if the name I say is wrong. I want you to twitch your head." He shows him a spoon, and says "spoon." No response. Not surprising. He shows him a ball and says "knife," and the boy's head twitches. A coincidence? But as the tests continued, it became clear that the boy understood the objects and their names. It was not the head twitching; it was the boy twitching his head. As a result of this discovery, an engineer built a device to let the boy move a cursor on a computer screen and select letters. Not only could he spell words, he could make sentences. His consciousness was freed from his almost inert body—a freedom made possible only by his brain and the experience of having mainstreamed in school to (amazingly) learn from the behavior of the teacher and the children around him. A truly heroic achievement.

In his book *Attunement*, architectural historian and theorist Alberto Pérez-Gómez (2016, p. 142) asserts that cognitive science has jettisoned any reliance on computer brain models. However, computer brain models—and computer models of cognitive processes more generally— play a continuing and central role both in cog/neuroscience in general and this book in particular, while also offering ideas for technological application under the banner of AI. For Pérez-Gómez, "embodied dynamicism" is a stance in cognitive science that arose in the 1990s. However, while much cognitive science has (often insightfully) conceived of cognition as a disembodied and abstract mental representation, "action-oriented perception" was central to Lettvin et al.'s (1959) "What the Frog's Eye Tells Frog's Brain," which in turn provided a basis for the symposium of Ingle, Schneider, Trevarthen, and Held (1967) that placed the study of vision firmly within the realm of behavior. Moreover, feedback linkage of organism and environment was central to Wiener's (1948) *Cybernetics* and was carried over into psychology by Miller, Galanter, and Pribram (1960) in *Plans and the Structure of Behavior*. Such studies provided a major stimulus for the emphasis on "action-oriented perception" in my book, *The Metaphorical Brain: An Introduction to Cybernetics as Artificial Intelligence and Brain Theory* (Arbib, 1972); while, as we have seen, Neisser's (1976) *Cognition and Reality: Principles and Implications of Cognitive Psychology* established the perception–action cycle. These are basic notions for this book.

Pérez-Gómez claims that

[n]eurobiology now recognizes the continuity of consciousness (sentience) in life, ranging from single-celled organisms to human self-consciousness. Despite obvious differences among different classes of biological entities, this realization is crucial: consciousness is . . . inherent in life.

This is erroneous in my opinion, and seems unhelpful. Better to concentrate on the further observation that in the case of humans, culture is no mere external addition or support to cognition; it is woven into the very fabric of each human mind from the outset. Symbolic culture, in particular the human linguistic, architectural, and urban environment, shapes the cognitive potentiality of the human mind. Stripped of culture, we would simply not have the cognitive capacities that make us human.

This is indeed a strong point of agreement—but then I must ask, "What is it about the human brain that uniquely enables us to develop human symbolic cultures that make possible the experience and design of human linguistic, architectural, and urban environments?" (I emphasize the plural.) This will be the central theme of Chapter 8, building on what we have learned in the preceding chapters. The crux for architecture is not what we share with cells and bacteria but rather the human capacity for "prereflective purposeful action and a reflective understanding of our place in the natural and cultural world" that cognitive science seeks to illuminate in partnership with neuroscience.

Our consciousness is often focused outward, but we are also capable of introspection—and at that time the relationships are mediated by "mental models" of real and imagined worlds. Anesthesia will block them. As noted earlier, the brain mechanisms supporting human consciousness may have evolved because our need to share our intentions with others to coordinate our activity led to processes in the brain that could sample activity across many brain regions to form a "précis," and this in turn offered an evolutionary opportunity for activity in different regions to become better coordinated through access to this précis.

But, yes, in general, we are continually interacting with the external world, and that includes the traces of what we have sketched or written. Our experience shapes our brains, our brains then shape our experience. The fact that our experience in great part involves the dynamics of our body's ongoing relationship with the world in no way displaces the brain from its role in providing the mechanisms that make this dynamics possible, whatever the extent of "consciousness" in that experience.

To continue, let's turn to a talk entitled, "Between Art and Science—Reality and Experience in Architecture and Art," in which Pallasmaa (2018) stressed the importance of a humanistic perspective in architecture. His comments are indeed highly relevant, but here I want to emphasize that connections between the humanist perspective and the realm of neuroscience are richer than this particular talk made explicit. Indeed, when the architect Robert Lamb Hart titled his book, *A New Look at Humanism—in Architecture, Landscapes, and Urban Design* (Hart, 2015), it was with the intent to alert architects to the importance of a humanism that embraces "the maturing sciences of human life."

Here are two quotes from Pallasmaa's talk:

I do not want to underestimate the cognitive and rational ground of building design, but I wish that the human capacities of feeling, atmosphere, intuition, memory, empathy and imagination were not underestimated, either.

Gaston Bachelard [1958] . . . came to the conclusion that science does not, and cannot, say anything meaningful about the reality of lived life, the human life world of sensory encounters and existential meanings . . . it can be articulated and mediated only through artistic and poetic imagery.

A major feature of the present book is to show how humanistic insights into feeling, atmosphere, intuition, memory, empathy, and imagination may be complemented and even enriched by the insights from neuroscience and the broader sciences of which it is part. Given this, I must strongly disagree with Bachelard's view that *only* artistic and poetic imagery can mediate our understanding of the reality of lived life.

Pallasmaa cites two neuroscientists, but only for their appreciation of art. Quoting Vittorio Gallese:

From a certain point of view, art is more powerful than science. . . . Being human squares with the ability to ask ourselves who we are.

Since the beginning of mankind, artistic creativity has expressed such ability in its purest and highest form.

I would rather say that artistic creativity is but one form, and leave aside questions of relative "height" or "purity." Consider, for example, the impact on our understanding of "who we are" wrought by the hypothesis of Copernicus that the Earth revolves around the sun, or the new understanding of our relation to other animals that flowed from the work of Darwin and Wallace. I would claim that modern advances in neuroscience are beginning to offer a similarly potent transformation in our understanding of "who we are."

Quoting Semir Zeki:

Most painters are also neurologists [. . .] they are those who have experimented upon and, without even realizing it, understood something about the organization of the visual brain, though with the techniques that are unique to them.

Zeki is simply wrong—or, at least, willing to blur the line between neurology and psychology. Yes, painters and sculptors have over the centuries developed great insights into the phenomenology of vision and so have helped lay the basis for a cognitive science of vision, but this in no way led them to insights into the actual inner workings of the brain. For an example of modern efforts to enrich such insights, one may note the books edited by art historian Ernst Gombrich and vision scientist Richard Gregory (Gombrich & Gregory, 1973; Gregory & Gombrich, 1973) that do indeed incorporate lessons from neuroscience.

Pallasmaa also quotes the Spanish neuroanatomist (many would say the greatest neuroanatomist), Santiago Ramón y Cajal, whom we "met" briefly in Figure 1.11:

If our study is concerned with an object related to anatomy or natural history, etc., observations will be accompanied by sketching, for, aside from other advantages, the act of depicting something disciplines and strengthens the attention, obliging us to cover the whole of the phenomenon studied. . . .

But Cajal does not claim the supremacy of art, or a neurological intuition for artists. Instead, he argues for the utility of drawing as a way of focusing observation in some scientific disciplines.[11] However, Cajal's drawings are still prized today for their beauty (Swanson, Newman, Araque, & Dubinsky, 2017) as well as the scientific insight they provide more than a century after his great work laid the foundation for our modern view of neural circuitry (Ramón y Cajal, 1899, 1911).[12] An example of Cajal's artistry in advancing science is provided by his drawing of a Purkinje cell of the cerebellar cortex (Figure 1.13). You may recognize the Purkinje cells in simplified form that Szentágothai included in his drawing of the neural architecture of the cerebellum. Many neuroscientists have accepted the challenge of seeking to understand the implications of this exquisite geometry for the cerebellum's contribution to action and experience (Eccles, Ito, & Szentágothai, 1967).

Pallasmaa advances the view that "[s]cience and art can be seen as opposite, *perhaps even mutually exclusive*, approaches to reality" (again, my italics) by recalling the work of James Turrell:

James Turrell has articulated experiences of light, and enabled us to see "tactile light" and "old light," cosmic light that has travelled thousands of light years through outer space before hitting our retina; this experience even permits us to touch time and sense infinity and eternity.

11. In this spirit, Mark Alan Hewitt gave the title *Draw in Order to See* to his cognitive history of architectural design (Hewitt, 2020). However, one might extend the title to *See in Order to Draw in Order to Understand and Thus See With More Understanding* . . . and so the cycle continues.

12. Cajal published the 1899 version in Spanish, *Textura del Sistema Nervioso del Hombre y de los Vertebrados*, but the 1911 version was in French, *Histologie du Systeme Nerveux de L'homme et des Vertebres*. Cajal noted that, if one wished to gain an international scientific audience, one then had to publish in English, French, or German. The fact that the field has narrowed to English is in large part due to Adolf Hitler. This claim may seem shocking at first, but consider the impact of the mass emigration of scientists from Germany that was one side effect of his monstrous activities.

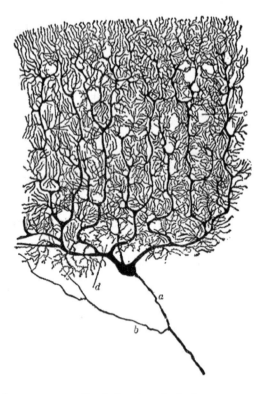

Figure 1.13 My favorite neuron: Cajal's drawing of a Purkinje neuron of the cerebellar cortex. (From Ramón y Cajal, S. [1899]. *Textura del sistema nervioso del hombre y de los vertebrados.* Madrid: Imprenta y Librería de Nicolás Moya.)

Yet it was science that taught us the awe of thousands of light years. The broad strokes of new science eventually enter into common parlance and thus may affect not only the way we experience our everyday lives but also the mindset that artists (and architects!) bring to their work, and the way in which "the general public" may come to appreciate them. Indeed, Pallasmaa is clear that science need not be destructive of our appreciation of art:

> Science has occasionally even been accused of robbing the world of its sense of magic and poetic wonder through offering explanations that only appeal to reason. Already in 1817 the poet John Keats

blamed scientists like Isaac Newton for destroying the poetry of the rainbow.[13] However, we need not to be supporters of either science or art [alone], as we can have confidence in both realms, each one with its own specific intentions and tasks. *I do not believe that neuroscience could destroy the poetry of architecture.* Do not science and art ultimately both approach the mysteries of the world, human consciousness and understanding and the enigma of our existence in the world? [My italics.]

I agree. The aim of this book, however, is to go further, supporting the positive assertion that neuroscience can enhance the poetry of architecture as well as meet the practical challenges of factoring an enriched understanding of the experience of architecture into design. And, indeed, Pallasmaa has been one of the leading architects supporting the rapprochement between the two perspectives, as witnessed by his organization of the Helsinki workshop published as *Architecture and Neuroscience* (Tidwell, 2013) and his co-editing of *Mind in Architecture: Neuroscience, Embodiment, and the Future of Design* with Sarah Robinson (Robinson & Pallasmaa, 2015).

Two-way reduction

The architectural historian Harry Mallgrave, whose book *The Architect's Brain: Neuroscience, Creativity, and Architecture* (Mallgrave, 2009) provided a major stimulus for developing my own engagement in the A↔N conversation, stresses that architecture is predominantly a "whole body" experience—a multisensory, emotional, hormonal, and phenomenal one grounded in the entire bodily organism—and that culture is highly

13. Quoted in Dawkins, R. (2004). "Bar codes in the stars." In H. Broecher (Ed.), *Olafur Eliasson: Your lighthouse: Works with light 1991–2004* (p. 13). Wolfsburg: Kunstmuseum Wolfsburg/Hatje Cantz Verlag.

integrated with that experience. I agree, but Mallgrave (2020) further cites Thompson and Varela (2001) to the effect that:

> The nervous system, the body and the environment are highly structured dynamical systems, coupled to each other on multiple levels. Because they are so thoroughly enmeshed—biologically, ecologically and socially, a better conception of brain, body, and environment would be as mutually embedded systems *rather than* as internally and externally located with respect to one another. [My italics.]

My concern is with the "rather than." I argue that we must engage both viewpoints in conversation if we are to understand either. Holism must be "put in its place." The architect seeks to probe the mind of the client and the minds of potential users to come up with a new part of the built environment. Wholes must be divided into parts to understand them, even if the aim is to yield a new synthesis. If we wish to understand how people will perceive a building, how they will act in a building, and what memories they will have of the building, then the individual and the environment must be separated and the design of the latter developed in painstaking detail before they can be put together again. My task in this book is not to tell architects that they will fail unless they master cog/ neuroscience. There are too many great buildings—and humble but successful buildings—already in the world for that to be plausible. Rather my aim is to invite architects and neuroscientists—and all those who think about how they experience and behave within the built environment—to engage in a conversation between architecture and neuroscience to their mutual benefit, a benefit that cannot be gained if appreciation of the whole denies the need to analyze the parts and understand their interactions. Holism obscures understanding—we need the back and forth of analysis and synthesis. I cannot hope to delimit all the neuroscience relevant to "creating environments that are intriguing or compelling in some manner, environments that are adaptive to our organisms, environments that are restorative or restive, or more simply, environments that make us happy [rather than being] . . . dangerous, annoying, tedious, and injurious to [our] health" (Mallgrave, 2020), but I offer a range of ideas that will support further A↔N conversation.

To develop this rapprochement, I need to return to the earlier diagram,

Architecture ↔ Cognitive Science ↔ Neuroscience

to clear up misconceptions about the A↔N conversation. Some architects I have talked to fear that the aim is to reduce their task to plugging in algorithms to convert the program (in the architectural sense) into a completed design. But if we look at the recent successes in how AI supports humans in Web searches and so on, we see that the issue is not so much a restriction of possibilities—"this is the way you must do it"—but rather the challenge of developing tools to help us navigate a huge space of possibilities that in the past we would not have known about, and to help exploit those possibilities in an effective way while nonetheless responding to our own imagination and desires. Complementing such AI-centered issues, in an age of advancing computer technology, certain parts of the design process will require a back and forth between the architects' innovative perspective and the technologists' careful analysis. This is well exemplified in the use of structural engineering to assess the stability of structures.

For one example of how science can enrich our everyday "person-reality," consider the legacy of Copernicus. Our person-reality includes the observations that we stand on solid ground, that each day the sun rises and sets, and that in the night we see the stars and some of those are wanderers, the planets. Scientists seek to chart the patterns that underlie this person-reality by meticulously gathering data and analyzing them, perhaps using mathematics, to reveal a deeper reality that may violate common sense. We need not follow the details to incorporate key insights from the new scientific reality into an enriched understanding of our daily lives. We still say, "the sun rises," but we now know why we have that experience, and can understand much more besides, such as the changes explained by the finding that the Earth rotates on an axis that is tilted with respect to the ecliptic. Dramatically, these new insights also reshaped our view of our place in the Universe, and were long violently opposed by the Roman Catholic Church.

It takes time to develop an ever-better web of explanations and the facts to test it and to be explained by it, but these can both change our person-reality and answer fundamental questions about human existence. My strategy for linking neuroscience and architecture in this book is to examine aspects of the experience and design of architecture that *begin* to be understood within neuroscience. Different sciences look at the world at different levels and may seek to explain what occurs at one level by "reduction" to the more detailed understanding of lower levels: explaining biology in terms of molecular biology; explaining molecular biology in terms of chemistry; and explaining chemistry in terms of physics, for example. However, matter organizes itself into a hierarchy of entities whose dynamics at each level can be described approximately—and, often, more insightfully—without reference to lower levels. And yet at times that lower-level detail is necessary. Consider a rolling wheel. We observe its dynamics at "wheel" level—until a breakage forces a more detailed analysis.

Mary Hesse and I (Arbib & Hesse, 1986) stressed that since scientific paradigms change—consider how relativity theory and quantum mechanics have enriched the Newtonian paradigm (which still remains relevant for diverse applications)—one should think of a "conversation" between levels rather than a simple reduction of one level to the "truths" of a lower level. We called this approach "*two-way reduction,*" stressing that new insights at either the higher or the lower level may have implications for extending our understanding at the other level. My aim in this book, then, is to conduct a conversation between

The reality of persons in society and the (built) environment
and
The reality of the structure and function of brains

With the intermediaries of psychology and cognitive science
as further informed by insights into
Ecology and both biological and cultural evolution.

Of course, the very breadth of this framework makes clear that this book can only offer an entry into a vast enterprise that may occupy us for decades, even centuries, to come.

Dissecting phenomenology

To close this discussion, let's look at the surprising phenomenon of *hemineglect* or *unilateral neglect*. People with damage to the parietal lobe (an anatomical term explained in §1.4) on the right side of the brain may lose their awareness of the left side of their body. If they were putting on a shirt, they would put their right arm in its sleeve but would not dress the left arm. It could get even more bizarre. If the nurse asked the patient, "Mr. Smith, why didn't you put your shirt on this arm?" he might reply "Oh, I don't know what that arm is. Maybe the surgeon put it there as a joke."

Bisiach and Luzzatti (1978) in Milan showed that hemineglect may apply not only to the body in current actions but also to memory of the environment. They spoke of "unilateral neglect of representational space." Their subjects were two patients in Milan who were familiar with the plaza in front of the cathedral there, the Duomo. They said to them: "Imagine that you are standing in the Piazza Del Duomo, and you're looking at the Duomo. Tell me what you see." The patients would then describe in considerable detail the buildings on the right side of the Piazza. It appeared that they had lost memory of one half of the Piazza. But here's the surprise. The next instruction is, "Imagine yourself walking over to the Duomo, and then turn right around, and tell me what you see then." Now they describe the other side of the Piazza! The whole square is there in their memory, but because of the hemineglect, they can only recollect the half of it that is on the right in relation to their imagined perspective. Totally bizarre, but very interesting. Figure 1.14 shows an artist's reconstruction of the effect.

Such data do not offer a "plug-in" for work in architecture but do, I suggest, offer important notions for the *dissection of the phenomenology of architecture*. My hope is that, in the future, architects who know about how different processes combine to support what we normally take to be a seamless whole can learn how to differentially tap them to create desired effects. Yes, cognitive science often gives us an analysis of how behavior and experience (the realm of phenomenology) can become explicable if we address them in terms of several interacting processes without requiring us to localize those processes in the brain. In some cases, though,

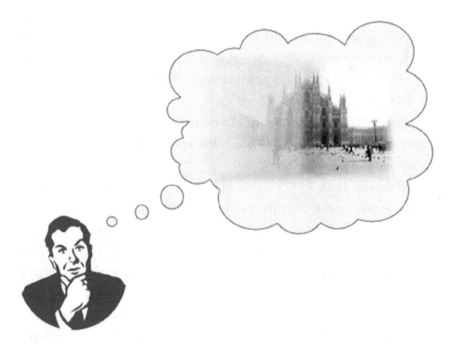

Figure 1.14 Hemineglect *in memory,* illustrating Bisiach and Luzzatti's (1978) report of two left-neglect patients who, when asked to imagine and describe from memory familiar surroundings (the Piazza del Duomo in Milan), omitted mention of left-side details regardless of the imaginary vantage point that they assumed. (From Bartolomeo, P., Thiebaut De Schotten, M., & Chica, A. B. [2012]. Brain networks of visuospatial attention and their disruption in visual neglect. *Frontiers in Human Neuroscience,* 6, 110. Public access.)

deeper insights will come from linking those processes to circuitry in specific regions of the brain—and attempting such linkages may force us to revise our original cognitive analysis and, in the process, improve our understanding of the phenomena we are assessing.

Great architecture has been created by architects who had remarkable intuitions about the effect of buildings on human experience and behavior but knew nothing about the brain as such. However, this does not imply that knowledge of the brain must therefore be irrelevant to future architecture. Brains certainly do exist, and we need to understand them—not necessarily in the service of better architecture, but certainly as a way to better understand ourselves, an understanding that can in turn enrich our appreciation of our place as humans in the environment, whether built or not.

REFERENCES

Arbib, M. A. (1972). *The metaphorical brain: An introduction to cybernetics as artificial intelligence and brain theory*. New York: Wiley-Interscience.

Arbib, M. A., Érdi, P., & Szentágothai, J. (1998). *Neural organization: Structure, function, and dynamics*. Cambridge, MA: MIT Press.

Arbib, M. A., & Hesse, M. B. (1986). *The construction of reality*. Cambridge, UK: Cambridge University Press.

Bachelard, G. (1958). *Poetics of space*. Boston: Beacon Press.

Bisiach, E., & Luzzatti, C. (1978). Unilateral neglect of representational space. *Cortex*, 14(1), 129–133. doi:10.1016/S0010-9452(78)80016-1

Brand, S. (1995). *How buildings learn: What happens after they're built*. London: Penguin.

Broca, P. (1861). Remarques sur le siège de la faculté du langage articulé, suivies d'une observation d'aphémie (perte de la parole). *Bulletins de la Societé Anthropologique de Paris*, 2, 235–238.

Broca, P. (1861/1960). Remarks on the seat of the faculty of articulate language, followed by an observation of aphemia (G. v. Bonin, Trans.). In G. von Bonin (Ed.), *Some papers on the cerebral cortex*. Oxford: Blackwell Scientific Publications.

Brodmann, K. (1905). Beitrage zur histologische Localisation der Grosshirnrinde. Dritte Mitteilung. Die Rindenfelder der niederen Affen. *Journal of Psychology and Neurology*, 4, 177–226.

Brodmann, K. (1909). *Vergleichende Lokalisationslehre Der Großhirnrinde In Ihren Prinzipien Dargestellt Auf Grund Des Zellenbaues*. Leipzig: Ja Barth.

Camargo, A., Artus, J., & Spiers, H. J. (2018). *Neuroscience for cities.* London: future-cities.catapult.or.uk.

Critchley, M., & Critchley, E. A. (1998). *John Hughlings Jackson: Father of English neurology.* Oxford: Oxford University Press.

Eberhard, J. P. (2008a). *Brain landscape: The coexistence of neuroscience and architecture.* Oxford, New York: Oxford University Press.

Eberhard, J. P. (2008b). A place to learn: How architecture affects hearing and learning. *ASHA Leader,* 13(14), 26–27.

Eccles, J. C., Ito, M., & Szentágothai, J. (1967). *The cerebellum as a neuronal machine.* New York: Springer-Verlag.

Gibson, J. J. (1979). *The ecological approach to visual perception.* Boston: Houghton Mifflin.

Gombrich, E. H. J., & Gregory, R. L. (1973). *Illusion in nature and art.* New York: Scribner.

Gregory, R. L., & Gombrich, E. H. J. (Eds.). (1973). *Illusion in nature and art.* New York: Scribner.

Hart, R. L. (2015). *A new look at humanism—in architecture, landscapes, and urban design.* Middletown, CA: Meadowlark Publishing.

Hewitt, M. A. (2020). *Draw in order to see: A cognitive history of architectural design.* San Francisco: ORO Editions.

Ingle, D. J., Schneider, G. E., Trevarthen, C. B., & Held, R. (1967). Locating and identifying: Two modes of visual processing (a symposium). *Psychologische Forschung,* 31(1 and 4).

Iriki, A., & Sakura, O. (2008). The neuroscience of primate intellectual evolution: Natural selection and passive and intentional niche construction. *Philosophical Transactions of the Royal Society of London B: Biological Science,* 363(1500), 2229–2241.

Kanaani, M. (2019). *The Routledge companion to paradigms of performativity in design and architecture: Using time to craft an enduring, resilient and relevant architecture.* New York and London: Routledge.

Laland, K. N., Odling-Smee, J., & Feldman, M. W. (2000). Niche construction, biological evolution, and cultural change. *Behavioral and Brain Sciences,* 23(01), 131–146. doi:10.1017/S0140525X00002417

Lamprecht, B. (2010). *Neutra: Complete works* (Edited by Peter Gössel; Preface and Editorial Assistance by Dion Neutra; Epilogue and Principal Photography by Julius Shulman). Köln: Taschen.

Leslie, T. (2010). Dankmar Adler's response to Louis Sullivan's "The tall office building artistically considered": Architecture and the "four causes." *Journal of Architectural Education,* 64(1), 83–93. doi:10.1111/j.1531-314X.2010.01102.x

Lettvin, J. Y., Maturana, H., McCulloch, W. S., & Pitts, W. H. (1959). What the frog's eye tells the frog brain. *Proceedings of the IRE,* 47, 1940–1951.

Mallgrave, H. F. (2009). *The architect's brain: Neuroscience, creativity, and architecture.* Chichester, UK: Wiley-Blackwell.

Mallgrave, H. F. (2020). Just what can architects afford? In B. Condia (Ed.), *Affordances and the potential for architecture* (pp. 38–59). Manhattan, KS: Kansas State Architectural Press.

Medawar, P. B. (1981, July 16). Stretch genes (review of Genes, Mind, and Culture: *The Coevolutionary Process* by Charles J. Lumsden and Edward O. Wilson). *New York Review of Books*.

Miller, G. A., Galanter, E., & Pribram, K. H. (1960). *Plans and the structure of behavior*. Holt, Rinehart & Winston.

Neisser, U. (1976). *Cognition and reality: Principles and implications of cognitive psychology*. San Francisco: W. H. Freeman.

Neutra, R. J. (1954). *Survival through design*. New York: Oxford University Press.

Odling-Smee, F. J., Laland, K. N., & Feldman, M. W. (2003). *Niche construction: The neglected process in evolution*. Princeton, NJ: Princeton University Press.

Pallasmaa, J. (2012). *The eyes of the skin: Architecture and the senses* (3rd ed.). Chichester, UK: Wiley.

Pallasmaa, J. (2018). *Between art and science: Reality and experience in architecture and art*. A talk at the Summer Course on Architecture and Neuroscience, NewSchool of Architecture and Design, San Diego, August 14, 2018.

Penfield, W., & Rasmussen, T. (1950). *The cerebral cortex of man: A clinical study of localization of function*. New York: Macmillan.

Pérez-Gómez, A. (2016). *Attunement: Architectural meaning after the crisis of modern science*. Cambridge, MA, and London: MIT Press.

Ramón y Cajal, S. (1899). *Textura del sistema nervioso del hombre y de los vertebrados*. Madrid: Imprenta y Librería de Nicolás Moya.

Ramón y Cajal, S. (1911). *Histologie du systeme nerveux de l'homme et des vertebres*. Paris: A. Maloine (English translation by N. and L. Swanson, Oxford University Press, 1995).

Robinson, S., & Pallasmaa, J. (Eds.). (2015). *Mind in architecture: Neuroscience, embodiment, and the future of design*. Cambridge, MA: MIT Press.

Smith, D. W. (2018). Phenomenology. In E. N. Zalta (Ed.), *The Stanford encyclopedia of philosophy*. https://plato.stanford.edu/archives/sum2018/entries/phenomenology/

Sullivan, L. H. (1896). The tall office building artistically considered. *Lippincott's Magazine*, 57(March), 403–409.

Swanson, L. W., Newman, E., Araque, A., & Dubinsky, J. M. (2017). *The beautiful brain: The drawings of Santiago Ramón y Cajal*. New York: Abrams.

Szentágothai, J., & Arbib, M. A. (1975). *Conceptual models of neural organization*. Cambridge, MA: MIT Press.

Tamari, T. (2016). The phenomenology of architecture: A short Introduction of Juhani Pallasmaa. *Body & Society*, 23(1), 1–4.

Thompson, E., & Varela, F. J. (2001). Radical embodiment: Neural dynamics and consciousness. *TRENDS in Cognitive Sciences*, 5(10), 418–425.

Tidwell, P. (Ed.). (2013). Architecture and neuroscience: A Tapio Wirkkala–Rut Bryk design reader (with contributions by Juhani Pallasmaa, Harry Mallgrave, and Michael Arbib). Espoo, Finland: Tapio Wirkkala Rut Bryk Foundation.

Tidwell, P. (Ed.). (2015). Architecture and atmosphere: A Tapio Wirkkala–Rut Bryk design reader (with contributions by Gernot Böhme, Tonino Griffero, Jean-Paul Thibaud, and Juhani Pallasmaa). Espoo, Finland: Tapio Wirkkala Rut Bryk Foundation.

Wernicke, C. (1874). *Der aphasische symptomencomplex.* Breslau: Cohn and Weigert.

Wiener, N. (1948). *Cybernetics: Or control and communication in the animal and the machine.* New York: Technology Press and John Wiley & Sons.

Zeisel, J. (2006). Inquiry by design: Environment/behavior/neuroscience in architecture, interiors, landscape, and planning. New York: W. W. Norton.

Zumthor, P. (2011). *Peter Zumthor Therme Vals.* (Essays: Sigrid Hauser and Peter Zumthor with translations by Kimi Lum and Catherine Schelbert; Photographs: Hélène Binet). Zurich: Verlag Scheidegger & AG.

Zumthor, P. (2012). *Thinking architecture* (3rd, expanded ed.). Basel: Birkhauser.

An action-oriented perspective on space and affordances

Architects design spaces. We visit them and contemplate them. We see, touch, feel, and respond emotionally to various aspects of them. We also use them: we act within and around them. The space offers perceptual cues, called *affordances*, for our various actions. We may (but only occasionally) call such action-related cues Gibsonian affordances in honor of J. J. Gibson, who pioneered their study. In general, our behavior within a building is not restricted to any one space or any one place within it or around it. Thus, we not only need affordances that we can recognize for various actions, but we also must find our way around these spaces to meet our various needs. As a result, navigation often extends beyond simply finding our way to a particular endpoint, providing paths that take us to a sequence of places where we can act and contemplate as need be as part of some ongoing behavior.

Stepping back from the specifics of architecture, we will explore in more detail not only the idea of an affordance but also the idea of an effectivity. What appears as an affordance for one person may not be an affordance for another because they lack the ability, the *effectivity*, to perform the cued operation. If one's intended action is to get from one floor of a building to another, the sight of a staircase may provide the affordance for actions that effect that transition, but for someone in a wheelchair it will not. In any case, it is important to distinguish affordances—perceptual cues—for an action from the physical apparatus (both outside the body and within it, including the capacity for neural control) that makes that action possible.

Within our overarching action-oriented framework, a visit to Lina Bo Bardi's São Paulo Museum of Art emphasizes that our *praxic actions*—motor interactions with the world around us, such as making our way around the museum—are integrated with *contemplative "actions,"* as when we stop to ponder a painting or sculpture. We may speak of *effective space* and *affective space*—of space as structured both for the effectivities of users within the building, and the emotional impact that the building can have on us. However, the architect's work does not end until these spaces are fully specified in terms of their embedding in the three-dimensional (3D) space around the site.

The visit also introduces the notion of *scripts*. Each script sets out the general rules for a particular kind of behavior, whether it be attending a birthday party or finding one's way around an art gallery or positioning oneself to contemplate a work of art. Such a script may suggest the places that a building must provide to allow people to act in a variety of ways. The architect may choose to let the building reflect familiar scripts or may devise novel scripts that transform the building's design but, preferably, nonetheless support the visitors' ability to adapt their familiar scripts to the novel experiences that the building offers.

A crucial focus for neuroscience is to explore how the brain links perception and action. Even though we perceive our interaction with the world as a unified melding of various senses and movements, neuroscience has shown that there are multiple *maps in the brain*—providing varied examples of the dissection of phenomenology. In addition to the *cognitive maps* that support wayfinding, there are diverse maps whose neural activity corresponds to aspects of some specific sensory or motor modality. Perhaps the most familiar of these are the *sensory homunculus* and *motor homunculus* that are played out over the two sides of the central fissure of the brain, but there are diverse specialized maps at the sensory and motor periphery that are linked to further brain regions that integrate them within our ongoing experience and behavior and emotions. This will be dramatically illustrated by showing how learning may adapt sensory–motor coordination in unexpected ways. In one example, people wearing inverting prisms came to adapt to the upside-down view of the world through repeated cycling through their town. In due course, the world came to appear the right way up—and yet, surprisingly, the lettering on the buildings still appeared upside down. I refer to this as an example of the *privacy of sensorimotor transformations*.

In one of several books encouraging us to go beyond visual perception in characterizing architecture, the Finnish architect Juhani Pallasmaa wrote of *The Thinking Hand*, emphasizing the way in which movements of the hand and tactile exploration could build up an appreciation of space that complemented the visual. But the hand alone cannot think—it is only through its coupling via the brain with diverse sensors and other effectors that it can become crucial to our thinking. Where some scholars emphasize *embodied cognition*—stressing how the body shapes cognition—I emphasize that our approach to action-oriented perception cannot succeed unless that body is animated by a brain of suitable complexity: embodied cognition meets *embrained cognition*. Hence our continuing emphasis on brains in bodies in the—social, built, and natural—environment.

This perspective on "the thinking hand" ties in with my work in modeling neural mechanisms that underlie the coordination of hand and eye. I approach this at two levels. The first introduces some basic ideas of *schema theory*, including the ways in which *coordinated control programs* can coordinate *perceptual* and *motor schemas*. In particular, we analyze how viewing the position and shape of an object can direct the motor control that rapidly brings the hand near to the object while *preshaping* the hand toward the size of the object, and how this initial rapid movement of arm and hand is refined as the hand invokes touch to establish a firm grasp of the object—a grasp that can in turn inform us further about the shape of the object or prepare us for further action. This analysis evokes the classic notion of the *body schema*, which assesses the position of the body and its multiple sensors and effectors in relation to the environment. Crucially, the body schema is an adaptable collage of perceptual and motor skills that can be invoked and adjusted depending on the current situation. For example, when holding a screwdriver, one's "body" ends not at the hand but at the tip of the screwdriver or even at the tip of the screw that is being driven.

In some cases, the basic psychological or cognitive analysis of schemas may be extended down to the activity of neural networks, and will let us introduce the notion of competition and cooperation as "the style of the brain," whether studied in terms of schemas or neural circuitry. This complements the "upward" challenge of understanding how such *schemas in the head* relate to *social schemas*—as in the way that our individual knowledge develops to incorporate focused patterns of generally accepted behavior and some (certainly not all) aspects of cultural systems like a language or religion or ideology.

Insights gained from the neurophysiological study of neurons engaged in monkey hand movements let us examine the "thinking hand" at the neural level. Most strikingly, we will discover a neurological distinction between a pathway (the *ventral "what" pathway*) that lets us recognize objects and their affordances in relationships that can provide the basis for (possibly conscious) planning of actions, and another pathway (the *dorsal "how" pathway*) that provides the (probably subconscious) fine matching of affordance-related details of the object to the motor control of the actions built upon it. For example, we may consciously decide to grasp a mug and drink from it but pay no conscious attention to the way in which the shape and size and position of the mug handle is transmuted into fine patterns of muscle coordination. Nonetheless, both are required to successfully complete the overall behavior.

To provide another perspective that may advance the A↔N conversation, the chapter concludes with a comparison, and a contrast, between the mental processes engaged by the architect in designing a building and by someone developing a computational model of interacting processes, whether at the schema or the neural level, that can both make sense of existing data from cog/neuroscience and support novel predictions that can inform the design of new experiments. Perhaps the most striking difference here is that once a building has been completed, post-occupancy evaluation may have less impact on the building itself than on the development of techniques that can be exploited in the design of other buildings. By contrast, new data may lead to a brain model that supersedes the previous model in the quest to understand and apply an ever-expanding pool of neuroscience data.

2.1. IN AN ART GALLERY: FROM WAYFINDING TO CONTEMPLATION

In our "visit" to the Therme at Vals, we saw how the practical—provide a doorway from one room to another—was blended with the aesthetic, marking one of those transitions by a heavy leather curtain that adds another dimension to the multisensory experience of those who use the thermal pools yet also enjoy the building itself and its relation to the valley that surrounds it. For a different experience, imagine that you are visiting an art museum. You want to go first to the exhibit of pre-Columbian art. For that, you have to get directions, perhaps in the form of a paper map sketching the layout of the museum, or (if the museum is familiar to you) you can consult the "map in your head," what we call a *cognitive map*. A third alternative is simply to explore and come upon the exhibit at random, but updating your cognitive map (more or less accurately) as you explore. In each case, you engage in what is called *wayfinding*, and this in turn raises considerations about what the architect does to help people find their way (Chapter 6).

What about within a particular room? The normal experience when you enter a room in an art gallery is that much of the space in the center is empty. There might be a statue or two or a couple of display cases in the

center, but most of the paintings will be around the walls. When you enter
the room, you might turn to read a description on the wall, and then go
to the left or right, following the wall until you've explored enough of the
room. If you are there to locate a particular artwork, many of the exhibits may not interest you. You walk by. For others, you stop. You develop
a strategy for viewing them. You approach and choose a viewing point.
You contemplate the object. Meanwhile, you have been avoiding obstacles,
benches, and other people, and choosing how to proceed.

Thus, we are back to the notion of affordances (i.e., the perceptions that
ground your strategies for movement and action), but now with affordances for locomotion complemented by something strangely different,
affordances for contemplation. All this poses challenges for the architect in
coming up with the form of the building and for the curator in coming up
with the setup for a particular event.

With this, let's look at one museum, the São Paulo Museum of Art,
that I have chosen because it defies almost everything I've just said about
exploring a museum (Figure 2.1). The architect was Lina Bo Bardi, who
was born in Italy but did most of her work in Brazil. As we approach from
the street, we are struck by the unconventional overall design, built like
a suspension bridge with much of the building suspended from the red
superstructure. Having seen this, our first job is to get safely across the
road, seeking affordances in gaps in the traffic and the time window they
offer, and then to get into the building. One might expect that for a building of this type and size, there would be a magnificent entryway, or at least
a conspicuous one, and architectural features that focus your attention on
how to approach it. Instead, Bo Bardi opted for devoting the ground level
to a public space where people can gather for meetings or demonstrations
or other social activity. It requires some visual exploration to discover to
the right of this space the affordances for entry offered by a staircase and
a lift, an elevator. Depending on how athletic you are, you can choose one
or the other to get up (you expect) to the exhibition floors. You are using
your general knowledge of buildings, whether consciously or not.

We get to the exhibit hall and discover that Lina Bo Bardi had a very
unusual idea about how to exhibit the art (Figure 2.2). Instead of being

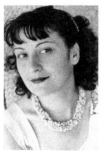

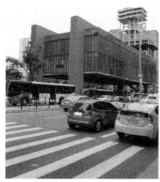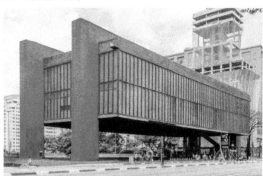

Figure 2.1 (*Top*) Lina Bo Bardi (1914–1992). (*Bottom*) São Paulo Museum of Art (the incomplete tower at right is part of another building). (*Left*) My photo to show the challenge of crossing the street. (*Right*) A clearer view of building access, via stairs and elevator at the far end. (*Top*: https://commons.wikimedia.org/wiki/File:LINA_BO_BARDI.jpg, SteveMagal, CC0, via Wikimedia Commons. *Bottom left*: Author's photo. *Bottom right*: https://commons.wikimedia.org/wiki/File:MASP_Brazil.jpg, Wilfredor, CC0, via Wikimedia Commons.)

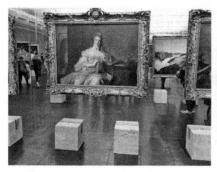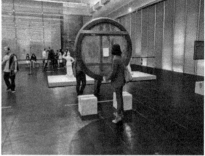

Figure 2.2 Lina Bo Bardi's unusual approach to exhibiting paintings. (Author's photos.)

hung on the walls, each painting is mounted on a big sheet of glass held vertical by being rooted in concrete blocks, creating a visual impression akin to floating in the air. Your affordances as a viewer are totally different from the usual wall-following. While standing in front of one painting here, you can look around to catch glimpses of others. Based more, perhaps, on an aesthetic rather than a wall-following criterion, you decide where to go next. The other strange feature is that the information about a painting is on its back, and so you develop another new strategy. Your attention is caught, you look, and then you say, "Well, what is this?" Maybe you go around the back, read the information, and then come around again to continue contemplating the painting. Or maybe you just move on to view another art work. Bo Bardi transformed a systematic exploration of one linear subspace at a time (moving parallel to a wall) to a more idiosyncratic exploration of artworks distributed across the two-dimensional (2D) space of the open floor (the only walls are external, where the windows are, with no art displayed).

Scripts

Discussing this particular museum makes clear that architecture may both build on conventions and defy them, with our behavior influenced in great part by general "scripts" of what to expect. Such scripts are built up through experience. Here, a *script* is a general plan for a certain type of behavior. Consider the different scripts for dining at a McDonald's fast food restaurant versus a fine restaurant. The first involves in-and-out fast consumption; the latter involves lingering over fine food and a bottle of wine (to be followed by a large tip). The "program"—the general specification of the restaurant for the architect—would, in part, specify which type of restaurant to design. The architect (in concert with the interior designer) would fulfill the program by designing a room that supports these scripts—with bright lighting and basic seating at McDonald's, and dim lighting and comfortable chairs at the fine restaurant. The notion here is that the successful architect must develop a sense of the scripts that will guide the behavior of users of the building, and that the design will have to accommodate activities that follow these scripts.

Back to Bo Bardi. In the first instance, getting into the place, she defies one convention, namely a conspicuous entryway for an important building, yet she lets you see the stairs or elevators that provide entry. In the second instance, she invites you to view paintings and their relationships in new ways. In other words, her design forces visitors to modify their usual scripts both for entering a large museum and for viewing the artworks. More general knowledge of public buildings may allow them to be surprised at the layout of the street level and yet give them the tools to solve the problem of gaining entry.

The term "scripts" entered the conversation between artificial intelligence (AI) and cognitive psychology with the publication of *Scripts, Plans, Goals and Understanding: An Inquiry Into Human Knowledge Structures* by Schank and Abelson (1977); but it was similar to the use of "frames" by the AI pioneer Marvin Minsky (1975) in "A Framework for Representing Knowledge," and by the sociologist Erving Goffman (1974) in *Frame Analysis.* You go to the doctor, and the receptionist asks, "How are you?" and you answer, "Fine, thanks," yet when the doctor asks you the same question, you say, "I feel terrible. I have this pain. . . ." What changed? You went from the greeting frame to the doctor–patient frame. In the same way, a building can frame the behavior of those who visit it, and offer spaces that support diverse scripts. Further, the scripts may be for social as well as individual behavior, and the purpose and mood of the people around them may change the script even within the same space—just contrast the mood in a church during a service, a wedding, or a funeral. The building supports the various scripts but need not be determinative—and the scripts may constrain the individual and/or encourage exploration.

To refine the earlier example, a "go-to-restaurant script" might include the requirement that one has the option to read a menu before deciding what to eat, that one places an order before one eats, and that one pays before one leaves. The reader can think of many different instantiations for this, and one might include specific options for "eat in" versus "eat out." Perhaps particularly worth noting for architects is that different actions may require different places in one subtypology rather than another. For example, where you order and where you eat may be separate places in a fast food restaurant yet the same place, your table, in another type of restaurant. Again, refining the general script, you might be required to pay before you get your food in one restaurant, and pay after you eat your food in another. In working with the client then, the architect may begin to provide further details in refining the program by reshaping generic scripts, and begin to think about the spatial layout that supports the different actions required in the more site-specific portion of the scripts. A further issue is that, in general, a building must support diverse scripts and that some spaces must be shared between the scripts, while others will not. For the restaurant example, consider linking spaces that support scripts for the diners, the waiters, and the kitchen staff.

A key issue, to which we return when sketching steps toward a cognitive (neuro)science of design in Chapter 10, is that a successful design for some typologies of a building or urban scene may go beyond provision of intended functions (as captured in the various scripts) to also allow the pleasure of exploration, or discovering new details, or personalization. Bo Bardi's "script-bending" emphasizes that scripts may be conventional or may challenge the user to acquire new behaviors, just as novel forms may offer users new experiences. Moreover, a building may succeed not only by satisfying the planned scripts but also (at least for certain typologies) by offering the user more or less free rein in creating scripts of their own.

But with this, I leave scripts awhile and focus on developing your understanding of affordances, expanding upon the first glimpse of them in Chapter 1, and embedding them within the frameworks of schemas and neural circuitry.

2.2. AFFORDANCES AND EFFECTIVITIES

We have already stressed the notion of multimodal experience within the action–perception cycle. Thus, when we focus on vision (whether here or in what follows), it is to introduce ideas that can be applied far more

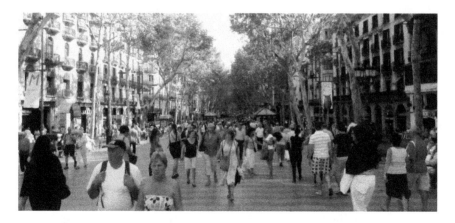

Figure 2.3 Las Ramblas in Barcelona. (Author's photo.)

broadly. The action–perception cycle provides the framework for our account of how the experience of space, and spaces, is integrated within our cognitive processes.

Conscious and subconscious dimensions of affordances

Imagine that you are walking down Las Ramblas in Barcelona (Figure 2.3). The striking yellow contrast at the center might grab your attention and, having saccaded (rapidly moved your gaze) there, you can recognize that a woman is wearing a yellow dress and has a handbag over her shoulder. But she's not somebody you know; she's just one person in the crowd. She merits no more than a glance as you walk along, perhaps going to a particular bar or to the Metro station, or—in the same spirit of contemplation that moves you in an art gallery—simply enjoying the architecture and the flow of people that constitutes the passing scene.

Whether contemplating, or walking toward a specific destination, your conscious perception can link directly to action. You may have to move to the left or the right to approach and greet a friend or take a closer look at an interesting shop front. But—and this is crucial—you may swerve to avoid a collision *even if you have no conscious awareness of who or what you were about to collide with.* In each case, we may talk about *affordances* for action, a notion made explicit by J. J. Gibson (1966, 1979)—using perception to trigger, or offer opportunities for, particular actions. In his honor, we (occasionally) call such action-related cues *Gibsonian affordances*—we will meet non-Gibsonian affordances in Chapter 4.

When walking hurriedly, for example, one might consciously notice a gap in the crowd and move toward it to exploit the opportunity to move faster than others. However, Gibson was more concerned with *subconscious* affordances, like *optic flow*—the world projects onto your retina, so there is a flow of features across the retina as you move, or as objects in the world move relative to you (Figure 2.4). He observed that when pilots fly into an airport, it is not conscious perception of the shape and position of the runway alone that guides their actions. The subconscious perception of optic flow plays a crucial role in determining when to level out and how to adjust speed when landing the plane (Gibson, 1955). Researchers following Gibson, like David Lee in Edinburgh, have shown how optic flow provides data the brain can use about a possible collision and time until contact (Lee & Kalmus, 1980). Compare driving down a long straight road. As you move forward, the visual scene "flows outward" across your retina, appearing to come from the horizon point on the road ahead, the *focus of expansion* (FOE, also known as the *vanishing point*). The FOE depends on your motion relative to the environment. If a car were approaching you on a side road, it would have a different motion relative to you and thus a different FOE (Figure 2.5). Moreover, the rate of the optic flow has the information needed to compute whether the car will hit you if it maintains its current course, and what the time to contact will be.[1]

---

1. A series of cerebral cortical areas devoted to processing visual motion were found that lie in front of the primary visual cortex (Brodmann area 17). In particular, the medial superior temporal area (MST) has neurons that are directionally selective and have receptive fields that cover large parts of the visual field. MST neurons respond to looming (expanding) and rotating stimuli and have activity that might be related to optic flow, particularly in determining heading, with sensitivity to shifts in the focus of expansion of radial motion and to the differences between the movement speed in the center and periphery of the full field motion (Wurtz, 1998). These studies show that neural ingredients for computing optic flow are available in

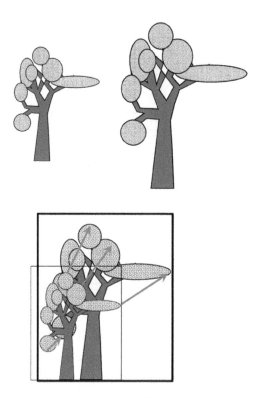

Figure 2.4 If, as we walk forward, we recognize that a tree appears to be getting bigger, we can infer that the tree is in fact getting closer. However, J. J. Gibson emphasized that we do not need object recognition to make such inferences. Much information about the position, orientation, and overall movement of the organism relative to its environment can be picked up by low-level systems. The *bottom* figure indicates the retinal displacement of four features of the image from the first view to the second. However, as one walks, the tree gets steadily closer. *Optic flow is* the time-varying pattern traced as each local feature of the scene creates a trajectory of retinal images.

Back then to your walk down Las Ramblas. There may be something in your periphery that you're not even conscious of, but the brain determines there's going to be a collision in a couple of seconds from a certain direction and you change direction without a conscious thought as

the brain, but do not demonstrate the neural circuitry of the brain that computes time until contact. However, there are many computer algorithms for these computations, and they are of great importance for the development of driverless cars.

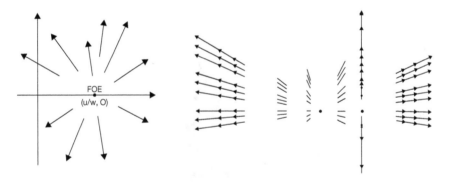

Figure 2.5 (*Left*) Optic flow flees the FOEfocus of expansion). (*Right*) The FOE is based on the relative motion of observer and environment. Here we see two flow fields—one for the background, and another (vertical) on a collision course with observer. (From Arbib, M. A. [1989]. *The metaphorical brain 2: Neural networks and beyond.* New York, Wiley-Interscience.)

to that affordance offered by the optic flow. It may be that you'll later get an indignant phone call from a friend who says, "Hey, why did you snub me?" . . . but you were just subconsciously avoiding a collision.

In discussing how people behave, it is important to distinguish these *two senses of affordance*, the conscious and the unconscious, whether the affordances are for locomotion or other actions. We recognize a doorway as offering an entrance to or exit from a room or building, but if we decide to go through that doorway, the unconscious affordances shape our trajectory, as when we duck our head if the doorway is low. If a door is designed for use by the general public, then it should be designed to offer prominent visual cues, perhaps even including explicit signage as to where it leads, as a way of aiding the user's conscious decision about whether to go through that door. If the door is designed only for staff, it should be inconspicuous so that few members of the public will be tempted to use it. However, in addition to advertising relevant affordances that may be consciously noted, there is the challenge of establishing the "unconscious affordances," as in determining the tread in a flight of stairs, or in ensuring that a doorway will be wide enough to allow for ease of passage under expected density of use.

The notion complementary to affordances is that of *effectivities*, the actions that one can actually perform. Affordances are related to what it is we can do. An affordance for locomotion is different from an affordance for flying. If I were a bird traversing Las Ramblas, I might fly up to go over the head of an obstacle to avoid a collision, but as a human I have to keep walking. A staircase offers affordances to most people, but not, for example, those confined to wheelchairs. Similarly, most humans can grasp objects and use them in diverse ways for which many other creatures (e.g., cats, frogs) do not have the effectivities—though birds can use a different effector to achieve a similar effectivity, using their beaks for becculation when, for example, they manipulate materials to build a nest.

Each object has an associated set of affordances; but *for each person these depend on their set of effectivities*, and the coupling may change with experience as one masters new skills and adjusts old ones. Conversely, an object may "reveal" different sets of affordances for different tasks—e.g., lifting a cup versus stroking a cup versus drawing a cup. And each action is accompanied by different expectations (multisensory: visual, haptic, and maybe more) for each type of action. Of course, humans being humans, we might consciously recognize affordances for creatures (actual or imagined) with affordances different from our own—as when an architect designs a dovecote to accommodate the flying and nesting of doves. But this brings us back to one of the themes of the A↔N conversation: understanding how people (rather than doves) very different from the architect might use a building, and what criteria of performance need to be addressed. For a home for people with Alzheimer's, an understanding of memory loss may help with understanding how to provide affordances to help people find their way to the dining room or bathroom. For a kindergarten, the small size and limited knowledge of the children is complemented by their energy and curiosity. What must the architect know to build a space that encourages learning and enjoyment, rather than providing a "storage area" to keep the children out of the way until their parents are finished at work each day?

Back to Las Ramblas again. You didn't intend to look at the woman in yellow but couldn't avoid glancing at that central splash of yellow against the background. Certain things or motions pop out of the image and grab attention, whereas others can only be found by searching. If I ask, "Where is the M?" in Figure 2.3, it may take you a while to find it. If someone had said, "Meet me at the Metro," then maybe this M would catch your attention *top-down*, based on your intention rather than the basic properties of the image, and then you might move over to read the sign to see whether it helps you get to the Metro station.

Multiple maps in the brain

Neuroscience employs the word "map" in two principal ways: "cognitive maps" and "maps in the brain" of the current spatial disposition of perceptual stimuli or of parameters for action. Cognitive maps link directly to a phenomenon well-known to architects: the design of buildings and towns to support wayfinding (Chapter 6). But here we focus on a notion specific to the study of the brain—the way various "spaces" of the external world, like the current visual input hitting the retina, or the pattern of pressure on the skin, are initially encoded in different groups of neurons, and yet interact with each other in the brain to give us that integrated sense of our immediate environment. These diverse representations gain their coherence because there is a repertoire of actions that we have learned to coordinate.[2]

I see an object. I want to pick it up. For my action to succeed, my estimate of where the object is in my locomotor space must enable me to get to a place where it is in my reaching space, and meanwhile I move my arm in anticipation and shape my hand to successfully pick it up in a manner smoothly coordinated with my locomotion. This in turn involves expectations as to how the object will feel when I grasp it, and this may lead in turn to a tightening of the grip if the object is felt to be slipping, or a relaxation of pressure if the grip on a fragile object feels too hard. This only works because these multiple representations have become tuned so that they work together for a whole range of actions. Our learning develops

2. Groh (2014) offers a highly readable (but lengthy) introduction to these two kinds of map in her book *Making Space: How the Brain Knows Where Things Are.*

couplings of affordances and effectivities—we acquire new actions only as we learn to recognize opportunities for carrying out those actions as well as what the effects of those actions will be.

Figure 2.6 shows the two best known maps *in* the brain, the *motor homunculus* ("little human") of primary motor cortex (BA 4) and the *somatosensory homunculus* of the primary somatosensory cortex (BA1). (Recall the Brodmann areas [BAs] of Figure 1.9.) The space represented in each homunculus is that of the body surface or musculature, not of the external world with which we interact. The use of the term *homunculus* is misleading. Neither "little human" is capable of perception or cognition— they are simply vivid pictorial descriptions of the brain maps that constitute the somatosensory and motor portals of cerebral cortex.

The *somatosensory homunculus* shows that neurons in different parts of somatosensory cortex are tuned most strongly to respond to stimuli affecting different parts of the body, with nearby neurons responding best to nearby patches of the body surface. The *motor homunculus* shows that stimulation of different regions of motor cortex will affect muscles in different parts of the body. The homunculi were introduced into neurology by Wilder Penfield and Edwin Boldrey (1937), who summarized the results of electrical stimulation of cerebral cortex under local anesthesia of 126 patients whose skulls had been opened for brain surgery. By working with awake patients, they could rely on the patients' verbal report of elicited movements and tactile sensation. The form of each homunculus indicates the amount of cortical area dedicated to motor or somatosensory functions of each body part—the sensory and motor representations of the hand being especially notable. However, the diagram obscures the fact that there is some functional overlap between stimulation fields rather than an orderly sequence of segregated areas.[3]

3. Catani (2017) celebrated the 80th anniversary of Penfield and Boldrey's seminal paper by re-examining the authors' findings and clarifying the substrate that generated the homunculi. Gandhoke, Belykh, Zhao, Leblanc, and Preul (2019) sought to assess the accuracy of this pictorial means of showing cortical representation, and concluded that the homunculi, if truly drawn according to cortical mapping evidence, could never have been recognized as nearly humanoid—and yet, they note, it is because of these pictures that they have attained their educational and practical longevity.

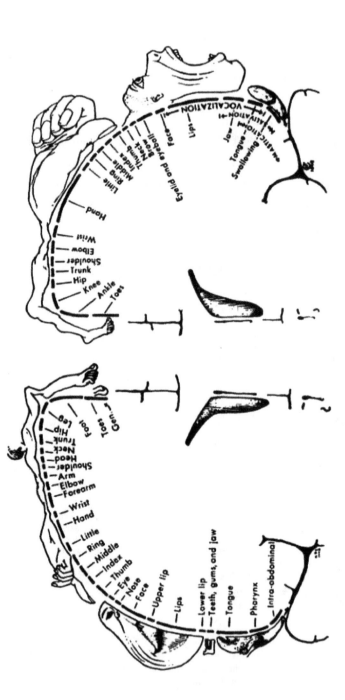

Figure 2.6 The somatosensory (*left*) and motor (*right*) homunculi. Note the large regions devoted to the hand in both maps—both finer sensitivity and greater precision of motor control—compared with the entire body surface and limbs. However, these "homunculi" are just two of the maps in the brain. They say nothing, for example, about the distribution of acuity in vision or audition. The areas marked "eye" do not register visual stimuli—they relate to the sense of touch of the eye and the control of the eye muscles. (Reprinted from Gandhoke, G. S., Belykh, E., Zhao, X., Leblanc, R., & Preul, M. C. [2019]. Edwin Boldrey and Wilder Penfield's homunculus: A life given by Mrs. Cantlie [in and out of realism]. *World Neurosurgery, 132*, 377–388, with permission from Elsevier. Their figure 4 is based in part on Penfield, W., & Rasmussen, T. [1950]. *The cerebral cortex of man: A clinical study of localization of function.* New York: Macmillan.)

Both these maps are called *somatotopic* because the activity of each cell corresponds to a place (Greek *topos*) on the body (Greek *soma*). However, it is easy to misunderstand the limited nature of these two "maps." They indicate, for example, how sensitive our hand is as an organ of touch, and how subtle the hand is in the many muscles that allow refined control of its many "degrees of freedom" of movement, but other brain regions are required to transform visual signals into the control of the hand in grasping an object, let alone coordinate the two hands in skilled manipulation.

In early stages of visual cortex, we find maps of the way in which visual stimuli activate neurons in the retina. Several brain regions a short distance (in terms of neural connection paths) employ a *retinotopic code*: the position of activated neurons corresponds in distorted form to position on the retina whose stimulation will activate the cell. The distortion here is that the fovea, subtending only a few degrees, occupies as large a portion of the map as does the visual periphery. The *superior colliculus* in mammals is a visual area in the midbrain that has a retinotopic map such that stimulation at one place will trigger a reflex movement to foveate its *receptive field*, the region of space that would stimulate the corresponding position on the retina. The superior colliculus also contains a retinotopic map of both sound and body—so that we can *saccade* (make a rapid eye movement to attend visually) to the source of a sound or an itch on our bodies. This mammalian structure corresponds to the *tectum* in other creatures such as frogs. In frogs, stimulation at a point in the tectum will cause the frog to snap as if there were a fly in the retinotopically encoded direction.

Close to the sensory periphery, the maps are dominated by the sensory surface—as in the retinotopic maps, or the somatotopic (body–place) map of the somatosensory "homunculus." As we move further through the circuitry, we find that *action-oriented spatial reference frames* support the brain's organization of sensory and motor data relevant to specific types of action (Arbib, 1997; Colby, 1998). There are representations that we can use when walking around, but there are also representations of *peripersonal* space, the space within reach. However, there are many more central regions of the brain that carry out complex computations, and are not structured as "maps in the brain" of either a sensory or motor periphery.

Our conscious experience gives us the "illusion" of a unified experience of the world around us—but only because these diverse representations in the brain interact with working memory and other dynamic representations. For example, because the retina has only a very narrow fovea, what we perceive as an overall scene is, in fact, the integration of multiple peripheral "sketches" with the details that build up through multiple foveations. Our brain integrates visual maps with those for sound, touch, and other senses and then, as the action–perception cycle proceeds, must translate these data into the diverse maps that control the action of the arm, the shape of the hand, the movement of the eyes, locomotion, and much more. The invitation to the architect is, again, to "dissect phenomenology"—to understand how different design features may differentially affect different maps in the brain, and then orchestrate them to make the building affect the user in appropriate ways, in terms of how it performs in both utilitarian and aesthetic terms.

The "privacy" of sensorimotor transformations

Maps can change with experience. For example, the child must continually re-coordinate visual maps with motor maps (relating affordances to effectivities) to successfully grasp a target within reach as that reach expands from birth into teenagerhood. As a more focused example, Tom Thach's group at Washington University in St. Louis (Martin, Keating, Goodkin, Bastian, & Thach, 1996a, 1996b) studied what happens when people put on prisms that shift the visual field to left or right and then throw a ball at a target. On the first throw, the ball goes wide, but with repeated throws the error gets smaller and smaller. Take the prisms off, and the error returns—in the opposite direction. You need a specific part of the cerebellum to be intact to make the shift, but the fascinating discovery was that the cerebellum does not learn to shift the visual field *as a whole*. It shifts the visual data for different actions. A person who had been wearing these prisms and learned how to compensate for an overarm throw might nonetheless throw off-target for an underarm throw! There is "privacy of sensorimotor transformations"—different transformations of perceptual maps for different tasks—and yet your brain can often assemble the information from the multiple maps after they are properly tuned in relation to each other, for whatever it is you have to do.

An even more intriguing example comes from Ivo Kohler's (1963) study of people who wore inverting prisms (initially, they saw the world upside down) and had to learn how to safely ride a bike through town. Subjects reported that they were able to navigate more and more successfully through town before they began visually experiencing the town as looking "right side up." Surprisingly, though, they reported that at this stage, even though the buildings seemed oriented correctly, the lettering on signs still appeared upside down—further dramatic evidence of the "privacy of sensorimotor transformations," here with different neural linkages from vision to navigation and to reading.

Space is defined by actions

The word *geometry* comes from the Greek *ge* (earth) + *metro* (measure). In high school, you may have studied Euclidean geometry, where straight lines can be parallel, going on forever and never meeting, an idealization of measuring the farmer's fields. You may have even studied Cartesian geometry, the inspiration of René Descartes, where the geometry meets algebra, with 2D Euclidean space measured out by an (x,y) coordinate system defined relative to two orthogonal axes, or a 3D space marked out with (x,y,z) coordinates. The surface of our planet, though, when idealized as a sphere, has "straight" lines defined by great circles—so all lines meet. The geometry of the Earth, unlike the geometry of the earth of the farmer's field, is non-Euclidean. When the architect lays out the construction drawings for a building, the geometry is often Euclidean, and the computer used may well keep track of Cartesian coordinates.

But when Louis Kahn says, "Architecture is the thoughtful making of spaces. It is the creating of spaces that evoke a feeling of appropriate use," it is not the space of Euclid or Descartes or their successors to which he refers. It is to notions of space very much in the spirit of this book. It is space defined by actions—indeed, by the affordances of such actions. The space of a room may be defined by how we move to get from one place to another, and the significant places in the room—defined not only by the architect but also by the current disposition of objects and other people in the room—are defined by the affordances they offer. Of course, it is more complex than that. The height of the ceiling within a cathedral or the height of its steeple are defined not by any chance that we will ascend, spiderman-like, to the ceiling or to the top of the tower, but rather by the way we must tilt our head to direct our gaze upward, and this indeed may tie back to experience we have of outdoor spaces measured against the height of trees or hills we have climbed.

The space of architecture, then, is not the 3D space in which we may imagine the building to be embedded, but rather a disposition of surfaces in relation to each other that support our actions, whether they be praxic or social, but also support our contemplation of the building from within, or as viewed from the outside, or the vistas that the building frames of the landscape or townscape beyond. We might speak of *effective space* and *affective space*—of space as structured by the effectivities we can exercise within the building, and the emotional effects that the building can have on us. And, indeed, like Einstein's notion of space-time, architects must envision the scripts that will link space, time, and memory in the experience of, and behavior within, the buildings they design. Having said this, though, I stress that *the architect's work does not end until all the surfaces that define the effective and affective spaces of the building are fully specified in terms of the 3D space around the site where the building will be constructed*, and that here the tools of Euclidean and Cartesian geometry may play the crucial role in transforming these relationships into the specifications that will shape the building process.

With this, the time has come to exemplify why architects might be interested in the hand and to develop our understanding of the visual and tactile control of hand movements, in tandem with a growing understanding of the relation between schemas and neural circuitry in developing the cog/neuroscience end of the A↔N conversation.

2.3. THE THINKING HAND

Taliesin West, near Scottsdale in Arizona (the original Taliesin is in Wisconsin), was the winter home of Frank Lloyd Wright, who was considered by himself and many others to be the greatest American architect of the 20th century. Sarah Robinson, an architect who had trained at Taliesin West (long after Wright's demise), had published a book, *Nesting: Body, Dwelling, Mind* (Robinson, 2011), in which she had begun to explore some of the ways in which psychology, phenomenology, and, to some extent, neuroscience could inform architectural thinking. Building on these themes, she organized a meeting at Taliesin West on *Minding Design: Neuroscience, Design Education, and the Imagination* in November of 2012.[4]

Having been invited as one of the four keynote speakers at the 2012 meeting, with Pallasmaa being the first, I chose as the architectural "hook" for my talk Pallasmaa's *The Thinking Hand: Existential and Embodied Wisdom in Architecture* (Pallasmaa, 2009), a book that I had already read and admired. It provided a phenomenological view of the role of the hand both in interacting with the world and in bringing a tactile component to the experience of architecture. Consider, for example, a door handle. Whatever its visual appearance, it should feel "good" when grasped, but also be designed to facilitate the action of opening or closing the door. Pallasmaa also stressed the role of the hand in sketching as a means to bring the body into the design process. These themes, it seemed to me, linked well to themes of my book *How the Brain Got Language* (Arbib, 2012), which focused on the idea that the path to human language was, initially at least, through manual gesture, which then recruited and helped elaborate the vocal system as a means of expression, with cultural evolution undergirding the long transition from "protolanguage" to language (more on this in Chapter 8). Today,

4. The co-edited volume *Mind in Architecture: Neuroscience, Embodiment, and the Future of Design* (Robinson & Pallasmaa, 2015) includes several chapters based on presentations from the Taliesin West meeting. This book remains one of the best resources for getting an entrée into the A↔N conversation.

even when speaking, co-speech gestures of our face and hands are a crucial part of our performance and may provide emotional and other shading that better captures the attention of our audience. Moreover, Deaf people[5] learn and use signed languages as readily as the rest of us learn spoken languages.

This section, then, is in some sense a souvenir of one of my first extended A↔N conversations. The value for me was that I could learn so much about architecture from reading Pallasmaa's books (and the conversation has flourished in person and by email since), not in the manner of passively accepting "the truth," but rather in seeing ways in which my knowledge could be increased by what he was saying while also stimulating me to say something new in seeking to align what I was learning with what I already knew from my previous experience in neuroscience and elsewhere. And so the give-and-take continues. I hope our spirit of mutual respect shines through, and that many of you will, informed by what you learn from this book, have many fruitful A↔N conversations of your own.

In what follows, I extract some statements made by Pallasmaa in his book, and then address what is added by analysis of how the brain mediates the coordination of eye and hand.

1. *The knowledge and skills of traditional societies reside directly in the senses and muscles, in the knowing and intelligent hands, and are directly embedded and encoded in the settings and situations of life.*

The debate here is over the use of the word "directly." This book explores the role the brain plays in linking the senses and the muscles, exemplified in linking vision and touch to the control of hand movements in action and perception.

---

5. The capital "D" in Deaf signifies that not only are the people deaf, but also they belong to a community of deaf people who can communicate freely through possession of a shared nonvocal language.

2. *The hand is crucial to the evolution and manifestations of human
intelligence.*

Just as the Deaf community shows that people may make rich use of
language without hearing, so may people who lack hands exhibit normal
intelligence. Nonetheless, the use of hands is a core expression of intelligent interaction with the world for most people; and manual praxis and
gesture played a key role in the development of human brains to the point
that they could support symbolic behavior, language, and . . . architecture. My EvoDevoSocio approach to language origins in Chapter 8 will
emphasize how the brain's linkage of eye and hand has changed not only
with the biological evolution that shaped the brain and body (including
the hand) of early *Homo sapiens* but also with the cultural evolution that
transformed human societies, environments, and technology in the tens
of millennia that followed.

3. *Human consciousness is an embodied consciousness. The world is
structured around a sensory and corporeal center.*

Certainly, the architect is much concerned with how humans—brains in
bodies—interact with the environment. However, language and abstraction support human development in a manner that need no longer be
linked only to that embodied core. The practice of architectural design
yokes the embodied, the symbolic, and the aesthetic.

4. *Learning a skill is not primarily focused on verbal teaching, but
rather the transference of the skill directly from the muscles of the
apprentice through the act of sensory perception and bodily mimesis.*

However, verbal teaching serves to help the learner understand the
overall structure of a skill and—combined with pointing—to direct attention to key affordances and actions. Observing the teacher cannot directly
inform the muscles of the apprentice—only long practice can modify the

brain's synapses to yield skilled performance, and the teacher's verbal
feedback may play a crucial role.

5. *This capacity of mimetic learning is currently attributed to mirror
   neurons.*

Here, Pallasmaa does bring in the role of the brain. Indeed, mirror
neurons have been a major concern of my research since the 1990s as
part of a collaboration with Giacomo Rizzolatti, Hideo Sakata, and Marc
Jeannerod. The discussion of mirror neurons will be taken up in Chapter 5
in relation to brain systems "beyond the mirror."

6. *Architectural ideas arise "biologically" from unconceptualized and
   lived existential knowledge rather than from mere analyses and
   intellect.*

But why "rather than" and why "mere"? Depending on what we are
doing, our embodied intuitions may be dominant, yet on other occasions,
our formal analyses are crucial. I think Pallasmaa is railing here—and it
is important to do so—against a view that reduces architectural design to
a rational process of design-by-algorithm that dispenses with the role of
imagination. My aim is not to downgrade the experience architects bring
to their craft, but rather to see how it integrates embodiment and rationality to do better than either might alone. "Half-forgotten images" factor
into this "pre-rational" phase, but what emerges is then subject to critical
analysis, as we shall see in our steps toward a cognitive (neuro)science of
design in Chapters 9 and 10.

2.4. THE THINKING HAND AND ITS SCHEMAS

The time has come to get a better sense of how schema theory provides a
cognitive level of analysis that can bridge between phenomenology of a
particular behavior and experience and its dissection in terms of neural
processes. Using the discussion of *The Thinking Hand* as motivation, the

analysis in this section will be at the schema level, which we will extend to consideration of the body schema, followed by a broad discussion of schema theory in §2.5 and then a neural perspective in §2.6 that incorporates data on both brain anatomy and neuronal activity.

A coordinated control program for the reach-to-grasp

Marc Jeannerod, a neuropsychologist at Lyon in France, and his colleague Jean Biguer studied humans reaching to grasp objects (Jeannerod & Biguer, 1982). Figure 2.7 shows the shape and position of the hand at various points in the reach-to-grasp. The arm transports the hand

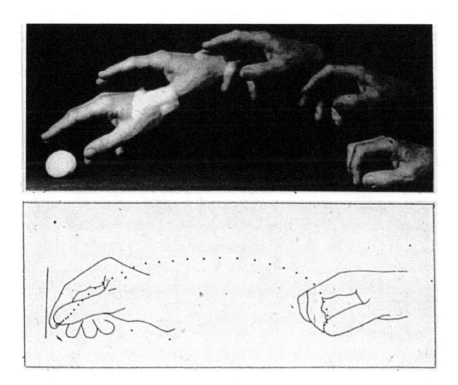

Figure 2.7 The hand preshapes for an affordance. (*Top*) Preshaping of the hand while reaching to grasp a ball. (*Bottom*) Positions of the thumb-tip traced from successive frames in reaching to grasp a pencil-like object shows a fast initial movement (large spacing) followed by a slow completion (small spacing) of the grasp. (Photo and diagram courtesy of Marc Jeannerod.)

along a "safe" trajectory that avoids bumping along the table or leaving the hand ill-positioned for the grasp. Meanwhile, the hand begins to *preshape* to arrive at the ball with a little safety margin so that the hand can then enclose and complete the grasp. In line with our multisensory theme, note that the relevant sensory system is vision until the final phase, but that the final shaping and positioning of the hand is under the control of tactile feedback guiding contact with the object.

Hearing Marc talk about these results at a conference in 1979 inspired me to develop a schema-based analysis of the process involved. Figure 2.8 shows the initial model (Arbib, 1981), defining the integration of *perceptual schemas* (visual analysis of the object in relation to the hand) and *motor schemas* (to control the coordinated movements of arm and hand). I call it a *coordinated control program* because it combines aspects of a *control system* (providing signals to control movement) with the *computer scientist's notion of a program* that specifies the scheduling of various operations.

In my experience, architects find such figures as daunting as I find floor plans for buildings. My architect friends tell me they can look at floor plans and readily imagine the experience of walking through the building. Let's see if we can look at Figure 2.8 together and get a sense of how information "flows" through the network. One crucial difference is that, unlike a person walking through a building, schema diagrams involve information (data, or control signals) traversing the layout along many arrows ("corridors") or schemas ("rooms") at a time. Information spreads out, with multiple interactions occurring as action is linked with perception (and, in general—but not in this example—with current internal state).

Perceptual schemas. At the top, we see three perceptual schemas. In this example, they process visual input to provide three affordances: first, the location of the object, and then, *after this is determined*, its size and orientation.

The crucial point is that the perceptual schemas here serve to encode parametric details of the affordances to be exploited by

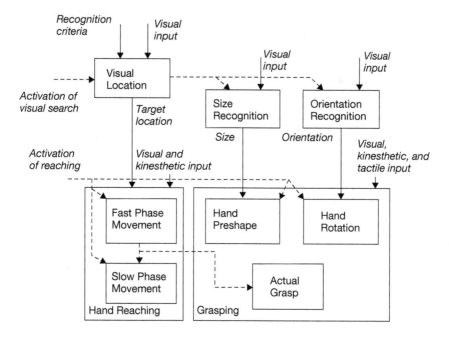

Figure 2.8 A coordinated control program for reaching to grasp. At the *top*, three perceptual schemas gather the visual data needed to establish the location, size, and orientation of the object to be grasped. At the *bottom*, there are motor schemas for controlling the arm (hand reaching) and the hand (grasping). The inner structure of the motor schemas is described in the text. Two kinds of data are transferred. *Dashed lines* indicate activation signals, which tell a schema to start processing; *solid lines* indicate transfer of data to schemas so that they can act on the appropriate parameters. (Adapted from Arbib, M. A. [1981]. Perceptual structures and distributed motor control. In V. B. Brooks [Ed.], *Handbook of physiology—The nervous system II. Motor control* [pp. 1449–1480]. Bethesda, MD: American Physiological Society.)

the motor schemas that provide the effectivities for completing the task.[6]

Motor schemas. Recognition of visual location activates motor schemas to control the arm in reaching toward the object; recognition of size

---

6. My figure was for many years widely used in courses in kinesiology. However, like many models, it serves only as a first approximation, to be improved or rejected as research proceeds. In my group, for example, we came up with an improved model that could yield mid-course corrections if changes in the position or shape of the object were detected early enough in the trajectory (Hoff & Arbib, 1993).

and orientation triggers the motor schema to control grasping. Crucially, though, each of these motor schemas has *subschemas*:

- The *Reaching schema* involves first a motor schema that rapidly brings the hand near to the object; on completion, this triggers a second motor schema that controls a slow movement that completes the reach under visual and tactile control.
- The *Grasping schema* starts with the simultaneous activation of two motor schemas: one for preshaping and the other for orienting the hand appropriately for the targeted affordance of the object (what might be appropriate for a door handle is not so for a ball). The transition from fast to slow movement in the Reaching schema then signals transition within the Grasping schema to the *Actual Grasp* (or *Enclose*) motor schema, which, in general, will complete the grasp under tactile rather than manual control.

The analysis corresponds to the notions of feedforward and feedback. The principle of *negative feedback* is familiar from the example of the thermostat: detect an error and change so as to reduce it. Thus, during the actual grasp, visual feedback may help adjust the position of the hand relative to the object before contact is made but, more important, tactile feedback is employed in adjusting finger positions and forces to ensure a firm grip. The problem with using feedback alone, though, is that it is relatively slow: each movement must be monitored and the current error sent back to the brain for analysis before updated instructions are sent to adjust activity of the muscles. *Feedforward* avoids feedback and so is much faster, but it requires learning—in the present case, to transform the visual analysis of the distance between the initial position of the hand and the object into a feedback-free trajectory that will enable the arm to accelerate the hand toward the object but then decelerate it to a near stop for the transition to feedback control.

Motor schemas may thus be sophisticated *adaptive* control systems, with learning here required to adjust the schema's *internal model* of the relation between vision and action. This notion was already implicit in our earlier example of throwing darts. Note there that an error signal is received (how far the dart is from the bullseye) only after the throw is complete. It is thus useless for control of the ongoing movement by negative feedback. Instead, we talk of *learning feedback*—the error signal is exploited by a learning system that adjusts the relevant sensorimotor transformation for future use.

Grasping exemplifies the multisensory nature of much action—combining vision and touch for its successful completion. Vision, combined with learning, helps one both direct a rapid arm movement to bring the hand close to the object and preshape it in relation to the *chosen affordance*—lifting a mug by the rim versus the handle is an example of such a choice. Touch only works up close, providing the feedback needed to complete a firm grasp on the selected part of the object.

The reach-to-grasp is but the first stage in a vast range of human skills, from throwing a ball to manipulating objects, to using and making tools, and to specifically human skills in writing and sketching.

Tools and the body schema

Henry Head and Gordon Holmes (1911) applied the term *schema* somewhat differently.[7] We have seen that a brain lesion in the parietal lobe on the right side of the brain can cause hemineglect that may apply not only to the body but also to "unilateral neglect of representational space" in memory of the environment. The study of hemineglect was part of what motivated Head and Holmes to introduce the notion of the *body schema* by saying that

---

7. Head, a neurologist, is one of those people who rejoice in having a name that fits with their profession. Similarly, for many years the standard textbook in neurology was edited by Russell Brain, later Lord Brain. As a historical aside, later editions were edited by Roger Bannister—he was the first human to run a 4-minute mile but went on to become a neurologist.

Anything which participates in the conscious movement of our bodies is added to the model of ourselves and becomes part of those schemata: a woman's power of localization may extend to the feather of her hat.

Clearly, this was written in a very different age in which neurologists knew ladies who wore hats with long feathers on them. Perhaps you have had the experience that if you are wearing a hat, probably not with a feather on it, and you come to a low doorway, you may duck your head subconsciously to go through the doorway even though without the hat you would not have done so—you automatically adjust your body schema to the affordances of the building in relation to your current "configuration."

A classic study from Moscow (Fukson, Berkinblit, & Feldman, 1980) showed that at least part of the body schema can be served by spinal circuitry without any involvement of the cerebral cortex. They took a frog whose spinal cord had been cut off from its brain by severing the pathways joining them. When they put some irritant on its forelimb, the frog would wipe away the irritant with its hind leg—and this wiping movement remained accurate even when the experimenters changed the position of the forelimb: "The spinal frog takes into account the scheme of its body during the wiping reflex."

Tool use reminds us that the body schema does not specify just where the physical body effectively ends, but also how a using a tool changes affordances and effectivities—the body schema is modified functionally as well as extended spatially. As it is being picked up, the tool is like any other object being manipulated. But once the tool is held properly, the "end effector" is transferred from the hand to some part of the tool, and the affordances and effectivities are now with respect to the tool, not the hand (Figure 2.9). Arbib, Bonaiuto, Jacobs, and Frey (2009) referred to this as the *distalization of the end-effector*, while offering some analysis of the brain mechanisms involved. But it is still the hand that has to be controlled: visual attention is directed to the end effector, but haptic feedback is still provided via the hand even though its meaning depends strongly on the phase of the current

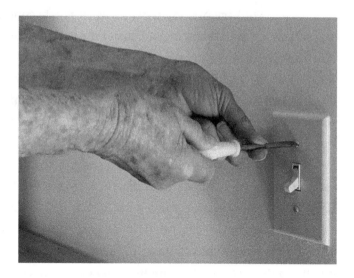

Figure 2.9 Distalization of the end effector. In using a tool, the body schema extends to the "business end" of the tool, and while the tool is in use, it is the tool that provides the hand's effectivities and thus sets the relevant affordances. Consider the relation of the screwdriver to the slot in a screw head. (Author's photo.)

task. If I am writing with a pen, I have new effectivities to make marks on the paper, but to control the actions thus afforded, I do not directly sense the pressure of the pen tip on the paper, but instead get an indirect measure via the pressure of the pen on my hand, transduced from the tip of the pen—haptic feedback augmented by visual feedback as my writing unfurls on the page.

In short, the body schema changes with one's circumstances, whether one is wearing a feather-tipped hat or using a tool. Given our discussion of multiple maps in the brain and the "privacy" of sensorimotor transformations, we see that the body schema is in fact a *dynamic assemblage of perceptual and motor schemas* that can be differentially deployed depending on the tools we are using or the clothes we wear and also with the tasks we are engaged in. Moreover, the body schema is not only dynamic in its assemblage but is also a learning system, making adjustments both in the tuning of the various schemas and in the patterns of their coordination. Returning to the schema diagram of Figure 2.8, note that the young child will not have the linkage of these schemas as an innate coordinated control program, but must have learned to master the various component skills *and* the way they are coordinated.

The relevance to the architect is that the inhabitant's body schema proceeding out from the body is complemented by what we might call the *environment schema*, incorporating certain affordances that the surroundings provide for our effectivities. For example, placement of windows may serve both to offer affordances for seeing what is outside the building and, with the possible help of internal lighting, help the user locate relevant affordances for action inside the building. If a long corridor has a central strip of carpet with a strip of stone or wooden flooring exposed on either side, then the change in both sound and foot-feel may supplement visual cues in keeping users from bumping into the walls. In the same vein, the German town of Augsburg, reacting to two occasions when pedestrians were hit by the quiet electric street-trains while looking at their phones (they had no visual awareness outside peripersonal space), installed ground-level traffic lights to warn people who are looking down at their screens that a tram is approaching or when the normal traffic light turns red (Figure 2.10).[8]

Think of the building as a set of tools for living, a sort of inside-out robot or collection of such robots. We learn to use a room or a building by adjusting our body schema not only to the tool in our hand but also to the complementary tools provided by the changing interface with the building. If the building itself is endowed with a range of actions, then we may begin to learn how architecture might indeed be influenced by what we know of human interaction through social neuroscience. The slogan *out from the body and in from the building* offers something deep for us to pursue and understand better. *Can we speak of the body schema of the building?* A topic for Chapter 7.

8. https://www.thelocal.de/20160422/german-city-creates-floor-traffic-lights-for-smartphone-addicts

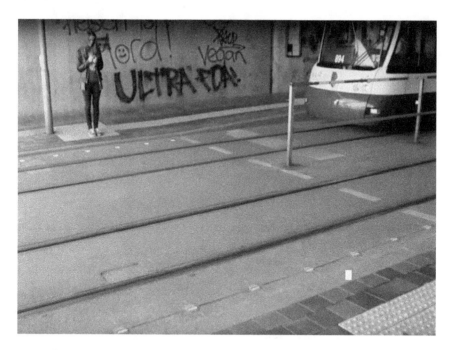

Figure 2.10 Solving a problem with cell phones in Augsburg. Flashing red lights in the sidewalk may catch the attention of downward-attending cell phone users when a street-train is approaching. (Screenshot from https://www.youtube.com/watch?v=3Va9EpF9_hY, with permission from the newspaper *Augsburger Allgemeine*.)

2.5. SCHEMAS: UP TO SOCIETY; DOWN TO NEURONS

We have now got a feel for affordances and effectivities in both locomotion and manipulation, with examples of linking perceptual and motor schemas in the reach-to-grasp. The notion of body schema has made explicit how our effective movements depend on an updated knowledge (often implicit) of how the various parts of the body, possibly extended by clothes and tools, relate to the environment. We now look at perceptual and motor schemas in some generality and then proceed both "upward" to social schemas that provide a distributed representation of the knowledge shared to varied extents by the members of a culture or community and "downward" to neurons.

Schemas in the head

The notion of *schema* is often traced in modern philosophy to Kant (2003 [1781]) and (as we have just seen) in neurology to Head and Holmes (1911). Influenced by Head and Holmes, Frederic Bartlett's book *Remembering* (Bartlett, 1932) stressed that we cannot recall what happened in total detail. Rather, memories are encoded in terms of familiar knowledge, or schemas, so that some information may be lost or distorted. Consider the game where people are seated around a table. One person whispers a little story to the next, and that person repeats it to the next, and so on around the table. Then the last person tells the story out loud and the first person bursts into laughter because, even though each person has tried to repeat the story they heard, recoding it in their own scripts/schemas has changed some of it, and the overall changes may indeed be drastic. We will see a pictorial version of this in §3.6.

Schemas played an important role in the analysis of child development offered by Jean Piaget (1952, 1954). In particular, Piaget stressed the role of learning. In a given situation, children may or may not be able to deploy their current knowledge. Piaget spoke of *assimilation*—making do with existing schemas—versus *accommodation* in cases where one may need to acquire new schemas to better mediate behavior (or thought) in the current situation and henceforth in related situations.

My own quest has been for a general framework for schema theory that links cognitive science, neuroscience, and sociology. Let's first consider *basic schema theory*, exemplified in the reach-to-grasp figure (Figure 2.8). The action–perception cycle demands that we integrate patterns of perception, *perceptual schemas*, with patterns for action, *motor schemas*. Consider recognizing an apple (a piece of fruit, not a computer). What we observe about it may depend drastically on what we intend to do with it. Taking a walk through an orchard, we may pause simply to admire an apple, or to pick it. In the latter case, we observe it more closely to assess whether it is ripe but not too ripe, and we must further assess its shape and location before we can successfully grasp and pluck it. Quite a different linkage of perception is required if we are to peel the apple or to eat it, and the latter brings the mouth as well as arm and hand into play and adds taste and smell to the senses of vision and touch. All this gives us a sense of the active engagement and disengagement of diverse schemas as the action–perception cycle continues—notions that apply equally to study of how people experience the built environment and how consideration of this may factor into design.

Activation of perceptual schemas may encode (whether consciously or subconsciously) the presence of certain affordances, but other perceptual schemas may report on the identity of objects or actions, even the characteristics of overall scenes. A *schema assemblage* combines an estimate of environmental state with a representation of goals and needs. The *internal state* is also updated by knowledge of the state of execution of current plans made up of motor schemas. Other schemas are involved further from the sensory or motor periphery.

Design can affect these variables. Good lighting may help a person see and avoid obstacles, but dim lighting is more appropriate in a theater where attention to the performance should not be distracted by the immediate surroundings of the audience. Similarly, design can affect the "needs" of a person, as when an aroma increases a sense of hunger to attract that person to purchase food, or an attractive vista distracts someone from a current errand to gaze out the window. In other words, we may be strongly motivated and seek affordances that will let us satisfy that need, but affordances—and other environmental factors, such as undue heat or cold, or glare—that attract our attention may divert our activity into other paths.

Schemas can be organized into larger structures that (while still schemas) have also been called *frames* and *scripts*, as we saw in our discussion of Bo Bardi. Another example will give a further sense of this general idea: The *Birthday script* includes generic plans that, for the guest, include actions like "give present" and "sing 'Happy Birthday,'" and for the honoree will include actions like "open presents" and "blow out candles." This frame or script sets certain expectations and limits on the order of the different actions (don't attempt to blow out the candles if they have not yet been lit) and how to respond to different contingencies (there may not be any candles on the cake), but still provides much freedom for choosing different courses of action within (or close to) that general script.

In discussing Bo Bardi's art museum in São Paulo, we saw the complementarity between the scripts that the architect seeks to support by her design, and the scripts that users develop to guide their behavior in the finished building. You can extend this by thinking through the ideas of schema and script as they apply to your daily routine in your own home, and how the design (architecture/interior design/landscaping) both constrains and supports your activities. As another exercise, consider occasions when you need to acquire novel but related perceptual and motor schemas—as so often happens when trying to figure out the shower controls in a hotel bathroom.

Finally, note the culture-dependent nature of these scripts. For example, the "entering a house" script includes wiping your feet on the doormat in Europe but removing your shoes in the genkan entryway in Japan. Such differences in script have implications for the architect, of course, whose design must accommodate them.

Competition and cooperation is "the style of the brain"

For now, I leave action aside, and focus on purely visual perception. Consider the painting by René Magritte, a Belgian surrealist, as shown at left in Figure 2.11. Activation of visual schemas for sky, castle, and mountain *cooperate*. Although a castle could be on a plain with a forest behind it, our experience with views of castles is consistent with the castle being positioned atop a hill or mountain with the sky for backdrop, as in the view of Edinburgh Castle at right. Thus, we have no problem seeing a castle atop a mountain in this painting.

But Magritte is a surrealist. He is not content with giving us a "mere" picture, and indeed the painting we have just examined is only the top part of his painting "Le château des Pyrénées" (1959) shown in Figure

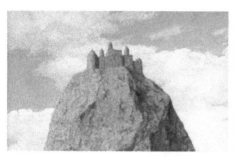
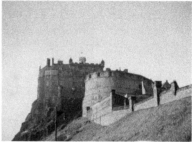

Figure 2.11 (*Left*) Magritte's castle. (*Right*) Edinburgh Castle. (*Left*: See acknowledgement in Figure 2.12. *Right*: Author's photo.)

2.12. Here, we see that the part we have already examined is only "locally" realistic. The bottom half shows, perhaps, a massive boulder falling into the sea. For the central object, two interpretations, two schemas, are now in *competition*—mountain versus boulder. Put the two together, and the painting becomes unrealistic, surrealistic. The local realism is battling global constraints, and in this case there is no overall, coherent, interpretation of the image.

My point here is not to claim the relevance of Magritte's castle for the study of architecture. Rather, it is to help us understand the processes at work in our visual perception that resolve different hypotheses about what we are seeing. Often, these processes proceed to completion without our conscious awareness. The Magritte painting, by undermining a coherent resolution, makes it easier to bring these processes to the level of conscious analysis.

As we will see in detail in Chapter 3, our perception of a scene involves the interaction of processes that proceed in two directions. *Bottom-up* processes (processing "up" from local visual features toward the overall interpretation of the scene) are those based on local stimuli—we might recognize a patch of an image as being an image of cloud because of its color, shape, and texture. But our perception of the scene may also involve *top-down* processes (*down* from the emerging high-level interpretation— recognition of one part of a scene may affect recognition of another), as when our expectation of meeting a friend may cause us to see the face of a

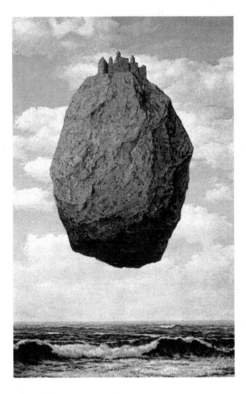

Figure 2.12 René Magritte (1959) "Le château des Pyrénées." (© 2020 C. Herscovici/ Artists Rights Society [ARS], New York.)

---

passerby as that of the friend until a closer look, more detailed bottom-up processing, reveals that we are mistaken.

Schema instances may agree ("mountain" and "castle"; or "boulder" and "sea")—we say they *cooperate*: the relation between them increases the "confidence level" of the other. Other schema instances may *compete* (it is unlikely that the same region of the image could be interpreted as both a mountain *and* a falling boulder): increasing activation of either reduces the confidence level of the other. This dynamic pattern of competition and cooperation may proceed until the confidence level of a critical mass of schema instances may pass some sort of threshold or consensus to constitute the current interpretation of the scene (much more on this in §3.4). This is one of the reasons that we say that *competition and cooperation (aka cooperative computation) is "the style of the brain."*

With most scenes in everyday life, we can settle on a single interpretation (usually based on selective attention to only some of the details) that can form the basis for our further action. With Magritte, we have to settle for paradox. He paints in a style that ensures you will be very confident of what you are seeing locally, but with no way to avoid incoherence overall. The resulting frisson of paradox gives his work the charge for which he is famous. Escher drawings often share this property of "locally coherent; globally incoherent." Some have suggested that this also characterizes London's modern skyline as contrasted with Rome's, though not all observers would agree.

The architect, understanding this, can decide whether a given architectural space is to offer a straightforward interpretation that can frame the user's behavior (as might be the case in the public spaces of a hospital) or yield a visual cacophony that may stimulate confusion but whose resolution is the challenge sought by the visitor (as may be the case in an entertainment space).

These observations set the stage for the more rigorous analysis of the competition and cooperation of visual schemas in §3.4, where we will see that a fuller analysis requires us to consider *schema instances* (to be explained there) and not just schemas. We will see that perception itself is a process of *construction*, building (perhaps subconsciously) a more or less coherent interpretation from different local hypotheses (the schema instances) about what is going on in different parts of the image. Those that are coherent will cooperate and work together; those that are not will compete. In general, this coherence will spread to all parts of the scene that we attend to, unlike a Magritte painting where that search for coherence remains unfulfilled.

From schemas in the head to social schemas

We are not solitary creatures. We are shaped not only by our interaction with the physical world but—especially—through our social interactions, interactions that depend not only on our underlying biology but

(EvoDevoSocio) the culture in which we are raised. The notion of *social schemas* captures something of the way in which the society around us influences who we become. Architecture is then both shaped by such schemas (the current cultural milieu) and can help shape its further cultural evolution.

The work with Mary Hesse on our book *The Construction of Reality* (Arbib & Hesse, 1986) opened up the social dimension to complement my work on schema theory exemplified above. Her study of the history and philosophy of science had led her to investigate the "social construction" of science (Hesse, 1980). How is it that astronomers became convinced that the Earth moves around the sun, rather than vice versa? How is it that physicists came to adopt the probabilistic view of the world offered by quantum mechanics, yet still saw Newton's view of a deterministic world as a limiting case? Mary's studies led her to understand that it requires prolonged social interaction, combined with innovative experiments and novel theorizing, for a group of people to change their worldview, what Kuhn has called a *paradigm* (Hesse, 1980; Kuhn, 1962).

My choice of the title *The Construction of Reality* for our collaboration was inspired in part by Jean Piaget's *The Construction of Reality in the Child* (Piaget, 1954). Working with Mary helped me better appreciate *The Social Construction of Reality* (Berger & Luckmann, 1966). We worked together to develop a shared epistemology—a theory of how we know about the world—broad enough to integrate my brain-centered account of schemas with her view of knowledge as something that emerges within and across a social group. The outcome was to extend schema theory to include not only the individual's *internal* schemas ("schemas in the head"), as discussed previously, but also *social schemas*.[9] The latter do not necessarily exist in any one place and may not even be grasped within the mind of any single individual, but are instead emergent from the diverse patterns

9. Social schemas are similar to *collective representations* (Durkheim, 1915). However, they are somewhat different from *memes* as defined by Richard Dawkins in his book *The Selfish Gene* (Dawkins, 1976) as "a new kind of replicator . . . a unit of cultural transmission, or a unit of imitation," an idea developed with great enthusiasm by Susan Blackmore (1999). To see the difference, consider the English language as a social schema. Individual words and catch phrases may enter and drop out of use within a community as transient memes.

of behavior exhibited by individuals within the society, with each individual having interiorized the social schema in terms of somewhat different "schemas in the head." For example, each reader of this book (unless in translation) has a knowledge of English, yet may find some words and some grammatical constructions I employ unfamiliar, without denying that we are both employing the English language.

Cultural evolution operates more on an "ecology" of social schemas, a Great Schema if you will, that frames whole patterns of social behavior even as elements within it change over time. There is no one place that defines the English language as a whole. Rather, each native English speaker grows up in a society in which English is spoken and discovers that certain words and phrases are used in certain contexts. Each child thus gets a highly personal sample of what can be said (and, later, written) in English. Fragments of language come linked with related situations in statistical patterns. Certain words appear together in distinctive ways to describe what is going on, to provide instruction, to fulfill requests, to express endearment, and so on. But out of that, the child's brain is able to build up internal schemas—based on changes in connectivity and other parameters within the brain's neural networks—to recognize words, understand what they mean, and build up constructions that fit the words together to gain pragmatic success in using words to get milk or tell mummy "I love you," or to accomplish other things of importance to the young child.

Here, social schemas augment the regularities of interaction with the physical world (how to eat an apple and what sensations of touch and taste to expect, or the way an object will fall if you let go of it, and so many more) to allow the child, and then the adult growing up, to build their own personal network of "schemas in the head." This includes not only fairly pragmatic schemas—how to get milk, how to recognize whether a dog is friendly—but also social constraints—what is "proper" behavior, how to behave in a restaurant or in class or at the dining room table, and so on.

In short, then, social schemas provide part of the vocabulary in which we can talk about our EvoDevoSocio perspective. The EvoDevo part teaches us that the genome of each human is indeed distinctively human—it will under most circumstances guide the growth of a person who shares a range of "normal" human capacities for perception, action, emotion, and sociality. But it also emphasizes that the way we develop depends greatly on our social "niche," both in the family and in terms of larger groups such as those defined by language, religion, and ideology as well as a range of more specific customs. We can view this niche as the dynamic product of cultural evolution—the result of a process of niche construction heavily constrained by social dynamics (Socio).

This, of course, has diverse implications for architecture. A house (or the larger area of which it is part) must address the basic human needs for assuaging hunger and thirst and eliminating waste products. However, social schemas can provide crucial constraints on the way even basic needs are met—while further architectural drivers are more culturally specific. Relevant variations may vary from the simple matter of what to do with shoes at the entryway of a home or office, to complex constraints on the relation between men and women. For example, laboratories in a university in Saudi Arabia had to be designed for use by men and women at different times, with entrances from different passageways to ensure no mingling between them (Ken Kornberg, personal communication). In neither of these examples does knowledge of the brain seem *directly* relevant, but further analysis can offer a historical and anthropological account of the emergence of the social schemas involved, taking into account the biologically under-written range of possibility for developmental trajectories. Social neuroscience will increasingly reveal what it is about the human brain that makes social schemas possible, and how they may shape individual behavior while also providing the basis on which new social schemas may emerge.

In his book *The Architect's Brain: Neuroscience, Creativity, and Architecture*, Harry Mallgrave (2009) offers a history of architecture with an unusual twist. He explores the cognitive style of each architect in this historical review and asks what one might infer about the brains of those architects as they practice their craft. No biological evolution separates the brains of these architects, but each approaches architecture differently because their brains have been shaped by their development within a distinctive cultural and personal milieu.

An architect asked me: "Is it really the brain that changes? Isn't it simply the following of human life to change styles, art and cultures, to follow trends and simply to evolve with the technology?" I think there is a key misunderstanding here that I began to address in discussing two-way reduction in §1.5—we enrich our understanding of both brain and person by seeking relations between them. Palladio could not have designed the buildings that he did had he been born in China, or a century or two earlier. But, equally, Palladio could not have developed buildings and architectural ideas that we still admire today had he not been endowed with a brain that supported a range of visuomotor skills and a rich memory and imagination. He both reflected and changed the social schemas shared by architects in his place and time. We can seek a purely biographical account of his cultural and personal particularities, and that may be as close as we can get to an understanding of his particular genius, exploring the experience and the memories that contributed to his achievements. Indeed, I offer essays of this kind for Jørn Utzon and Frank Gehry in Chapter 9. But this is a book on the A↔N conversation, and so in Chapter 10 I begin to probe the general principles of brain operation linking memory, imagination, and more that enable architects (and many others) to exploit their biological and cultural inheritance, filtered through their own individual experience and development, to make their own contributions. A rich conversation must go both ways—this particular study may be less a case of what neuroscience can offer to help the architect, and more a way in which architecture may challenge neuroscience to seek new understandings.

From schemas in the head to neurons and synapses

Having moved "up" to social schemas, we now move "down" to neurons. "Basic" schema theory studies schemas for a cognitive account of action, perception, and other cognitive functions as dynamical, interacting systems underlying mental and overt behavior. This provides an appropriate language for cognitive science. However, one needs a *neural schema theory* to move on to the data from neurophysiology, lesion studies, and brain imaging as we test hypotheses on (i) how schemas are related to neural mechanisms distributed across diverse regions of the brain and/or (ii) how neural circuitry may implement the schema's dynamics, continuing our theme that the brain is a system of systems.

Our brains do not provide a simple stimulus–response chain from receptors to effectors (though there are such reflex paths in the spinal cord). Rather, the vast network of billions upon billions of neurons is interconnected in loops and tangled chains so that signals entering the net from the receptors interact there with the billions of signals already traversing the system, both to modify activity within the system and to yield the signals that control the effectors. In this way, the central nervous system enables the current actions of the organism to depend not only on its current stimulation and present intentions but also on the residue of past experience expressed in the activity and changed structure of its network.

Different parts of the brain may have very different neuron types and/or "architectures." Consider the two drawings in Figure 2.13 (half of Figure 1.11). Without being in any sense concerned about these fine details in our present conversation with the architecture of buildings, we can see that the neuron types and the patterns of connectivity are very different. This makes clear that *there is no such thing as a typical neuron*. Nonetheless, it is helpful to examine a "basic neuron" abstracted from a motoneuron of mammalian spinal cord.

A number of ramifying branches called the *dendrites* protrude from the cell body to form a major part of the *input* surface of the neuron. There also extrudes from the cell body, at a point called the *axon hillock*, a long fiber called the *axon*, which generally branches into the so-called *axonal arborization*. Certain "boutons" on the axon impinge upon other neurons or upon effectors. The locus of this interaction is called a *synapse*, and we say that the cell with the bouton *synapses upon* the cell on which it impinges, and refer to these cells as the *presynaptic neuron* and *postsynaptic neuron*, respectively.

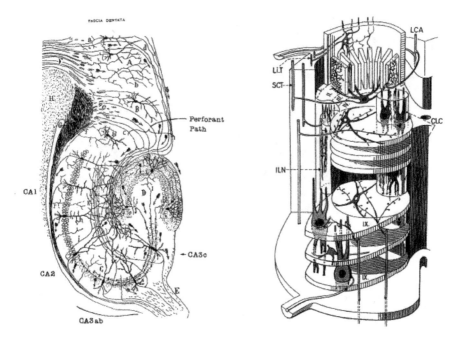

Figure 2.13 Schematizations of core neural circuitry in two brain regions, showing the different types of neurons in each, as well as the very different "architecture" of their arrangement. (*Left*) The "seahorse" cross section of hippocampus (Ramón y Cajal). (*Right*) Spinal cord (Szentágothai). These diagrams appeared earlier as half of Figure 1.11. (From Arbib, M. A., Érdi, P., & Szentágothai, J. [1998]. *Neural organization: Structure, function, and dynamics.* Cambridge, MA: MIT Press.)

We can best imagine the flow of information as shown by the arrows in Figure 2.14. Most synapses tend to "communicate" activity to the dendrites or soma of the cell they synapse upon, whence activity passes to the axon hillock and then as a "spike" of activity down the axon to the terminal arborization. We say the neuron "fires" each time a spike is generated. The axon can be very long indeed. For instance, a neuron that controls the big toe is rooted in the spinal cord and thus has an axon that runs the complete length of the leg. We may contrast the immense length of the axon of such a neuron with the minute axon lengths of neurons packed into several layers in the retina.

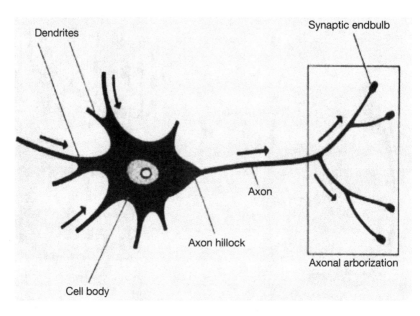

Figure 2.14 Schematic view of a neuron. Activity from receptors or other neurons modifies membrane potentials on the dendrites and cell body. The effects of these changes converge upon the axon hillock where, for appropriate spatiotemporal patterns of incoming activity, a pulse of membrane potential will be propagated along the axon, branching out into the axonal arborization to activate the synaptic endbulbs that modify the membrane potential of other neurons, or of muscle fibers or glands, in turn. (From Arbib, M. A. [1972]. *The metaphorical brain: An introduction to cybernetics as artificial intelligence and brain theory*. New York: Wiley-Interscience.)

The effect of a spike arriving at a synapse may be *excitatory*, making the postsynaptic neuron more likely to fire or, conversely, *inhibitory*, tending to make it less likely to fire. At the axon hillock, the propagated effects of many different synaptic inputs will converge, so that even if these changes are themselves small, the total contribution (across possibly thousands of input neurons, though some neurons have only three or four inputs) by which excitation exceeds inhibition in some time period may be large enough to fire the neuron. It may take the excitation from many inputs overwhelming inhibition to fire a neuron. Thus, differential changes in the weights (strengths of influence) of the input synapses can greatly affect the set of input patterns that will cause a neuron to fire. This is why *synaptic plasticity* plays a central role in many theories of the neural mechanisms of learning and memory (§5.3). We may also speak of *neuroplasticity* for these and other neural changes.

Some synapses can emit a chemical substance called a *neuromodulator* that can modulate the way the postsynaptic neuron behaves in diverse ways other than excitation or inhibition. (More on this in §4.2.)

Excitation and inhibition provide, at the neural level, the cooperation and competition that we earlier declared, when analyzing dynamics at the schema level, to be the "style of the brain." And, of course, this "style" persists as we move up to the level of people interacting with each other both within and between groups.

Single-cell studies of activity in neural circuits. It is possible to record the activity of single neurons during different tasks, but this can rarely be done in humans—only if the results are needed during neurosurgery as part of determining how to cut the brain in a way that will reduce damage to the patient after recovery (recall the work of Penfield that led to the discovery of the motor and somatosensory homunculi), or in the development of neuroprosthetics. Thus, most of our detailed data on neural circuitry come from microelectrode recordings from nonhuman animals, especially monkeys and rodents but also from diverse other species ranging from frogs to songbirds. We will examine data on early visual processing in the brains of frogs, cats, and monkeys in §3.2, but here let's briefly examine a study of the rat hippocampus.

Figure 2.13 (left) showed the neural circuitry in a cross section of rat hippocampus as drawn by Santiago Ramón y Cajal. Figure 2.15 (left) captures the classic finding by John O'Keefe and Jonathan Dostrovsky (1971) of what are called *place cells*. The delicate tracery shows the path of a rat running around a square arena, while the red dots show where the rat was when a *particular* cell fired—the red dots delimit the *place field* for the place cell. Clearly, one cell does not specify the rat's location with much precision. However, a key notion from neuroscience is that of a *population code*. It takes a group of neurons for the brain to precisely encode information. If we imagine a group of cells with different but overlapping place fields, then their joint activity would specify

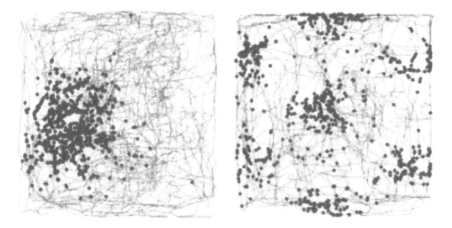

Figure 2.15 Tracery shows the trajectory of a rat in a recording enclosure. The *red dots* show (*left*) where a single *place cell* in the hippocampus fired and (*right*) where a *grid cell* in the medial entorhinal cortex fired as a rat moved around the enclosure. Whereas most place cells have a relatively compact firing region, the *place field*, the firing fields of a grid cell (at least for an animal in a simple enclosure) form a periodic hexagonal matrix tiling the entire environment available to the animal. At present, there has been little mention of the grid cells in the A↔N conversation, so in this volume we will ignore them and discuss only the place cells. (Adapted from Witter, M. P., & Moser, E. I. [2006]. Spatial representation and the architecture of the entorhinal cortex. *Trends in Neurosciences*, 29(12), 671–678, with permission from Elsevier.)

that the rat is in the region in which their place fields overlap. Using more place cells yields more precision in specifying location. The brain can exploit this principle in mediating the action–perception cycle in diverse behaviors, not just navigation.

Neuroscientists may focus on one region of the brain in a monkey or a rat or other lab animal and see what the cells are doing there during a particular task, or use brain imaging in humans to associate active brain regions with performance of a task. However, each part of the brain receives input from other parts of the brain and sends output to yet other parts of the brain; and there are return pathways. Thus, the data are always samples from a larger system. The further catch, of course, is that across evolution, the brains of different species change as much as their bodies do. Thus the extent to which details of non-human brains yield insight into the working of human brains will vary from system to system, and may remain open to lively debate. In particular, rats and humans have different brains, different bodies, and different behaviors. Thus, we cannot simply take the data that has built on O'Keefe's studies to explore the circuitry in which place cells are embedded in the rat brain and "plug it in" to an account of the circuitry that underlies the blobs in fMRI studies of the human brain.

The work of John O'Keefe inspired an immense outpouring of work on place cells and the hippocampus by many researchers. This work then spread to analysis of neurons, such as head direction neurons, in various areas connected to the hippocampus. The most famous sequel was the work of Edvard and May-Britt Moser who found in the entorhinal cortex, a major input region to the hippocampus, neurons they called *grid cells*. In simple arenas, at least, these cells were somewhat like place cells, but instead of having a place field in one connected part of the arena, a grid cell would be activated when the rat was in a place near any point on a hexagonal grid (see Moser, Kropff, & Moser, 2008, for a review of "Place Cells, Grid Cells, and the Brain's Spatial Representation System"). Indeed, this work was considered so significant that the Nobel Prize in Physiology or Medicine 2014 was awarded one half to John O'Keefe, the other half jointly to the Mosers "for their discoveries of cells that constitute a positioning system in the brain." This prize recognized both a paradigm shift in the study of cognitive neuroscience, and some of the amazing insights that followed from it concerning how the world is represented within the brain.

I will explore the relevance of place cells, the hippocampus, and neighboring regions to wayfinding in Chapter 6 (see Epstein, Patai, Julian, & Spiers, 2017, for an overview of "The Cognitive Map in Humans: Spatial Navigation and Beyond"). Chapter 10 will address the human hippocampus's role, in concert with other brain regions, in mediating episodic memory and imagination. However, in neither of these chapters have I found it necessary to discuss the role of grid cells when seeking a rapprochement with the experience and design of architecture. This remains a challenge for future A↔N conversations.

2.6. THE THINKING HAND AND ITS BRAIN

We continue discussion of *The Thinking Hand,* but now bringing in neural schemas, attending to details about the brain gleaned from recording from single neurons in monkeys that complement lesion and brain imaging studies in humans.

In §2.2, I stated that "We recognize a doorway as offering an entrance to or exit from a room or building, but if we decide to go through that doorway, the unconscious affordances shape our trajectory, as when we duck our head if the doorway is low." We shall now see (but focusing on hand movements rather than locomotion) that this distinction is realized in separate pathways in the monkey and human brain—another entry in our quest to "dissect phenomenology." We examine two pathways that link primary visual cortex to premotor cortex (Figure 2.16). The *dorsal pathway* (think of the dorsal fin atop a shark) travels up to the parietal lobe and then across to *premotor cortex* (which lies in front of primary motor cortex, and sends key signals to it). The *ventral pathway* goes down to the

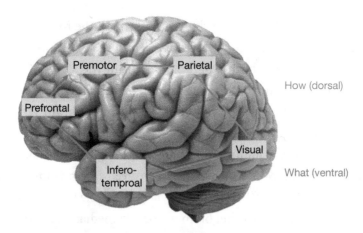

Figure 2.16 The ventral and dorsal pathways for visual control of hand actions. The ventral pathway analyzes the scene to enable the prefrontal cortex to determine "what" to do; the dorsal pathway then fills in the details of "how to do it," passing affordance parameters to premotor cortex to adjust motor schemas for the selected actions.

inferior (i.e., lower) part of the temporal lobe and then up through the *prefrontal cortex* (PFC; the frontmost part of frontal cortex).

The ventral path is the "how" system. Goodale, Milner, Jakobson, and Carey (1991) studied a patient with a lesion of the ventral pathway. They would, for example, show her various cylinders and ask her to tell them how wide each was. (Note that knowing that something is a cylinder tells you nothing about its size.) She could not state its width, whether in speech or pantomime—the overt declaration of width did not correlate with its actual value. Yet when they asked her to pick up any one of the cylinders, she did so with a perfect correlation between the maximal width of the preshape and the diameter of the cylinder. The width was available for carrying out the action on the dorsal pathway (thus named the "how" system), but not available to stating "what" its value was.

The dorsal path is the "what" system. Conversely, Jeannerod, Decety, and Michel (1994) studied a patient who had a lesion of the dorsal pathway. She was able to reliably report on the size and even pantomime it (the ventral pathway is thus called the "what" pathway—she could state *what* the width was). However, when reaching to grasp a cylinder, she could not preshape her hand based on visual cues. Instead, she would just keep her hand at its maximal extension until it hit the object; she would then use the sense of touch to enclose and successfully grasp the cylinder.

We turn from human neuropsychology to neurophysiological studies of the macaque monkey from both Hideo Sakata's group at Nihon University in Tokyo and Giacomo Rizzolatti's team in Parma in Italy to augment the human studies by Jeannerod and others to learn more about the underlying circuitry of manual control (see Jeannerod, Arbib, Rizzolatti, & Sakata, 1995, for an overview). Based on functional magnetic resonance imaging (fMRI) studies, neuroscientists believe that, in manual control, macaque circuitry has much in common with the human brain. There are, of course, differences as well, but these are not relevant here. I will show how a computational model, the FARS model (named for the modelers Fagg and Arbib and the neurophysiologists Rizzolatti and Sakata) built on these data to offer a more detailed analysis of the dorsal and ventral pathways, and to offer new insights into the handling of affordances (and the affordances of handling). In §2.7 I will discuss the general notion of a "computational model" in neuroscience as distinct from a "physical model" in architecture to draw parallels between design in architecture and in the design of brain models.

I devote the rest of the section to linking macaque neurophysiology to the computational model. Although several of my architect colleagues like to skip such material, I hope that many of you will persevere, at least skimming the material to glean some of the details at first reading. In any case, please resume reading after the double lines for a review of the key "take home messages."

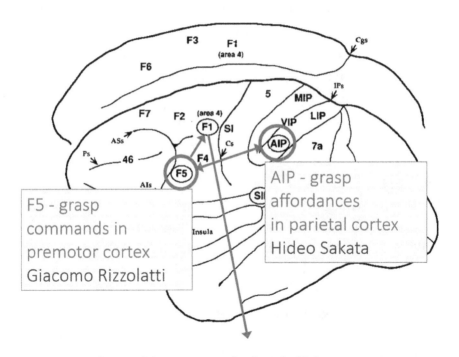

Figure 2.17 A side view of the macaque monkey brain highlighting two regions crucial to the visual control of hand movement. Region AIP is associated with visual processing that extracts affordances of an object for grasping, and area F5 in premotor cortex contains neurons that set up motor schemas for grasping and send their codes to primary motor cortex F1 to set up detailed instructions to the muscles. (Adapted from the macaque brain template in Jeannerod, M., Arbib, M. A., Rizzolatti, G., & Sakata, H. [1995]. Grasping objects: The cortical mechanisms of visuomotor transformation. *Trends in Neuroscience*, 18[7], 314–320.)

Studying the dorsal pathway, Sakata's group found that an area called AIP in parietal cortex (Figure 2.17) encodes the affordances of objects for grasping, while Rizzolatti's group studied the region they call F5 in premotor cortex.[10]

The ventral path contains an area called inferotemporal cortex (IT, the lower part of the temporal lobe) associated with recognizing what an object is. While IT will show distinctive neural activity to distinguish the identity of a small cube from that of a small sphere, AIP in the dorsal pathway encodes both objects in the same way because each provides the affordance for using a precision pinch.

For hand movements, Sakata's area AIP sends data to the region F5 in premotor cortex where Rizzolatti's team found cells that fired when the monkey carried out a particular kind of grasp: one neuron might fire vigorously during a precision pinch but not for a palmar grasp or vice versa; another might fire for tearing paper but not for breaking peanuts.

A crucial note: In Chapter 5, we will discuss the seminal discovery of "mirror neurons" by the Rizzolatti group. Not all neurons in F5 are related to hand movements, but among those that are, *mirror neurons* fire both when the monkey executes a certain type of action and when observing a similar action performed by another. In the present section, though, we concentrate on *canonical neurons* that are active when the monkey executes an action but not when the monkey is just observing actions.

Just as we noted in §2.2 that the brain "maps" the world in many ways, this linkage of parietal affordances to motor schemas occurs for other

---

10. It is not important here to know what these abbreviations stand for, but for those who care to know, here is the explanation. There is a groove (neuroanatomists call it a sulcus) in the parietal cortex, called the *intraparietal (IP) sulcus*. Region AIP is at the anterior (front) end of IP; LIP (the lateral part of IP) is at the side of it. The F in F5 stands for frontal, but the number 5 is no more meaningful than the numbers Brodmann assigned to his areas—F5 is the fifth region in the way the Parma group numbered regions of frontal cortex. Similarly, the Parma group called primary motor cortex F1, though most people denote it M1.

types of action as well. For example, the cortical area LIP near AIP provides a retinotopic map that registers possible targets for saccades and sends these to a frontal region called the frontal eye field to determine which target to saccade to.

The FARS model (Fagg & Arbib, 1998) offers an account of how various brain regions cooperate in allowing a human or a monkey to look at an object, figure out how to grasp it, and have the motor cortex send the signals to the muscles that will cause that grasp to be performed. It provides explicit hypotheses on how the interactions between the dorsal ("how") and ventral ("what") streams cooperate to activate the canonical neurons in F5 that determine the current grasp. Some brain regions are modeled at the schema level (dynamic "sketches" of what the region contributes), while in other regions the neural networks have been specified in detail. The complete model has been implemented on computers to yield interesting simulation results, but here we just look at FARS in conceptual terms. Nonetheless, I encourage you to use the two FARS figures to get some sense of what is involved in a computational model of how certain brain regions work together to support a range of functions.

The dorsal stream of FARS (Figure 2.18) processes visual input about an object to extract affordances. It is the part of the brain that is operative when the goal is to pick something up, irrespective of what the object is, or its use. Inspired by Sakata's data, the model includes area cIPS (another region of the dorsal stream) to provide information about the position and location of patches of the surface of the observed object. These data are processed by AIP to recognize what different parts of the object are opposed to each other such that they can between them support a stable grasp, thus extracting affordances for the grasp system, which are then passed on to F5. This generalizes the case considered by Jeannerod and Biguer—for a ball, any grasp across diametrically opposed patches of the spherical surface will do, so choosing an affordance for the ball reduces to selecting the size and orientation for the grasp.

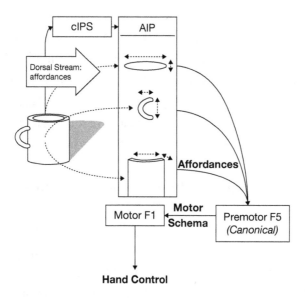

Figure 2.18 The dorsal stream part of the FARS (Fagg-Arbib-Rizzolatti-Sakata) model, which takes input from the primary visual cortex and processes it via, especially, areas cIPS and AIP of parietal cortex. AIP does not "know" the identity of the object but can only extract affordances (opportunities for grasping the object considered as an unidentified solid), indicated here by portions of the object that are particularly graspable. Here, and in Figure 2.19, there are "boxes" connected by arrows. Each box is labeled with a function; some boxes are also labeled with the names of brain regions. The association of a function with a brain region, or the claim that an arrow represents connections between the two indicated brain regions, will in general be based on available neuroscience data, but in some cases will represent hypotheses that suggest new neuroscience experiments.

Crucially, design of the FARS model emphasizes that visual input might activate AIP codes for more than one affordance, while an affordance might activate F5 codes for more than one type of grasp. To address this, the circuitry had to include a *winner-take-all* (WTA) mechanism, a neural network to select just one of the affordances encoded in AIP and/or just one of the motor schemas compatible with the selected affordance(s). This process would result in area F5 sending the code for the selected motor schema to primary motor cortex, area F1, to commit the network to a single course of action. The goal has thus been narrowed from "grasp this (unspecified) object" to "grasp this affordance of the object using this specific grasp." It was then the task of F1, working in concert with other brain regions, to command the appropriate pattern of coordinated movement of arm and hand to achieve this goal. (We did not include this command pathway in the FARS model because that is handled by other neural models.)

The full model (Figure 2.19) brings in the ventral stream. It now addresses the case where the agent has a more specific goal—for example, to drink coffee from the mug. In contrast to the dorsal stream, the ventral stream from primary visual cortex to inferotemporal cortex, IT, is able to recognize what the object is. This information is passed to PFC, which can then, on the basis of the current goals of the organism and the recognition of the nature of the object, bias AIP to select the affordance appropriate to the current task. This prefrontal processing is modeled schematically; other models assess neurobiologically plausible neural networks for implementing PFC's functions, but this book will not present any of them.

For example, if we see a mug just as an obstacle in the way of our getting hold of a magazine underneath it, we might grab the mug by the rim to lift it out of the way; but if we plan to sip coffee from the mug, the odds are that we will grasp it by the handle. As we saw in Figure 2.18, the dorsal (how) stream doesn't "know" what that object is, but it can recognize affordances for grasping. The ventral (what) stream recognizes the object as a mug and reports this to PFC, and PFC has access to working memory, which can answer, for example, "Is there coffee left in the mug?" and assess motivation, for example, "Do I need another shot of caffeine?" If the answer to both is "yes," PFC could come up with the plan to pick up the mug by the handle to get some coffee, and this would lead to gating only the affordance for the handle from AIP to get to F5 to set up the action, inhibiting the other affordances.

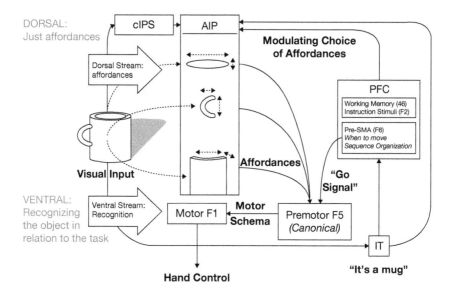

Figure 2.19 The full FARS model. If F5 relied only on the dorsal stream to activate a motor schema, it would choose the "most graspable" affordance. However, the FARS model also brings the ventral stream into play: inferotemporal cortex (IT) identifies the object and its meaningful parts; prefrontal cortex (PFC) then uses this identification of the object, in concert with task analysis and working memory, to help AIP select the appropriate affordance from its "menu." Given this affordance, F5 can then select an appropriate motor schema and instruct primary motor cortex to forward its execution.

The FARS model exploits data from *monkey* physiology to gain insight into how various brain regions cooperate in allowing a *human* to look at an object and grasp it.

You don't have to remember what FARS is the acronym for, so long as you get the idea that it is our neural model of visual control of grasping that illustrates the more general integration of "what" and "how" in diverse behaviors.

The FARS model will act as a reference point in Chapters 5 and 10, not because of its details but because it illustrates several key ideas: The most important point is to reinforce the notion that behavior involves both high-level (possibly conscious) decisions and (frequently subconscious) tuning of motor schemas to match subtle details of the body schema and the external world. The FARS model, based on the F5 canonical neurons, shows the importance of object recognition (IT) and "planning" (PFC) in modulating the selection of affordances in the determination of action. We thus begin to understand that many different neural populations must work together for the successful control of behavior.

Extrapolating from what is actually "in" the FARS model from manual control to behavior more generally: perceptual schemas can analyze the disposition and affordances of objects in the environment and then pass parameters onward to motor schemas to coordinate these schemas in successfully carrying out the task. Different affordances (registered in posterior parietal cortex) would be selected by the ventral path for action (as determined in premotor cortex) depending on the current task; fine-tuning for motor schemas to exploit that affordance would then be provided by the dorsal path.

2.7. DESIGN IN ARCHITECTURE AND IN BRAIN MODELING

To extend the intuition gained through the introduction of the FARS model for the reach-to-grasp (or to encourage you to repeat the attempt to gain it), and to set the stage for later brain-inspired modeling, I argue that both architects and brain modelers exploit many similar cognitive processes in their different design challenges.

Reminder: For an architect, the *program* is the initial specification of requirements for a building; for the computer programmer as well as the brain modeler, the program is the detailed set of computer instructions that will achieve the specifications. The word "model" also has different connotations. For the architect, a three-dimensional model captures some current aspects of the form of a building as it takes shape during design. For the neuroscientist, a computer model of the brain ultimately takes the form of a computer program that provides detailed instructions for running computer simulations to test the model. However, neuroscientists also use the word "model" in a second sense. The rat may be considered a "model" of the human for studying a variety of processes such as those involved in navigation. Similarly, we have just seen that the monkey can serve as a model animal for the study of the visual control of eye movements and hand movements.

Back to computational models of brain function. We check whether, when we provide the simulation program with codes for the *current inputs and internal states* of an animal (or a subsystem under study), the *computed output* will match observed data or offer unexpected results. In the latter case, we may need to update the model, or we may be able to offer new predictions to be tested by experiments (Arbib, 2016; Arbib & Bonaiuto, 2016). For the FARS model, the encoded inputs represented the location and affordances of the object; the internal state included the current location and shape of the hand, as well as specification (rather sketchy in the current implementation) of the current task and working memory, and the output is the reach-and-grasp trajectory.

Whereas an architect's floor plan describes a building that is relatively static (although it will provide a stage on which people behave and interact), a computational model of the brain provides a dynamic map of a changing system that is continually reconfiguring itself, changing state, so that its response to new inputs depends on the current state to both produce measurable outputs and to update the state. In other words, a computational model (unlike most physical models of buildings) underlies a dynamic map of a changing system. It is more akin to the computer program that generates a dynamic weather map whose output of cloud patterns and likelihood of rain can depend on diverse further "state variables" such as the geospatial distribution of temperature at different levels of the atmosphere. Even if we do not see them on the screen, the weather map is based on these state variables that the computer program exploits to support predictions of how the weather will change.

In the schema model of Figure 2.8, each box represented a schema, and the arrows between them represented flow of data as well as activation signals. Moreover, the model was based on human behavioral data. The FARS model was based on both human data (lesion data that distinguished between the dorsal and ventral streams) and monkey data. There, the boxes generally correspond to known regions of the brain, and the model will (for at least some of the boxes) provide computational models of neural network dynamics so that runs of the simulation can be used to compare simulated neural firing with that observed in behaving monkeys. In a model like FARS, each region:

1. Corresponds to a region in the monkey (or other) brain, or represents a relevant function whose localization in the brain is irrelevant to the scope of the model; and
2. Contains state variables and algorithms or modeled schema dynamics or neural net dynamics for how the internal state will change as inputs come in (whether sensory inputs, or from other regions) and outputs go out (whether to control overt behavior or affect other regions).

For some of the schemas that serve the behavior we are studying, we may not know much about where they are implemented in the brain or what neural networks are involved. In that case, it becomes a module in the program that is described computationally, but without the computations being linked to neurobiological processes. We have a schema model akin to our previous model of reach-to-grasp. However, the schema model becomes a brain model when, as in FARS, various regions in the model come with hypotheses on what part of the brain they correspond to. Moreover, we may have hypotheses about how their function might be achieved by biologically plausible neural networks whose behavior can be tested against neurophysiological data.

In later chapters, I will offer various brain models both at the schema level (such as the VISIONS model of §3.4) and in terms of the interaction of circuitry and/or schemas in various brain regions (as in the model of learning in the mirror neuron system in §5.4, and the models of the role of hippocampus and other brain regions in navigation in §6.3). All this leads up to IBSEN (an acronym for *Imagination in Brain Systems for Episodes and Navigation*) in Chapter 10, a cognitive neuroscience model (currently conceptual, rather than implemented for computer simulation) of processes ongoing in the brain of an architect working on a problem of architectural design.

As part of the A↔N conversation, the IBSEN model will offer fresh ideas to architects concerning the relation between memory and imagination, and a framework to be further developed in response to their ideas on their design procresses. I will offer no *immediate* payoff of this attempt for the architect, but will argue that this case study of designing a brain model will offer conceptual rewards, advancing the claim that using neuroscience to dissect phenomenology can benefit the design of buildings intended to affect the experience and behavior of users of the building. More specifically, the modeling will offer ways to move beyond the current neuroscience database to set challenges for further neuroscience research that will yield answers relevant to the role of imagination in design considered as a process of mental construction.

Given this, the following parallel may deepen insight into the A↔N conversation:

The architectural design process involves not only imagining an overall image of the intended building (based on site, typology, program, and more) but also developing fragmentary representations to address site analysis, contextual analysis, forms, scripts, and the necessary affordances, and so forth, as one develops details on the way to the final design. Parts of the high-level design are reassessed as the linkages between different parts are related to the developing details and the emerging concept of the whole. And so the process continues. The result is a building whose success will be measured by the satisfaction of its later users (perhaps with some exceptions, such as prisons, where social aims may prevail over individual ones).

To take a domestic example: You may ignore the bathroom while you focus on the design of the kitchen. Later, you can return to the design of the bathroom and assess whether or not the recent design decisions for the kitchen affect its design. This may be unlikely, whereas there may be strong interaction between the designs of the kitchen and the dining room, with repeated cross-reference as design of each proceeds. Nonetheless, there will be separable subproblems within the design of each, even as one moves toward a coherent design for the house as whole.

Developing a large-scale model in computational cognitive neuro-science may start with an interest in certain brain regions and certain cognitive functions (including those defined by examples from everyday experience and behavior, but enriched by the insights that clinical studies and brain imaging may offer), and then ask how the phenomena may be understood by models worked out at the schema and/or neural network level and then (going beyond the conceptual level to which this book is restricted) implemented on a computer as the basis for detailed simulations. These simulations can be used to test the model against available neuroscience data and to make predictions to be tested by future experiments.

The "images that come to mind" for the brain modeler are of two main kinds:

1. There will be relevant empirical data gleaned from diverse sources. These will be consistent in some ways but not others, and even more damagingly, the published interpretation offered for the data will often not match the rigor with which the data are gathered. In a neuroscience paper, the methods employed to gather data may yield carefully analyzed results—and yet the narrow focus of the experiment and the lack of training of the researchers in computational approaches to neuroscience may flaw their ideas on the general implications of the studies.

2. Even more important "images" will be provided by prior models, but these prior models may address different subproblems of the overall problem—for example, an analysis of visual mechanisms for color perception and another for form perception may lack

key mechanisms to explain how the two are integrated—and even those that suggest ideas for the same subproblem may agree in some ways, but not others, and may address related phenomena and data sets, but not necessarily those most relevant to the problem at hand (Arbib, Plangprasopchok, Bonaiuto, & Schuler, 2014).

A major distinction between the architect and the brain modeler is that the *modeling–experiment cycle* is central to cognitive neuroscience, whereas the *design–experiment cycle* remains highly limited in architecture. Evidence-based design and post-occupancy evaluation can in part address the latter deficit. However, the challenge remains to focus on a small number of key variables relevant to many different architectural situations, and then design an experiment (to be conducted by architects working with cognitive scientists or, probably less often, neuroscientists) to test predictions and gather data about their relationship. In any particular design problem, the architect and consultants might then be able to sample the accumulated body of data (recall John Eberhard's vision in *Brain Landscape*). Most of the focused studies will reveal relations between only a few variables, and the data may in fact be valid only for a limited architectural context. The challenge will then be to assess which of these focused data sets can indeed offer ideas that can be marshalled—whether or not with the help of computers—to address the challenges of a current design project.

REFERENCES

Arbib, M. A. (1981). Perceptual structures and distributed motor control. In V. B. Brooks (Ed.), *Handbook of physiology: The nervous system II. Motor control* (pp. 1449–1480). Bethesda, MD: American Physiological Society.

Arbib, M. A. (1997). Modeling visuomotor transformations. In M. Jeannerod (Ed.), *Handbook of neuropsychology, Vol. 11, Sect. 16: Action and cognition* (pp. 65–90). Amsterdam: Elsevier.

Arbib, M. A. (2012). *How the brain got language: The mirror system hypothesis.* New York & Oxford: Oxford University Press.

Arbib, M. A. (2016). From neuron to cognition: An opening perspective. In M. A. Arbib & J. J. Bonaiuto (Eds.), *From neuron to cognition via computational neuroscience* (pp. 1–71). Cambridge, MA: MIT Press.

Arbib, M. A., & Bonaiuto, J. J. (Eds.). (2016). *From neuron to cognition via computational neuroscience*. Cambridge, MA: MIT Press.

Arbib, M. A., Bonaiuto, J., Jacobs, S., & Frey, S. H. (2009). Tool use and the distalization of the end-effector. *Psychological Research*, 73(4), 441–462. doi:10.1007/s00426-009-0242-2

Arbib, M. A., & Hesse, M. B. (1986). *The construction of reality*. Cambridge, UK: Cambridge University Press.

Arbib, M. A., Plangprasopchok, A., Bonaiuto, J. J., & Schuler, R. E. (2014). A neuroinformatics of brain modeling and its implementation in the brain operation database BODB. *Neuroinformatics*, 12(1), 5–26. doi:10.1007/s12021-013-9209-y

Bartlett, F. C. (1932). *Remembering: A study in experimental and social psychology*. Cambridge, UK: Cambridge University Press.

Berger, P. L., & Luckmann, T. (1966). *The social construction of reality*. Garden City, NY: Doubleday.

Blackmore, S. J. (1999). *The meme machine*. Oxford: Oxford University Press.

Catani, M. (2017). A little man of some importance. *Brain*, 140(11), 3055–3061. doi:10.1093/brain/awx270

Colby, C. L. (1998). Action-oriented spatial reference frames in cortex. *Neuron*, 20(1), 15–24.

Dawkins, C. R. (1976). *The selfish gene*. Oxford: Oxford University Press.

Durkheim, E. (1915). *Elementary forms of the religious life: A study in religious sociology* (J. W. Swain, Trans.). London: Macmillan. (Original work published in 1912)

Epstein, R. A., Patai, E. Z., Julian, J. B., & Spiers, H. J. (2017). The cognitive map in humans: Spatial navigation and beyond. *Nature Neuroscience*, 20(11), 1504–1513.

Fagg, A. H., & Arbib, M. A. (1998). Modeling parietal-premotor interactions in primate control of grasping. *Neural Networks*, 11(7–8), 1277–1303.

Fukson, O. I., Berkinblit, M. B., & Feldman, A. G. (1980). The spinal frog takes into account the scheme of its body during the wiping reflex. *Science*, 209(4462), 1261–1263.

Gandhoke, G. S., Belykh, E., Zhao, X., Leblanc, R., & Preul, M. C. (2019). Edwin Boldrey and Wilder Penfield's homunculus: A life given by Mrs. Cantlie (in and out of realism). *World Neurosurgery*, 132, 377–388. doi:10.1016/j.wneu.2019.08.116

Gibson, J. J. (1955). The optical expansion-pattern in aerial location. *American Journal of Psychology*, 68, 480–484.

Goffman, E. (1974). *Frame analysis*. New York: Harper and Row.

Goodale, M. A., Milner, A. D., Jakobson, L. S., & Carey, D. P. (1991). A neurological dissociation between perceiving objects and grasping them. *Nature*, 349(6305), 154–156.

Groh, J. M. (2014). *Making space: How the brain knows where things are*. Cambridge, MA: Harvard University Press.

Head, H., & Holmes, G. (1911). Sensory disturbances from cerebral lesions. *Brain*, 34, 102–254.

Hesse, M. B. (1980). *Revolutions and reconstructions in the philosophy of science.* Bloomington: Indiana University Press.

Hoff, B., & Arbib, M. A. (1993). Models of trajectory formation and temporal interaction of reach and grasp. *Journal of Motor Behavior*, 25(3), 175–192.

Jeannerod, M., Arbib, M. A., Rizzolatti, G., & Sakata, H. (1995). Grasping objects: The cortical mechanisms of visuomotor transformation. *Trends in Neuroscience*, 18(7), 314–320.

Jeannerod, M., & Biguer, B. (1982). Visuomotor mechanisms in reaching within extrapersonal space. In D. J. Ingle, R. J. W. Mansfield, & M. A. Goodale (Eds.), *Advances in the analysis of visual behavior* (pp. 387–409). Cambridge, MA: MIT Press.

Jeannerod, M., Decety, J., & Michel, F. (1994). Impairment of grasping movements following a bilateral posterior parietal lesion. *Neuropsychologia*, 32(4), 369–380.

Kant, I. (2003 [1781]). *Critique of pure reason* (J. M. Meiklejohn, Trans.). New York: Dover Publications. (Original work published in Riga in 1781)

Kohler, I. (1963). The formation and transformation of the perceptual world. *Psychological Issues*, 3(4), 165–166

Kuhn, T. S. (1962). *The structure of scientific revolutions.* Chicago: University of Chicago Press.

Lee, D. N., & Kalmus, H. (1980). The optic flow field: The foundation of vision [and discussion]. *Philosophical Transactions of the Royal Society of London. B, Biological Sciences*, 290(1038), 169–179.

Mallgrave, H. F. (2009). *The architect's brain: Neuroscience, creativity, and architecture.* Chichester, UK: Wiley-Blackwell.

Martin, T. A., Keating, J. G., Goodkin, H. P., Bastian, A. J., & Thach, W. T. (1996a). Throwing while looking through prisms. I. Focal olivocerebellar lesions impair adaptation. *Brain*, 119(4), 1183–1198.

Martin, T. A., Keating, J. G., Goodkin, H. P., Bastian, A. J., & Thach, W. T. (1996b). Throwing while looking through prisms. II. Specificity and storage of multiple gaze-throw calibrations. *Brain*, 119(4), 1199–1211.

Minsky, M. L. (1975). A framework for representing knowledge. In P. H. Winston (Ed.), *The psychology of computer vision* (pp. 211–277). New York: McGraw-Hill.

Moser, E. I., Kropff, E., & Moser, M.-B. (2008). Place cells, grid cells, and the brain's spatial representation system. *Annual Review of Neuroscience*, 31(1), 69–89. doi:10.1146/annurev.neuro.31.061307.090723

O'Keefe, J., & Dostrovsky, J. O. (1971). The hippocampus as a spatial map: Preliminary evidence from unit activity in the freely moving rat. *Brain Research*, 34, 171–175.

Pallasmaa, J. (2009). *The thinking hand: Existential and embodied wisdom in architecture.* Chichester, UK: John Wiley & Sons.

Penfield, W., & Boldrey, E. (1937). Somatic motor and sensory representation in the cerebral cortex of man as studied by electrical stimulation. *Brain*, 60(4), 389–443.

Piaget, J. (1952). *The origins of intelligence in children.* New York: Norton.

Piaget, J. (1954). *The construction of reality in the child.* New York: Norton.

Robinson, S. (2011). *Nesting: Body, dwelling, mind.* Richmond, CA: William Stout Publishers.

Robinson, S., & Pallasmaa, J. (Eds.). (2015). *Mind in architecture: Neuroscience, embodiment, and the future of design*. Cambridge, MA: MIT Press.

Schank, R., & Abelson, R. (1977). *Scripts, plans, goals, and understanding: An inquiry into human knowledge structures*. Mahwah, NJ: Lawrence Erlbaum Associates.

Witter, M. P., & Moser, E. I. (2006). Spatial representation and the architecture of the entorhinal cortex. *Trends in Neurosciences*, 29(12), 671–678. doi:10.1016/j.tins.2006.10.003

Wurtz, R. H. (1998). Optic flow: A brain region devoted to optic flow analysis? *Current Biology*, 8(16), R554–R556. doi:10.1016/S0960-9822(07)00359-4

A look at vision, and a touch more

In his essays of the 1920s, *Vers une Architecture* (1927 English translation, *Towards a New Architecture*), Le Corbusier derided much of the architecture of his time and reveled in what he considered a new engineering aesthetics offered by the way in which the function of airplanes, cruise ships, and automobiles seemed to dictate their evolving forms. Nonetheless, he used the example of the Parthenon to argue that, no matter what engineering aesthetics might offer, the architect would add emotional dimensions that the engineer could not, thus creating an architectural aesthetics. This chapter begins, then, by building on Le Corbusier's observations to discuss the challenges of balancing the practical and the aesthetic in designing and judging the performance of a building—developing a performative architecture. Here, I will use the term aesthetics in relation to judgment of the emotional impact of a building. From this perspective, beauty is just one aspect of aesthetics, one that has fostered much disagreement between architects. Nonetheless, there is a growing research area of neuroaesthetics that seeks to probe the way in which people judge the value of art and architecture.

The further aims of this chapter are threefold: to advance our understanding of vision at the neural and schema levels; to consider the implications of such studies for the aesthetic judgment of visual form; and to remind ourselves that vision is but one of the modes of perception that are important for our experience within the built environment.

Our approach to neural circuits for vision will expand the study of visual circuits that are in many ways similar to our own, specifically neural circuits in the monkey, to embrace those in the frog. The contrast between these systems will provide one demonstration of the way in which the A↔N conversation can be enriched by studies of species far removed from the human. In particular, we will see that early visual processing in the frog is directly linked to capturing prey and avoiding predators whereas, in contrast to such *action-oriented perception*, the early stages of the primate visual system are *general-purpose*, extracting features of the visual scene that can then be analyzed in diverse ways by other areas of the brain.

We then take a brief detour to look at learning and memory in a general perspective that distinguishes *working memory* (a version of short-term memory relevant to our current behavior), *episodic memory* (which provides the basis for autobiographical memory of various significant episodes of our lives and the way they fit together and whose processes can be grossly impaired by damage to the hippocampus and surrounding regions), *procedural memory* (the memory that serves the development of our various skills), and *semantic memory* (the memory of diverse facts). We exemplify some of these ideas as we turn to VISIONS, a classic computationally implemented model of the perception of visual scenes. Although it was developed as an early approach to the artificial intelligence (AI) of vision, VISIONS nonetheless exemplifies some of the principles of brain operation captured by our schema theory, especially the *competition and cooperation* of schema instances in *constructing* an interpretation of the current scene. At any time the current assemblage of schema instances provides a working memory of the emerging understanding of the scene, exploiting the perceptual schemas that are held in long-term semantic memory. Such schema instances become laden with a range of parameters that express something of the size, shape, color, and other features of the objects as seen in the parts of the image they may interpret, and do so with varied precision and accuracy. Of course, we may notice aspects of the scene that do not seem of immediate relevance, while failing to see some that are crucial—an experience we well know from searching for a lost object only to discover after long effort that was "hidden in plain sight." Nonetheless, all such experiences have a chance to affect our visual memory. Going beyond the processes explicitly modeled in VISIONS, the success and failure of our interpretation of a scene in terms of the actions that we build upon it may provide feedback that the brain can exploit not only in forming episodic memories but in modifying semantic and procedural memories as well, both extending the stock of visual schemas and refining their linkage to motor schemas.

With this, we finally come to the aesthetic judgment of visual form. Our understanding of lower level mechanisms of mammalian vision will provide one perspective on what makes a visual scene attractive to a human observer. Complementing this, an account of how the frog brain may mediate action-oriented perception of the spatial relationship between prey and barriers will give us some sense of what might be the deep evolutionary underpinnings of the aesthetic relationships guiding the placement of forms within an overall architectural display.

To close the chapter, we note how the art historian Ernst Gombrich exploited a somewhat different version of schema theory in his forays into collaborative studies with psychologists of art and illusion. We then explore how the lessons gained in this chapter about visual perception may also prove relevant to multimodal action-oriented perception in general. As a dramatic example, we explain how it is that a blind artist developed the ability to paint pictures whose spatial layout, coloring, and depiction of objects make sense to those of us who can see the result. Moreover, we extend the earlier exposition of VISIONS to sketch a conceptual outline of MULTIMODES, a cognitive model that extends the principles of schema interaction from vision to the linkage of perception and action more generally, while expanding the focus from snapshots of scenes to the perception of episodes extended in time.

3.1. ENGINEERING AND ARCHITECTURAL AESTHETICS

Each architect, and indeed each user, will have strong criteria for judging the success of a building, and, to a first approximation, we may distinguish "aesthetic" and "utilitarian" Criteria. However, the judgment of aesthetic success varies widely from architect to architect, and Yael Reisner emphasizes "a troubled relationship" between architecture and beauty (Reisner & Watson, 2010, pp. 12–13). Some of the architects she interviews see beauty as an essential part of their design practice, whereas others deny that it plays any role. This emphasizes that our understanding of the brain does not yield formulas for "how architecture must be done" but rather enriches our understanding of how experience yields the diverse tastes of architects, and of the users of their buildings. Reisner quotes Juhani Pallasmaa as saying, "the discipline of architecture is 'impure' in the sense that it fuses utility and poetics, function and image, rationality and metaphysics, technology and art, economy and symbolization." Reisner concludes that the artistic (aesthetic) facet of architecture is often undermined in favor of pragmatic (utilitarian) requirements of the discipline; others might point to cases where an overemphasis on visual impact has led to inadequate attention to a building's utility.

Although many architects would deny that "beauty" is an architectural criterion, I will nonetheless use "beauty" to describe one aspect of "meriting positive aesthetic judgment." When we use the word "beautiful," our judgment may be widely shared (the beauty of a sunset) or shared by relatively few (the beauty of a mathematical proof). These two examples makes clear that the word "beauty" places almost no restriction on the neural mechanisms required for its recognition, but in §3.5 we will examine examples of how studies of visual neurophysiology have informed the analysis of certain forms of beauty.

The claim that "beauty is in the eye of the beholder" needs two immediate qualifications. First, most of us appreciate the beauty of certain pieces of music and certain natural sounds, such as, perhaps, the sound of a babbling brook or the songs of certain birds. And, of course, blind people, too, have a strong aesthetic sense. Thus, we need not only the eye of the beholder but also the ear of the listener—and then why not invoke touch, smell, and taste as well? Second, the spirit of this book requires us to assess *the eye of the beholder* in the same way that we played variations on the notion of *the thinking hand* in Chapter 2, where we explored how the brain mediates the relation between eye and hand.

To illustrate how variously different architects may trade off utility and aesthetics in seeking to meet the constraints of a given program, consider the three top entries for design of the Sydney Opera House (Figure 3.1). The program specified the site (Bennelong Point) and called for two

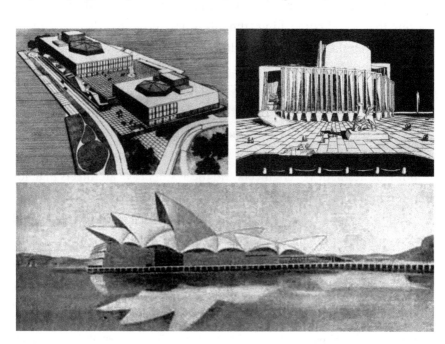

Figure 3.1 The top three entries in the competition for design of the Sydney Opera House. (*Top left*) The third-place entry. (*Top right*) The second-place entry. (*Bottom*) Utzon's winning entry (as visualized by Arthur Baldwinson). (From the *Sydney Morning Herald* of January 30, 1957; with permission.)

auditoriums. In the third-place entry, the auditoriums are in two separate buildings. The second-place design is sculpturally interesting, and has a central core housing the stage machinery for both auditoriums. However, Jørn Utzon won the competition. His winning design will be discussed at length in §9.2 to help ground steps in Chapter 10 toward an integrated cognitive neuroscience of the experience and design of architecture. Here, though, the point is that the practical demands of the program were met by such divergent designs.

In his *Ten Books on Architecture* (Rowland & Howe, 1999), Marcus Vitruvius emphasized three themes as being central to the design for a building: *firmitas* (strength), *utilitas* (functionality), and *venustas* (beauty). We are concerned here with the balance between utilitas and venustas. Vitruvius believed that a timeless notion of beauty would emerge from universal laws of proportion and symmetry, with the key example of proportional perfection offered by human proportions. This latter notion is not one that I find compelling (though it has certainly influenced many architects), but the challenge of endowing a building with a sense of what Vitruvius calls "eurythmia," a graceful and agreeable atmosphere, is an enduring one.

To address this, we turn to Le Corbusier's position as summarized in the 1927 translation of his essays *Vers une Architecture*—revealing the apparent (and enduring) inconsistencies in the way he declares his admiration for both the aesthetics of engineers and the aesthetics of architects that, for him, reaches its highest expression in the Parthenon. Le Corbusier[1] found inspiration in three types of machine—the ocean liner, the airplane, and the automobile—for a new aesthetic, the aesthetic of the engineer:

1. Here, "Le Corbusier" is shorthand for "the Le Corbusier who wrote *Vers une Architecture*," with no consideration of how the works and writings of Le Corbusier changed in later years. My remarks are based on the 1927 English translation (Le Corbusier, 1927) of *Vers une Architecture*—a collection of seven essays published (with one exception) in the magazine *L'Esprit Nouveau* beginning in 1921. Le Corbusier co-owned *L'Esprit Nouveau* with the painter Amédée Ozenfant, who claimed that the essays were based on conversations the two had had together. The 1927 translation has been criticized for its change of style and alterations to the text; a new translation (Le Corbusier, 2007) is said to be closer to Le Corbusier's intentions.

The Engineer, inspired by the law of Economy and governed by mathematical calculation, puts us in accord with universal law. He achieves harmony. . . . The tool is the direct and immediate expression of progress; it gives man essential assistance and essential freedom also. We throw the out-of-date tools on the scrap-heap . . . we must learn to see in an airplane not as a bird or a dragon-fly but *a machine for flying* [my italics]. . . . When a problem is properly stated, in our epoch, it inevitably finds its solution. To wish to fly like a bird is to state the problem badly. . . . To invent a flying machine having in mind nothing alien to pure mechanics, that is to say, to search for a means of suspension in the air and a means of propulsion, was to put the problem properly.

However, an airplane must satisfy many needs beyond "flying" alone, so this function does not determine its solution. Le Corbusier himself showed a picture of the Farman "Goliath" *bombing machine* as well as various other planes from around 1920, just as attention was turning to planes that could carry tens or hundreds of passengers. Even then, the designs were diverse, mainly biplanes but with some monoplanes and even triplanes, and land planes and sea planes with varied shapes of fuselage. The engineering aesthetic forced attention to wing lift and aerodynamic shaping, but much else seemed little constrained by "pure" engineering.

Le Corbusier used the grain elevators of the United States and Canada to support the notion that engineering was creating a new aesthetic with "the creations of modern industry yielding more and more buildings and machines, in which the proportions, the play of their masses and the materials used are of such a kind that many of them are real works of art, for they are based on 'number,' that is to say, on order."

At times, he seems to be suggesting that if only houses were built according to engineering principles—"a house is a machine for living in" (more on this in §7.1)—they would satisfy our aesthetic needs. But is the engineering "aesthetic" simply the successful combination of firmitas (strength) and utilitas (functionality)? At times, Le Corbusier seems to suggest that this in itself creates venustas (beauty). At other times, he seems to see beauty as the province of the architect alone.

> The Architect, by his arrangement of forms, realizes an order which is a pure creation of his spirit; by forms and shapes he affects our senses to an acute degree and provokes plastic emotions; by the relationships which he creates he wakes profound echoes in us, he gives us the measure of an order which we feel to be in accordance with that of our world, he determines the various movements of our heart and of our understanding; it is then that we experience the sense of beauty.
>
> Architecture is the masterly, correct and magnificent play of masses brought together in light.

The Parthenon provides Corbusier's ideal of the architectural aesthetic:

> Little by little the Greek temple was formulated, passing from construction to Architecture. One hundred years later the Parthenon marked the climax of the ascending curve. Each part is decisive and marks the highest point in precision and execution: proportion is clearly written therein. Phidias the great sculptor, made the Parthenon. There has been nothing like it anywhere or at any period. (Le Corbusier, 1927, p. 139)

Moreover, Le Corbusier seems to break away from the engineering aesthetic completely when he says of the Parthenon that

> it is no longer a question of customary use nor of tradition, nor of constructional methods, nor of adaptation to utilitarian needs. . . . No question of religious dogma enters in; no symbolical description, no naturalistic representation; there is nothing but pure forms in precise relationships. (Le Corbusier, 1927, p. 211)

Here Corbusier casts aside any notion of "a temple is a machine for worshipping in" (or some such) and celebrates the Parthenon purely for its form. Continuing, I find Corbusier's use of "mechanical" aberrant in discussing the Parthenon:

> We are in the inexorable realm of the *mechanical*. There are no symbols attached to these forms: they provoke definite sensations; there is no need of a key to understand them. Brutality, intensity, the utmost sweetness, delicacy and great strength. And who discovered the combination of these elements? An inventor of genius. These stones lay inert in the quarries of Pentelicus, unshaped. To group them thus needed not an engineer, but a great sculptor. [My italics.]
> (Le Corbusier, 1927, p. 211)

For me, despite this appeal to the *mechanical*, Corbusier's words exclude the Parthenon from the collectivity of airplanes, ocean liners, and automobiles that motivated his declaration of a new age of engineering aesthetics. Indeed, he offers a pejorative view of the "machine for X" he has lauded elsewhere:

> Clear statement, the giving of a living unity to the work, the giving it a fundamental attitude and a character: all this is a pure creation of the mind. This is everywhere allowed in the case of painting and music; but architecture is *lowered* to the level of its utilitarian purposes: boudoirs, W.C.'s, radiators, ferro-concrete, vaults or pointed arches, etc., etc. *This is construction, this is not architecture. Architecture only exists when there is a poetic emotion.* [My italics.]
> (Le Corbusier, 1927, pp. 214–215)

> It is quite true that *the architect should have construction as least as much at his fingers' ends as a thinker his grammar.* And construction being a much more difficult and complex science than grammar, an architect's efforts are concentrated on it for a large part of his career; but he should not vegetate there. The plan of the house, its cubic mass

and its surfaces have been dictated partly by the utilitarian demands of the problem, and partly by imagination, i.e., plastic creation. Here at once, in regard to the plan and consequently in regard to whatever is erected in space, the architect has worked plastically; he has *restrained* utilitarian demands in deference to the plastic aim he was pursuing; *he has made a composition.* [My italics.] (Le Corbusier, 1927, pp. 217–218)

But is "restrained" the right term? I suggest that there is no a priori form given by utilitarian demands, and architects succeed to the extent they find the right balance between "poetic emotion" in the form and success in meeting the functional (utilitarian) demands of the program. Corbusier here stresses that "a building is a machine for X" cannot yield architecture (in the positive sense) unless the architect bends the utilitarian demands of those functions X to yield a "composition"—presumably using the word as one would for a musical symphony or a great painting. We return to the lesson of Figure 3.1, and the ringing words of Sullivan's expression of the flexibility inherent in his dictum that "form ever follows function."

Nonetheless, one may see in the Villa Savoye, for example, the coming together of Le Corbusier's commitment to the age of machines as well as

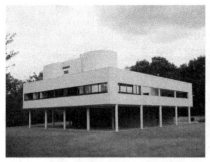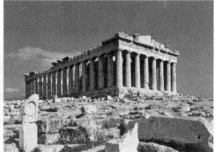

Figure 3.2 The pilotis of Le Corbusier's Villa Savoye (*left*) may be traced back to the columns of the Parthenon (*right*). However, with the introduction of the curtain wall and strip windows, they create a new aesthetic. (*Left*: en.wikipedia.org/wiki/File:VillaSavoye. jpg, Creative Commons Attribution-ShareAlike 3.0 license. *Right*: The Parthenon in Athens.jpg, photo by Steve Swayne, Creative Commons Attribution 2.0 Generic license.)

the classic ideal of the Parthenon, as the columns of the Parthenon become transformed into the pilotis that support the building (Figure 3.2). Curtis (2011) comments:

> The Villa Savoye itself is about many things—a utopian vision of modern existence, a "machine à habiter," a Purist language of form, a post-Cubist sense of space, a grammar for reinforced concrete— but it is also a distillation and abstraction of Classical Order and in some ways may be thought of as a machine-age temple. There is the ceremonial approach by car. . . .

Curtis (2011) further explores "the classical ideals of Le Corbusier." Rifkind (2011) adds that "Each new work transforms and completes its precedents through a critical process of interpretation." Here, one may recall not only Zumthor's "images come to mind . . . but all is new" but also Bartlett's linkage of the notion of schema to the way in which each retelling of a story is shaped in part not only by lapses in the memory of certain details but also by the crystallization of people's experience into different schemas and scripts that lead to a given episode (or writing or building) being read in different, possibly dramatically different, ways.

Even though Le Corbusier does not address his *apparent* inconsistency, we can happily embrace the challenge of combining the engineering aesthetic (function smoothly achieved) and the architecture aesthetic (touching the emotions). The successful architect modifies both in seeking a harmonious blend in which the form does not merely satisfy a basic functionality but also both enriches the experience of the specified functions and, perhaps, offers pathways for new experiences beyond those in the original program.

Although aesthetic judgment may invoke context and historical understanding to move beyond the immediate sensorimotor impact of a work, I do not insist that aesthetic judgment must involve explicit (e.g., verbally expressible) intellectualizing, analyzing, and theorizing. We can each look at a sunset and offer an aesthetic judgment: "That's gorgeous" or "That was disappointing." Of course, subconscious experience can encapsulate individual preoccupations, experiences, and cultural biases (although enjoying a sunset may reflect more primordial forms of appreciation), and that is why aesthetic experience is so subjective. What about judgment that something in a given genre is a "masterpiece"? Juhani Pallasmaa (personal communication) states that "[g]reat architects from Le Corbusier to Tadao Ando have internalized architecture through personal experience of historical masterpieces rather than learning the trade through theoretical and professionalist studies." Note, though, that the ability to "internalize architecture through personal experience of historical masterpieces" already depends on some guidance as to which buildings *are* historical masterpieces, and many of us will appreciate certain buildings more than others based on a more limited experience and analysis than that enjoyed by the "great architects."

Similarly, our sense of what is beautiful in paintings may develop as we view hundreds of paintings that have been selected for display in art galleries, but nonetheless our taste may vary from that of other people, agreeing with them on the merits of many works of art while disagreeing on others, even though many of us remain unable to put in words why one painting or building seems more beautiful than another. Robert Lamb Hart (personal communication), speaking for practicing architects, suggests that a client may find a building "beautiful" if it is "fit for purpose" and comes in under budget—"the beauty of the bottom line." However, repeating a design considered beautiful again and again decreases its aesthetic value—"joy incessant dulls the sense." It is no coincidence that companies spend money to have offices that express a distinctive identity. The beauty of nature rests in great part on its variety: each sunset and each glimpse of a stream running through the woods is beautiful in its own way within a general category of appreciation.

What I am struggling with as I write these lines is the distance between the basic idea of the action–perception cycle and intellectualized aesthetic judgment of an art object or a building. Our immediate situation is in general extended by episodic memory and our ability to plan far ahead— we may examine our current environment not only for how we will act now but also in terms of storing knowledge that may be of use later The aesthetic experience of a scene may be rooted in considerations such as, "The fruit on that tree is almost ripe. I must return here in two days to gather the fruit," but with cultural evolution allowing the leisured classes to abstract away an emphasis on practical implications. Perhaps Denis Dutton's (2009) *The Art Instinct: Beauty, Pleasure, and Human Evolution* may be relevant. For him, aesthetic taste is an evolutionary trait shaped by natural selection, with the human appreciation for art innate, and with certain artistic values being universal across cultures, such as a preference for landscapes that feature water and distant trees. Where he and I differ though, is when he takes this as contradictory to "social construction" rather than seeing such construction within an EvoDevoSocio perspective that grounds *cultural* evolution in the results of biological evolution intertwined with the idiosyncrasies of each person's development.

Balancing the practical and the aesthetic in performative architecture

The great American architect Louis Kahn is often quoted as saying:

> A great building must begin with the unmeasurable, must go through measurable means when it is being designed, and in the end must be unmeasurable.

But this applies to all buildings, whether or not Kahn would describe them as "great." Even from the start, the measurable and the vague are interacting in details of the site, the number and function of rooms, and other specifics of the program whether verbal or numerical. And yet, as the architect strives to make sense of these diverse (and possibly conflicting) demands, the actual shape of the building will be at first sketchy in both sense of the term. The form will morph in the architect's (or architects') imagination. A form that hugs the site or echoes the nearby buildings may compete with a form that stands in stark contrast to them. Aesthetics may favor a brutalist approach on one day and a curvaceous form the next; and perhaps the play of color may at times dominate the vaguely imagined geometry of the building. So, yes, at these early stages, the unmeasurable dominates, but the measurable still enters into the evaluation of the alternatives.

It is in the middle, as the design coalesces to the stage where construction drawings are to be produced, that measurements hold sway. The measurable comes to dominate as imaginative alternatives begin to yield to practicalities about the choice of materials, the cost of construction, and more, until the imagination is frozen in the details of plans and working drawings that make possible the physical construction of the building.

The details of construction then prevail until the project is complete. When the building is complete and the architect's and builders' work is done, many of the processes of construction will no longer be visible—the flesh covers the bones. The aesthetic impact, the atmosphere, the overall feel of the building will be unmeasurable—save, perhaps, through a careful cognitive science analysis. However, for those who live or work in the building, this will be complemented by more or less measurable factors that would play into a post-occupancy evaluation (were one to be made). Is that room too large or too small for its purpose? What are the energy demands? How would temperature vary across the seasons without use of HVAC? Does that lecture room have enough seats for the normal range of audience sizes, or too many? Does that art gallery allow enough people to view popular exhibits at the same time? What are the pluses and minuses of a factory's support of workflow? If the building looks attractive to many yet fails in the intended performative measures of its use and its experiential quality, then it has failed in its overall mission.

The design of a building will involve consideration of diverse criteria, both practical and aesthetic, and the tradeoffs between them may engage a partnership between architect and engineer rather than a notion that there are two separate aesthetics. From our current vantage point, we would note that architects must partner with engineers to achieve the forms they envisage (Saint, 2007) as, notably, Louis Kahn did with August Komendant to realize his unreasonable design for the Kimbell Art Museum of a Roman vaulted ceiling that was slit down the middle to let in light, just where the keystone should be. Komendant achieved this by redesigning the roof as a self-supporting, folded-plate structure of pre-stressed concrete.[2] Whether the final aesthetic effect is measurable or not, it will not exist unless it can be constructed. Here, it was the architect's aesthetic that shaped the form of that building, but it was the engineer's brilliance that made realization of that aesthetic possible.

The rest of this section offers a view of trading off between different design criteria that is informed by concepts from AI, suggesting strategies that move some of the unmeasurable into the domain of the measurable. You may choose to skip to the section's last paragraph without damaging your understanding of what follows.

Elsewhere (Arbib, 2019), I have linked the tradeoff between aesthetics and utility to the notion of *performative architecture* and the impact of computers on design. The concluding chapters of *Performative Architecture: Beyond Instrumentality* (Kolarevic & Malkawi, 2005) argue:

- Powerful computers and software can now be used to optimize structures with respect to numerically defined performance criteria.
- Performance criteria should be extended to include criteria like beauty that are not numerically definable.
- Performative architecture will engage a team of different talents.
- Architects will contribute a predominantly non-numerical feeling to design, seeking to describe spaces that inspire a range of human activities, assessing the impact of mood and feeling. They may seek to adapt the client's program to assess how people will respond to the completed building. Given an overall outline of a structural configuration, engineers will seek to realize it through computations that address factors like overall cost, thermal fluctuation, energy consumption, and more.

---

2. My thanks to Bob Condia for drawing my attention to the relation between Kahn and Komendant.

In pondering these claims, we realize that the building itself and the team of diverse talents that brings the design from the initial program to completion each form a *system of systems*. We will get another example of this perspective in §7.5 when we consider how a residential/medical/commercial complex in Singapore, Kampung Admiralty, integrates in diverse ways with its urban environment.

Rather than seeing beauty and utility as irreconcilable, I want to understand how tradeoffs are made between aesthetics and utility. Rationality alone cannot decide matters, and this will feed into the discussion (§4.2) of the relationship between emotion and cognition in human behavior. Indeed, the underlying issue is the selection of the criteria against which optimization or, perhaps better, *satisficing*, is to be assessed. In his book, *The Sciences of the Artificial* (Simon, 1969), Herbert Simon—an AI pioneer who received the Nobel Prize in Economics for his work on human organizations—noted that in most human decision-making, we do not do what is best (optimal) but what is good enough (satisfactory), perhaps because we lack the time or knowledge to determine what is best before we have to act. Thus, if we cannot make a building that is the most beautiful and the most useful (according to the criteria for these established by client or architect), we can at least seek to balance beauty and utility so that each is satisfactory, or even more so.

How are we to balance out the approach of diverse specialists working with the audience on diverse subsystems? In addressing this, an early concept from AI comes into play: that of *contracts* between subsystems of a system (Carl Hewitt, 1977). In a complex system, a particular subsystem will send requests or data to other subsystems, changing its behavior as it receives messages from them. The key point of a "contract" is that each system must be able to rely on the others' message without having to repeat their internal computations. In the same way, work on one part of a building will rely on certain specifications of another part of the building but not all the details; team members from different specializations must develop a shared understanding without mastering all the details of the other's expertise.

Even at the numerical level, there are major challenges here. There will rarely be a single value to optimize—for example, for HVAC, better insulation costs more, so one must trade off minimal cost for materials, M, and minimal projected energy costs, E. The AI technique of *constraint satisfaction* offers ways to balance out a variety of demands, where each desirable factor constrains the others. This is related to the method of competition and cooperation between schema instances in the system of visual scene understanding to be introduced in §3.4, but here the issue is to trade off between M and E. A parameter λ is needed to provide a measure of this tradeoff, and then seek to minimize $M + \lambda E$. For example, if λ is less than 1, this captures the notion that upfront materials costs are more important than long-term energy costs. The catch, of course, is that choosing λ is outside the remit of the computer or the engineer, and only communication with architect and client can determine this—but perhaps only after multiple simulations have charted the impact of different choices of λ.

But what about including "criteria like beauty that are not numerically definable"? One might have software that could design a surface to optimize some combination, C, of numerically well-specified design parameters—but there is no guarantee that the optimal form would be aesthetically pleasing. Well, what about defining a measure B of beauty for these surfaces, and then finding a tradeoff factor μ and then optimizing $C + \mu B$? The catch remains that B is non-numerical. One solution (no μ, no numerical B) would be to exhibit a range of examples with near-optimal values just of C, and have the architect rate them aesthetically, then use this to guide the final choice.

An alternative would be to train an artificial neural network to simulate the architect's rating of a set of forms as a basis for automating the evaluation of other forms, creating a computer means for supplying numerical B values. As an example of this, Li, Zhu, Zhao, Ding, and Lin (2020) applied deep learning to model aesthetic assessment, B, for a particular class of images, noting that people with different personalities will have different preferences. (The architect might ask: 2Bs or not 2Bs, that is the question.) In one study, a multitask learning network with shared weights was used to predict the aesthetics distribution of an image and five personality traits of people who like the image. In a second stage, based on the predicted personality traits and generic aesthetics of an image, an intertask fusion was performed to support prediction of an individual's personalized aesthetic scores on the image. While this study was unrelated to architecture, it offers a methodology that could be used to quantify how aesthetic values vary with design parameters for users with various personality profiles.

An intriguing question for our construction-based view of design is to assess the aesthetic impact when different structures are combined. Wang and Quan (2019) offer a provocative example in a very different endeavor, that of fashion: "A proper outfit should consist of different categories of items that are visually compatible and share a similar style," while taking personal aesthetic preference into account. They exploit both sequential learning and a deep aesthetic network to train an end-to-end model for composing aesthetic outfits automatically.

Having said this, let's note that such methods only make sense when an overall framework for a project has been worked out within which there is a (possibly large) range of parameters—some yes/no, others numerical—to be brought into some sort of balance. It seems highly improbable that a single parametric space could ever be defined in which the top three entries in the competition for design of the Sydney Opera House (Figure 3.1) could crystallize out as local optima!

All this, of course, raises further challenges. What of the client's tastes? What of the judgment of the typical user? And when it comes to aesthetics, how meaningful will the idea of "typical" be? Going even further, contrast designing for current tastes versus making a bold imaginative leap to something that may initially elicit negative reviews and yet will in time become widely admired. For example, when the Eiffel Tower opened to the public on March 31, 1889, many deemed it a disaster, a World's Fair gimmick that would, hopefully, be demolished after the Fair. Yet it persists today as a Paris icon.[3] Here, it would seem, there is no doubt that we pass from the measurable to the unmeasurable.

3. https://www.vox.com/2015/3/31/8314115/when-the-eiffel-tower-opened-to-the-public

Neuroaesthetics

There is now a burgeoning field of research on *neuroaesthetics*, exploring the connections between aesthetics (and especially the visual neuroaesthetics of artworks) and the human brain. I thus devote this section to two aims: (i) To offer pointers to some key books on neuroaesthetics literature, and (ii) to indicate the different path to neuroaesthetics that I develop in this volume. At the end of Chapter 5, I will review a number of papers from the neuroaesthetics literature to assess how they complement my approach to the A↔N conversation.

The Aesthetic Brain: How We Evolved to Desire Beauty and Enjoy Art (Chatterjee, 2014) offers a highly accessible, popular introduction to beauty and pleasure in their relation to the brain, but refers only once to architecture, describing a study (Kirk, Skov, Christensen, & Nygaard, 2009) whose analysis I will defer to Chapter 5. Kirk's study also appears to be the only architecture-related study in the edited collection *Aesthetic Science: Connecting Minds, Brains, and Experience* (Shimamura & Palmer, 2012), where it appears in a chapter by Ulrich Kirk himself on "The Modularity of Aesthetic Processing and Perception in the Human Brain." The collection *Art, Aesthetics, and the Brain* (Huston, Nadal, Mora, Agnati, & Conde, 2015) offers more rewards for the architect, containing five chapters that pay some attention to architecture, namely those on "Aesthetic Appreciation: Convergence From Experimental Aesthetics and Physiology," "Aesthetic Evaluation of Art: A Formal Approach," "Tension–Resolution Patterns as a Key Element of Aesthetic Experience: Psychological Principles and Underlying Brain Mechanisms," "Neurobiological Foundations of Art and Aesthetics," and "States, People, and Contexts: Three Psychological Challenges for the Neuroscience of Aesthetics." Since 2015, there have been further related books, including *Neuroaesthetics* (Skov, Vartanian, Martindale, & Berleant, 2018) and *The Arts and The Brain: Psychology and Physiology Beyond Pleasure* (Christensen & Gomila, 2018), but here I want to single out two books for special mention:

Feeling Beauty: The Neuroscience of Aesthetic Experience, by G. Gabrielle Starr (2013) uses the word "architecture" again and again—but only with the adjective "cognitive" or "neural." However, Starr develops a proposal for how aesthetic experience may rely on a distributed neural architecture linking brain areas involved in emotion, perception, imagery, memory, and language. This has features that overlap those in my cog/neuroscience approach to the experience and design of architecture. The integration of our two approaches poses one of the many challenges for future A↔N conversations. Further, Starr offers a humanist's assessment of how experience can reshape our conceptions of aesthetics and the arts and how individual differences in aesthetic judgment shape the varieties of aesthetic experience.

I close this book tour by returning to Yael Reisner, whose *Architecture and Beauty: Conversations With Architects About a Troubled Relationship* (Reisner & Watson, 2010) introduced this section. Her new collection, *Beauty Matters: Human Judgement and the Pursuit of New Beauties in Post-Digital Architecture* (Reisner, 2019), argues that interest in beauty is re-emerging in architecture. Her collection offers an interdisciplinary approach to this re-emergence, and combines discussions of aesthetics grounded in neuroscience, neuroaesthetics, mathematics, philosophy, and architecture with the analysis of the work of those international architects who are generating new aesthetics. Reisner notes that the term "post-digital" was introduced by computational designers and artists who accept that digital gains in architectural design are augmented by human judgment and cognitive intuition, a notion that accords well with our overall aim to balance beauty and utility, and the nod in the previous subsection to the integration of digital tools into performative architecture.

In §3.1 we established the challenge of developing an aesthetics that seeks to balance the demands of beauty and utility in architecture, all in the face of the notion that the evaluations will in general be subjective, challenging us both to understand that subjectivity and to seek shared underpinnings in the nature of human brains and bodies, each developed within and affected by varied social milieux. While much of the neuroaesthetics literature conducts studies at a cognitive level, in some cases complemented by functional magnetic resonance imaging (fMRI) studies, our quest is also to seek insight into the underpinnings at the level of the brain's neural networks.

In that spirit, §3.5 offers two examples at the neuro level: It first presents and assesses suggestions as to how the appreciation of beauty might be influenced by the early stages of visual processing in human cerebral cortex. It then jumps to the midbrain mechanisms of the frog visuomotor system to suggest how our appreciation of the proportions of architectural forms might be related to immensely ancient mechanisms linking vision to action. The sense here is that "good to go" as a judgment for successful action might underlie "good to go" as a judgment of aesthetic performance.

Chapter 4 will turn to the study of "atmosphere," the way in which buildings can exert an emotional influence over, or set the mood of, their users. Here, we bring into play the cog/neuroscience of the emotions, but with particular emphasis upon the transition from basic drives all the way to uniquely human emotions, including aesthetic emotions, that are intimately intertwined with human cognition. Another feature of the approach is to emphasize the transition from motion to e-motion by relating the affordances for action we have considered so far to the consideration of atmosphere as a "non-Gibsonian" affordance. I will also examine paintings by Turner and Constable whose analysis enriches our understanding of atmosphere, and I consider "inverting vision" as one component of the exercise of the imagination. Chapter 4 culminates with a critique of an exploratory fMRI study of "contemplative" spaces, pointing the way to future experiments.

Chapter 5 then brings us back to our concern with sensorimotor integration, but this time looking at how the neurons engaged in visual control of hand movements include *mirror neurons* that are engaged when the monkey executes a specific kind of manual action but also when the monkey observes an other executing similar actions. This leads into an assessment of to what extent such neurons in humans underwrite the capacity for empathy, and the extent to which empathy is related to the 19th-century German concept of *Einfühlung* as the active process by which we "feel ourselves into" objects of artistic contemplation. The chapter culminates with an exploration of the role of the motor system in the aesthetic appreciation of even a static work of art, as we envisage the actions of the artist in creating the work or the actions of the protagonists as seen in the work.

As throughout the book, the aim in offering these items to the A↔N conversation is to encourage other contributions, not to pre-empt them. They need to be fleshed out by architects and cog/neuroscientists who can link them to other developments in neuroaesthetics, especially those that take the interaction between aesthetics, utility, and the action–perception cycle seriously, and develop new experiments as well as case studies of diverse buildings.

But now we must learn more about vision.

3.2. NEURAL CIRCUITS FOR VISION

Where Le Corbusier links architectural aesthetics to the "play of masses brought together in light," emphasizing vision, we insist that architectural aesthetics must go far beyond the contemplation of visual form, emphasizing the multisensory experience of users moving through and around the building, acting and interacting as they do so. Nonetheless, it is to vision that we now turn, exploring both its neural underpinnings and its aesthetic potential. For our conversation to flourish, the reader needs to master some key findings about brain mechanisms that serve vision, at the levels both of neural activity in animal brains (this section) and of schemas (§3.4). The payoff will come with our foray in §3.5 into ideas on how beauty in art and architecture may be rooted in basic visual mechanisms.

In the earliest stages of visual processing, in the retina, receptors extract local information about the light reflected from surfaces in the world. But even within the retina, the signals from the receptors are transformed by several layers of neurons before reaching the ganglion cells, the output cells of the retina that send signals back to the brain. These and subsequent processes collate information from some neighborhood to come up with useful image descriptors.

Early in the process, we speak of "low-level vision," processing patterns of light covering small neighborhoods about a point. Eventually, "high-level vision" is to yield an overall action-oriented interpretation of the scene. For mammals, including humans, low-level vision provides an *intermediate representation* rich in explicit descriptors of edges and regions in the image. It is crucial to understand that these low-level "descriptors" are not available to our conscious perception; rather, they are patterns of neural activity that extract from sensory data various features that can be used to activate schema instances (as desctibed below), some of which will survive competition and cooperation to enter into our conscious perception. In an informal test to demonstrate this, I would ask my students to remember a list of words, but after a delay I would ask them which words were presented in cursive and which not. Perhaps 1 in 10 had noticed the difference (that is, activated a schema for recognizing whether a word was in cursive), yet all must have employed different low-level procressing to extract the letters and recognize the words. The intermediate representation encapsulates aspects of the visual array well-suited for interpretation of the image by processes whereby high-level vision can exploit the brain's (often implicit) knowledge of objects and the tasks to which they are to be put.

But visual processes differ across species in meaningful ways. To understand our own brains, it often helps to have a comparative analysis that shows in what ways our brains are similar to those of our evolutionary cousins—and to learn perhaps even more when we discover major differences. When I was an undergraduate at Sydney University, my primary passion was pure mathematics, but a reading of Norbert Wiener's classic book *Cybernetics: or Control and Communication in the Animal and the Machine* (Wiener, 1948), as well as studying the mathematics of computation, led me to a fascination with a new form of applied mathematics with strong links to biology and the brain. As part of this, I became friends with Bill Levick, then a Lecturer working on the neurophysiology of the cat visual brain. He introduced me to two classic papers on the neurophysiology of vision—one by a group at Harvard Medical School studying the monkey brain and the other by a group at MIT studying the frog brain (the basic anatomies are contrasted in Figure 3.3). I got to know researchers

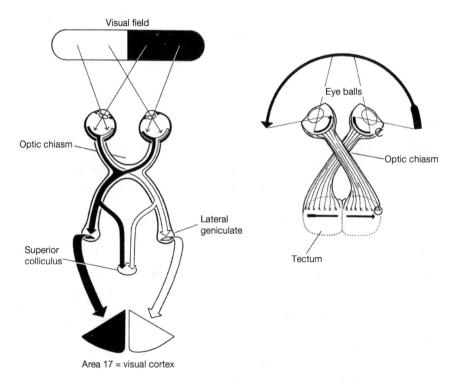

Figure 3.3 A comparison of the visual systems of mammals (e.g., monkey, or human) and frogs, clearly not to scale. The superior colliculus is the mammalian homologue of the frog's tectum, located in the mammal's midbrain, so we get here a glimpse of how greatly the evolution of neocortex has transformed the mammalian brain, demoting tectum from a primary role in frogs to a secondary role particularly associated with eye movements in humans. (*Right*) A drawing by Ramón y Cajal showing how each half of the visual field projects to the opposite (contralateral) side of tectum in the frog. (*Left*) Unlike the frog, mammals have forward-facing eyes, so that most of the visual field is seen through both eyes. The right half of the visual field projects to the left half of each retina, and the corresponding axons are sent to the left lateral geniculate (the visual area of the thalamus) and also to the left superior colliculus. Each half of the lateral geniculate projects to primary visual cortex on the same side (an ipsilateral projection). We speak of the collicular pathway to the midbrain and the thalamocortical pathway to visual cortex. (Adapted from Arbib, M. A. [1972]. *The metaphorical brain: An introduction to cybernetics as artificial intelligence and brain theory.* New York: Wiley-Interscience.)

from both groups while I was a graduate student at MIT, but the crucial point here is that these papers offered very different ways to think about the visual brain. This section will show how the two perspectives can be reconciled and (together with §3.4) will help deepen our appreciation of the relevance of neuroscience to architecture.

Feature detectors and information coding

An early success in the theory of low-level vision is provided by *lateral inhibition*, the structuring of a network so that neurons inhibit all but their closest neighbors. Such connections play a vital role in many different circuits, such as contrast enhancement. The grounds for understanding this phenomenon were laid by the physicist Ernst Mach in 1865 (see Ratliff, 1965, for an exposition, and much more on a subsequent century of research on lateral inhibition) and has been studied in touch as well (von Békésy, 1967).

Kuffler (1953) found ganglion cells (retinal output cells) in the cat retina that perform lateral inhibition. They have receptive fields, which to a first approximation are circular, with two regions. The rods and cones that influence the central region via interneurons have an excitatory effect (i.e., increasing the intensity of light falling on rods and cones connected to this central region increases the firing rate of the cell); while the surrounding annulus is inhibitory, so that if we turn up the intensity of light on the receptors there, we turn down the activity of the cell. This can act to enhance contrast. If the receptive field is near a boundary between light and dark regions, it will fire less than its neighbors on the dark side if the center of its receptive field is there, and more than its neighbors on the light side if the center of its receptive field is there. Figure 3.4 suggests how this works.

Lateral inhibition is just one of the low-level processes we may identify in animal visual systems. We will shortly document a number of others, but first we offer a more general perspective.

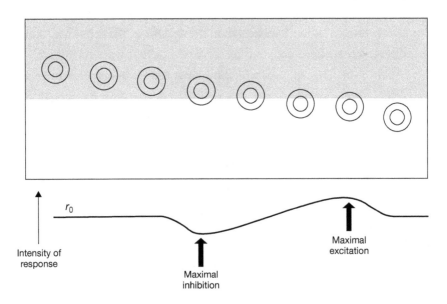

Figure 3.4 Mach bands explained. Each cell here has an on-center (stimulation there excites it) and an off-surround (stimulation there inhibits it). The intensity of response of these cells shows why there is a darker than dark band on one side of the border, and a lighter than light band on the other. (From Arbib, M. A. [1972]. *The metaphorical brain: An introduction to cybernetics as artificial intelligence and brain theory.* New York: Wiley-Interscience.)

Attneave (1954) was one of the first to bring Claude Shannon's breakthrough ideas on communication in the presence of noise (Shannon, 1948; Shannon & Weaver, 1949)—how to code messages before sending them, and decode them when they are received, to reduce the impact of noise in the intervening "channel"—into the study of vision. Shannon noted that whenever we have a priori information about an ensemble of "messages," we can use this to achieve an economy of description that would otherwise be unobtainable. For example, if arbitrarily complicated patterns of black and white dots were equally meaningful patterns of visual stimulation in our everyday lives, there would be no way of representing a visual scene more economically than by giving the light intensity at every point of the scene—a dot here, a white space there—rather than being able to focus on key curves or recognizable objects. However, as the success of caricatures of political figures attests, much of the information about a visual scene can be given by a few contours. Further, these contours are usually made up of relatively few segments—the intricate wiggles due to the presence of fur which perturb the curve of a cat's back are irrelevant to our recognition of the outline as being that of a cat, although our recognition of the texture of fur may add to our perception (see the comments on Barlow later).

Attneave constructed Figure 3.5 by finding the 38 points of maximum curvature from the contours of a picture of a sleeping cat and connecting appropriate points by straight lines. He thus forwarded the claim that the points of most importance in our recognition of form are those where a contour changes or comes to an end. Similarly, the architect in designing a skyscraper must assess whether the immense façade is (i) to be left as a uniform pattern of features with only the outline of the building offering a contrast; or (ii) whether to give form to the building by dividing that surface by distinctive forms or patterns of decoration, where the attention of the viewer can be drawn to patterns at different scales, as in the Chicago Athletic Club (recall Sullivan's tripartite division of tall buildings); or (iii)

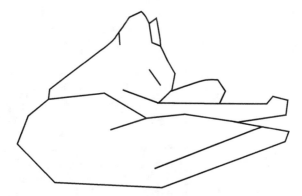

Figure 3.5 Attneave's sleeping cat. The drawing was made from a curvilinear drawing of a cat by connecting 38 points of maximum curvature by *appropriate* straight lines. Despite this drastic simplification, the resulting spatial arrangement of features remains recognizable as a sleeping cat. (From Attneave, F. [1954]. Informational aspects of visual perception. *Psychological Review*, 61, 183–193.)

one highly contrasting feature can (to the applause of some and the disdain of others) distract attention from other elements, as in the AT&T building of Philip Johnson and John Burgee.

These two examples (Figure 3.6) point us to the important notion of *segmentation*, of dividing a complex image into parts that may correspond to distinct objects or distinct patterns that may then be assembled to provide a more interpretable ensemble. The segmentation may be marked by explicit visual features or, as the "Chippendale top" of the AT&T building shows, may be imposed by the observer in an attempt to isolate meaningful, though not clearly demarcated, parts of the building or visual scene more generally.

The English neurophysiologist Horace Barlow (1959) approached the problem of visual preprocessing in a spirit akin to Attneave's, but in terms

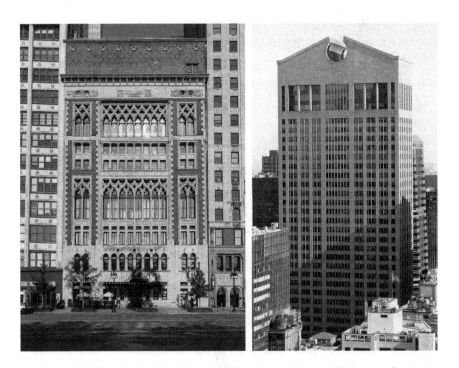

Figure 3.6 (*Left*) Chicago Athletic Association (now the Chicago Athletic Hotel). (*Right*) AT&T Building (now the Sony Building). (*Left*: © Alan Shortall, with permission. *Right*: Photo by David Shankbone, https://en.wikipedia.org/wiki/550_Madison_Avenue#/media/File:Sony_Building_by_David_Shankbone_crop.jpg, under the GNU Free Documentation license.)

of more strictly neural considerations.[4] Receptors transduce level of environmental energy into, say, frequency of axonal firing. Barlow asked how further layers of preprocessors might recode the input, making use of regularities in the normal environment, to "minimize the neural traffic." He hypothesized that the nervous system had evolved to ensure that a neuron's activity would only depart from its resting level if, in doing so, it would signal some property of the environment of potential importance to the animal. Rather than simply reducing information, the goal of preprocessing is to make *explicit* the information that the organism/robot needs for its action-oriented perception. As Attneave shows, preprocessing does not throw away the contour but rather recodes it in a form that is more compact and highlights data that may be useful in further interpretation.

Action-oriented visual preprocessing in frog

My own concern with neural studies of the linkage between action and perception goes back to the 1959 study of "What the Frog's Eye Tells the Frog's Brain" (Lettvin, Maturana, McCulloch, & Pitts, 1959), one of the papers that Bill Levick introduced me to. Surprisingly, we shall see (§3.5) that, in some ways, the frog's brain offers lessons for the architect that are missing in studies of the primary visual cortex of mammals, including monkeys and humans. This will thus offer another example of the paradox that the study of nonhuman brains is a requisite for fully understanding human brains.

A frog does not normally move its eyes save to compensate for head or body movements to maintain a stabilized image on its retina—as when on a rocking lily pad. Although frogs detect their prey solely by vision, they do not track their prey (though toads do) or search the visual field

---

4. It is worth a moment's reflection on where Barlow's 1959 article appeared—it was presented at a Symposium on Mechanization of Thought Processes. This is evidence of the early interaction between visual neurophysiologists and those who laid the foundations of AI that followed on the publication of Wiener's *Cybernetics* in 1948, which in turn built on developments in the 1930s and earlier 1940s.

for items of interest. They prey only on moving worms or insects, and their attention is never attracted by stationary objects. A large moving object provokes an escape reaction toward whatever region is darkest—but a form deprived of movement cannot be recognized as predator or prey. They seem to recognize their prey and select it for attack from among all other environmental objects because it exhibits a number of features such as movement, a certain size, some contrast, and perhaps also a certain color. They will not snap at a dead fly even when they are starving.

Lettvin et al. (1959) studied the common American frog, *Rana pipiens*. Jerry Lettvin, the neurophysiologist on the team, placed microelectrodes to record the reactions of different neurons, Humberto Maturana provided the neuroanatomy, while a neural network model (by Pitts & McCulloch, 1947) provided the conceptual framework for the study. Working at a time when computer graphics were not available for display of visual stimuli, Lettvin placed the frog so that one eye was in the center of a hemisphere (Figure 3.7) whose interior formed the experimental visual field. An electrode was so inserted into the frog that it could respond either to the activity of a single output cell, a ganglion cell, of the retina (by placing the tip of the electrode on the axon of that cell in the optic nerve) or to that of a cell in the tectum. By proper orientation of the animal, they could cover any desired part of the visual field and entirely control the input to the cells under study. The *receptive field* of each cell is the portion of the visual field in which stimuli could change the neuron's firing. Stimulating objects of various shapes and sizes were moved on the inner surface by means of a magnet moved on the external surface.

They discovered four different types of response in the retinal output cells, and these sent their axons to four different layers of synapses in the tectum, with the coding in the layers of the tectum being retinotopic, reflecting the spatial layout of the retina. One group of cells responded best to large objects moving in their receptive field, as if detecting a *predator* flying overhead. Another group (the so-called

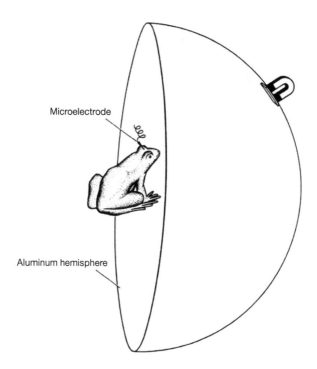

Figure 3.7 A magnet outside an aluminum hemisphere was used by Lettvin et al. to move visual stimuli inside the hemisphere. The frog's visual responses to the stimuli were then monitored by microelectrodes inserted into its optic tract or tectum. (From Arbib, M. A. [1972]. *The metaphorical brain: An introduction to cybernetics as artificial intelligence and brain theory*. New York: Wiley-Interscience.)

convexity detectors) responded best to small moving objects, as if detecting *prey*. As Lettvin et al. (1959, p. 1950) note, they discovered that:

> the [frog] eye speaks to the brain in a language already highly organized and interpreted, instead of transmitting some more or less accurate copy of the distribution of light on the receptors.

In other words, the eye is not a camera—it is already processing the image that it sends up the optic nerve, as suggested in their closing paragraph (p. 1951):

[T]he language in which they are best described is the language of complex abstractions from the visual image. We have been tempted, for example, to call the convexity detectors "bug perceivers." Such a fiber . . . responds best when a dark object, smaller than a receptive field, enters that field, stops, and moves about intermittently thereafter. The response is not affected if the lighting changes or if the background (say a picture of grass and flowers) is moving, and is not there if only the background, moving or still, is in the field. Could one better describe a system for detecting an accessible bug?

The crucial point: The encoding *in the frog retina* (but, we shall see, not in the monkey or human's) is such as to aid the animal in finding food and evading predators—frog vision is *action-oriented*.

There is to this day a tension between what can be attributed to single cells and what functions must be delegated to networks. Then as now, researchers who emphasize the accomplishments of single cells seek to isolate their "essential characteristics" (e.g., as bug detectors), while network theorists are happier to note the multidimensionality of cells, whose output varies to encode changes in contrast, depth, orientation, and so forth, all at the same time. My own group devoted much effort (Arbib, 1987; Cobas & Arbib, 1992; Didday, 1976, among many others) to developing an integrated model of diverse circuitry that we called *Rana computatrix* (the frog that computes) to address data on brain and behavior in frogs and toads by various researchers, including David Ingle (1968, 1983) and Peter Ewert (1987). Specifically, we showed how circuits in the tectum and other brain regions could convert visual recognition of a bug into the behavior of turning toward the bug, jumping toward it, and when close enough, snapping the bug up with its tongue and eating it. Conversely, recognition of a predator would yield escape behavior, turning and jumping in a direction that would take the frog away from the predator's trajectory. We even showed how the frog might detour to get to its prey if it had recognized both the prey and a barrier that obstructed its direct approach. We shall see that this may give us insight into visual neuroaesthetics.

General-purpose visual preprocessing in monkey

Let us now contrast the frog's *retinal* preprocessors with those in the *primary visual cortex* of cat and monkey, as discovered by David Hubel and Thorsten Wiesel at Harvard (Hubel & Wiesel, 1959, 1977) in work for which they later received a Nobel Prize. Building on the work of Kuffler (1953) on contrast enhancement cells in the retina, they recorded the response of single cells in primary visual cortex. They found "simple cells" responsive to edges at a specific orientation in a specific place in the visual field, and "complex cells," which respond to edges of a given orientation but in varying retinotopic locations. They also found hypercomplex cells, which respond to angles of specific size and orientation in varying locations (akin to the features posited by Attneave).

We have an interesting contrast here. The edge detectors in visual cortex found by Hubel and Wiesel serve generic feature extraction as the basis for further cortical processing (to be discussed in §3.4 in terms of schemas, rather than neurons). By contrast, Lettvin et al. (1959) found cells specialized to extract features relevant to the ongoing behavior of the frog even at the level of the retina. The latter is a clear case of action-oriented perception. However, the mammalian "edge detectors"—embedded now in a large mammalian cortex qualitatively different from anything in the frog brain—are "general-purpose." They are relevant to perception of a whole host of different scenes. Thus, many further brain regions are required to extract key data about the external world needed for the continuing action–perception cycle.

Figure 3.8 gives some sense of the complexity of the visual brain regions and their connections in the monkey brain. In forming this "spaghetti diagram," Felleman and Van Essen (1991) analyzed the monkey cortex to characterize regions of the brain whose neurons show different types of response to visual stimuli, and then traced the connections between them. They found that about 30% of the possible subregion-by-subregion connections are present. We will get into very few of the details shown here in the pages that follow. While this may come as a relief to the reader, it also gives some sense of the diverse interactions that enable mammalian

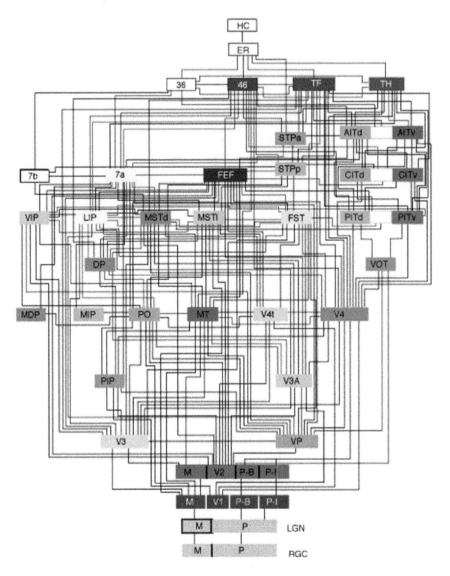

Figure 3.8 The "spaghetti diagram": a more complicated view of the visual system than we shall explore in this book, showing interconnections between brain regions associated with vision (Felleman & Van Essen, 1991). At the *bottom* of the figure, RGC = retinal ganglion cells, the output cells of the retina, and LGN = lateral geniculate nucleus, the region of the thalamus that sends signals from retina to primary visual cortex (V1 = BA 17), and vice versa. At the *top* of the figure, HC = hippocampus. All other "boxes" represent cortical regions. *Lines* show connections between regions. (From Felleman, D. J., & Van Essen, D. C. [1991]. Distributed hierarchical processing in the primate cerebral cortex. *Cerebral Cortex*, 1, 1–47, by permission of Oxford University Press.)

visual processing to serve action, cogitation, and contemplation in diverse ways—posing exciting challenges for future research on the neuroscience of vision and its entry into the A↔N conversation.

As we have just seen, Hubel and Wiesel found that neurons in V1, primary visual cortex, respond best to visual stimuli with an edge of a particular orientation. It requires competition and cooperation between these edge detectors for useful information to emerge. Neural networks can take local information about edges and integrate them to come up with good estimates for contours in the image: nearby cells that fire best for oriented edges that could join up in a continuous curve cooperate (increase each other's activity), while possibly discordant pairs of nearby cells compete (they tend to decrease each other's activity). Similarly, regions can emerge from assessment of continuity in variation of color or texture or depth or motion (features not assessed in the original Hubel-Wiesel studies, but explored in many subsequent studies)—and region growing and contour growing can compete and cooperate to yield a first-pass *segmentation of the image* into regions that are candidates for interpretation. These provide further examples of the Chapter 2 slogan: *Competition and cooperation is the style of the brain.* Unlike the style of computation desktop computers or tablets, this is a style in which many subsystems must interact repeatedly before a problem is solved. While the general mode of such computation has become increasingly well understood, an immense amount of work remains to be done—whether in teasing apart its neural mechanisms, or in finding its most efficient technological implementation to address specific tasks in AI.

Hubel and Wiesel suggested a hierarchy from retinal output via edge detectors to more complicated cells encoding shapes, and thence to encoded objects, and so on. Shortly after my arrival as a graduate student at MIT in 1961, Horace Barlow was visiting Warren McCulloch and explained the Hubel-Wiesel hierarchy to me, observing that this contour extraction enables you to recognize the face in a caricature. I then asked, "But then how do I see you are not a caricature?" This leads to a key observation. As we move up the hierarchy, our brain does not discard information from lower levels, but links parts of it to higher level representations—interpreting the former while giving meaning to the latter to yield an integrated view enriched by subtle undertones that can be brought to the fore by attention. Thus, *much about overall patterns of texture and shading and color can be preserved in the final percept even though most of the details of local features operated at a subconscious level to yield that percept.* Note that this "experiential aspect" includes the emotional shading present, whether this precedes or follows from the interpretive process. Once again, our phenomenological experience of a unitary consciousness proves to emerge from the interaction of diverse processes distributed across the brain.

Implications of studying nonhuman brains

In a classic set of four papers, Ingle, Schneider, Trevarthen, and Held (1967) showed that much insight could be gained into the mammalian brain by using the study of frogs to provide insight into key midbrain functions in mammals (e.g., by comparing frog tectum and mammalian superior colliculus)—a corrective to equating the brain with just the cerebral cortex. The ability of the frog to turn rapidly toward prey could be compared at a neural level to the ability of a mammal to make a saccade to direct the eyes to focus on a new visual target. Dean, Redgrave, and Westby (1989) would later carry this further by showing how the rat superior colliculus could also direct escape behaviors. These themes were later at the core of a book by Schneider (2014) on *Brain Structure and Its Origins in Development and in Evolution of Behavior and the Mind.* The study of the frog has also paid off in the study of mobile robots (Arkin, 1989, 1998) as part of a larger trend in neurorobotics inspired by studies of animal behavior (Prescott, Lepora, & Verschure, 2018), a theme that will recur in Chapter 7 when we consider buildings as "inside-out" robots.

Different animals live in different environments, have different behaviors (one might be a prey, another a predator), and have different capabilities for motor behavior. As a result, the information that they need about their world varies greatly. On this basis, we may hope to better understand the problem of vision if we can come to see which aspects of "visual system design" converge, and which differences are correlated with the differing behavioral needs of different species.

In the frog, we have seen that there are retinal cells well suited to provide input to a visual system that must detect small moving objects as prey, and large moving objects as predators. In the rabbit visual system, the retina contains movement-detecting cells specifically tuned for movement along the ground plane, which this lateral-eyed animal surveys in an almost 360-degree panorama. This visual streak provides the appropriate visual input for an "early warning system" for predators on the horizon. In the frontal-eyed cat, we find a retina more like that of primates, including humans, which seems to be concerned with "cleaning up the image" for contrast enhancement and motion detection.

The angle detectors "predicted" by our discussion of Attneave's sleeping cat have indeed been found in the visual cortex of cat but not in the frog's tectum. Why does this "prediction" fail for the frog? The following explanation seems plausible: The frog has a more limited visuomotor behavior than a cat or monkey, or human—the frog is irresponsive to stationary visual stimuli, but will snap at, or orient toward, an object moving in prey-like fashion, and will avoid a large moving object. *Thus, preprocessing at the ganglion cell level in the frog is already "action-oriented."* In the cat, on the other hand, even as "late" as the angle detectors of secondary visual areas, processing is "action-neutral."

Study of the frog can illuminate study of human vision by reminding us that no matter how important the emergence of cerebral cortex has been in expanding the range of human understanding, the midbrain mechanisms continue to be crucial partners in cerebral processes. It had long been believed by neurologists that a monkey (or human) without a visual cortex was blind. However, in a study evocatively called "What the Frog's Eye Tells the Monkey's Brain," Humphrey (1970) trained a monkey without visual cortex to pay attention to available visual cues, and after 2 years she was able to use these cues to grab at moving objects, and to use changes in luminance—such as an open door—for navigation. Crucially, though, delicate processes of pattern recognition were never regained.

Indeed, humans without visual cortex can also exploit visual cues in this way but, remarkably, with no awareness that they could see—this is known as *blindsight* (Weiskrantz, 1974). These basic reactive mechanisms in monkeys and humans provide a "platform" for more conscious visual perception. A human needs to combine the ability to react rapidly (jumping out of the way of an unexpected vehicle when crossing the street) with the ability to abstractly weigh alternatives (deciding on the best way to get to the next appointment). Evolution of the human brain has taken us from dedicated circuitry for every schema to the ability to acquire novel schemas distributed across *relatively* general-purpose machinery. The hedge "relatively" here is important. Advances in neuroanatomy have increasingly demonstrated that what were once thought to be large undifferentiated brain regions can in fact be discriminated into far smaller regions with distinctive patterns of input and output connections (Kaas, 2017). Presumably, each of these regions can access a distinct set of other regions (recall Figure 3.8 which only includes areas related to vision), and as these sets of subsets can be developed hierarchically, the result can be a "general-purpose" representation—but one that is distributed across more or less specialized partial representations each in a specific brain region, rather than being encoded in a single uniform computational medium.

Visual attention

As noted briefly before, the frog's tectum, mediating prey-catching and predator-avoidance, is the evolutionary homologue of the mammalian superior colliculus, which mediates the shifts of visual attention that may involve eyes alone, eyes and head, or even whole-body movements. The superior colliculus retains a frog-like ability to respond directly to external stimuli—like a glimpse of an unexpected movement—though not with zapping with the tongue. The key difference is that, in addition to reflex saccades, our saccades may be under top-down (cortical) control. Indeed, when we perceive a visual scene (as distinct, say, from orienting to a sudden noise or movement), a saccade is not an end in itself (look at this single point in the scene), but may involve integration of details from successive foveations to build up an overall (but still selective) appreciation of the scene. Such visual exploration and integration may serve immediate praxis, or current contemplation, or may serve to help accumulate details for memory and for long-term planning.

The task-dependent nature of such visual exploration was demonstrated in the laboratory by the Russian psychologist Alfred Lukyanovich Yarbus (1967), who monitored eye movements of subjects as they examined Ilya Repin's painting, "They did not expect him" (Figure 3.9).

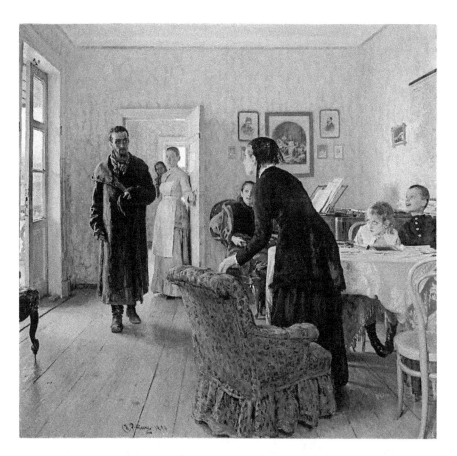

Figure 3.9 Ilya Repin's painting (1884–1888): "They did not expect him." (https://commons.wikimedia.org/wiki/File:Ilya_Repin_Unexpected_visitors.jpg. Public domain.)

Repin painted this when Russia was under the czar rather than the Communist Party, but even then, dissidents were sent to faraway prison camps. The painting shows a man who has just returned home from the camps, and his return was totally unexpected. We see him in the painting, but we also see the reaction of the family and servants to this surprising event. When Yarbus tracked subject's eye movements, he gave them instructions as to what to look for in the scene. Figure 3.10 shows the very different eye movement for three of the seven different tasks Yarbus used. For "give ages of the people," the scan locates the faces, and the bulk of the eye movements then explore them. For "remember the clothes worn by the people," the eye movements again locate the faces in the scene, but then move up and down below each face to look at the clothing, rather than maintaining focus on the faces.

The point of this study, consistent with our emphasis on action-oriented perception, is that perception normally involves a strong interaction between bottom-up cues that can draw attention to parts of the scene (as the bright

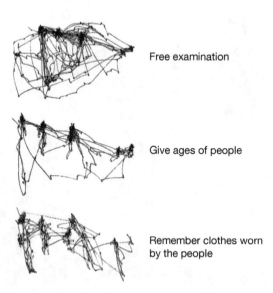

Free examination

Give ages of people

Remember clothes worn
by the people

Figure 3.10 The pattern of eye movements varies: three scans of the Repin painting under different instructions. (Adapted from Yarbus, A. L. [1967]. *Eye movements and vision*. New York: Plenum.)

yellow central region did in the view of Las Ramblas) and top-down cues based either on what one has already noticed about the scene (as in locating the faces to define where to examine the clothing) or the task one is addressing while examining the scene. In "real life," one always has certain expectations within the ongoing action–perception cycle, though one certainly has the ability for "priority interrupts" in response to unexpected events. Similarly, if you enter a room or building with a particular task in mind, you will direct your attention in terms of expectations of where you might find the affordances for completing that task. Of course, these expectations may not be met. An example: A task I gave to visitors to my office was "Find the stapler." They immediately directed their gaze to the surface of my desk, and with a "generic idea" of what staplers looked like, they rapidly found the stapler sitting there. But when I asked them to find the second stapler, most of them failed, unless I gave them the cue "look at the frogs on the bookshelves" (souvenirs given to me by visitors who recalled my long-ago interest in modeling the frog brain), and it was only by frog-by-frog analysis that they eventually found the other, unusual looking, stapler (Figure 3.11).

Let's consider the possible relevance of such studies to the architectural question of "how unexpected should a new design be?" Jerome Kagan (1970) studiedthe attention infants would pay to face-like stimuli (Figure 3.12). One-week-old infants show equivalent fixations to an achromatic representation of a human face and a meaningless achromatic design. Somewhere during the second month, the duration of attention comes under the influence of the infant's schemas. Four-month-old infants show markedly longer attention to the face than to the design, presumably because they have acquired a schema for human faces and the laboratory representation is moderately discrepant from that schema. However, if the representation of the face is too discrepant, fixation times are reduced.

All this led Kagan to formulate his discrepancy principle:

Discrepancy principle: Stimuli moderately discrepant from a schema elicit longer orientations than do either minimally discrepant (that is, familiar) events or novel events that bear no relation to the schema.

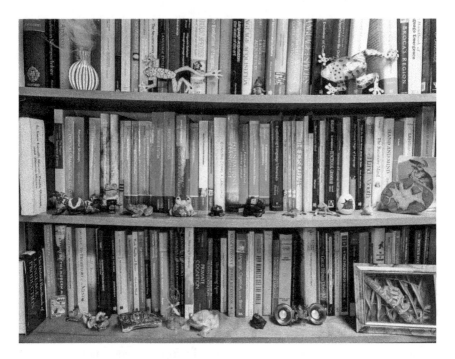

Figure 3.11 Where is the stapler? (Author's photo.)

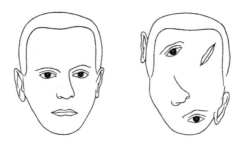

Figure 3.12 Stimuli such as those used by Kagan to assess attention and psychological change in the young child in grounding his discrepancy principle. (From Arbib, M. A. [1972]. *The metaphorical brain: An introduction to cybernetics as artificial intelligence and brain theory.* New York: Wiley-Interscience.)

The moral, one might suggest, is that if you wish to be successfully creative, your creations should be constrained by the discrepancy principle. And yet . . . the alternative is to do something so rewarding to others that they will have to follow. Here, briefly, we note the role of the critic—whether one whose influence is broadcast by the media, or a member of one's circle of friends—who may say, "This really merits your attention," or "Don't bother." And such influences may spread like a viral contagion to propel the novelty into a widely shared "vocabulary," or soon remove it from common discourse.

3.3. LEARNING AND MEMORY

What is memory for? As we develop, we master new ways to marshal various life experiences to handle new situations. The brain often acts "prospectively," using stored information to imagine, simulate, and predict possible future events and thus (consciously or subconsciously) choose a course of action that (based on our current knowledge, both explicit and tacit) seems likely to have a better outcome. However, there is no guarantee that particular memories will be either relevant or beneficial. Our biological evolution has given us learning mechanisms that "on average" may affect memories in ways that benefit us in the future, but encultur-ated humans living in a rich and complex environment will store diverse memories that may never be recalled, and others that can adversely affect our future behavior. Nonetheless, the understanding of the diverse forms of memory is crucial to both the experience and the design of architecture.

Crucially, buildings are often designed for people with very different brains from those of the architect, as we saw with Eduardo Macagno's take on "lifespan architecture." Brains mediate action, perception, cognition, and language. Learning and memory are crucial to the acquisition and deployment of the skills that employ these properties. General processes of maturation from infant to child to adolescent to adult will proceed along a genetically determined trajectory to the extent that the child develops in a "standard" environment, but our EvoDevoSocio framework reminds us that the cultural and physical milieu can ring changes, possibly drastic changes, on that trajectory. Variations from this trajectory include the traces of learning and memory based on the experience of each individual. Conversely, normal aging yields various indignities of both brain and body, including memory problems, but these are aggravated in diverse ways in neurological disorders such as Parkinson's disease and dementia. All these processes are studied in neuroscience at all levels, from genetics and molecular biology to behavior, and many of these findings have implications for the design of buildings that meet the needs of different populations.

An important distinction is that between *episodic learning*, forming traces in the brain of episodes in our lives, enabling us to recall something about them at a later date, and *procedural learning*, the acquisition of a new skill such as riding a bike. The list can be extended, such as memories for facts and faces. The cerebral cortex is implicated in all of these, but subcortical structures pay an essential role as partners in memory formation, with the hippocampus proving essential to episodic memory, while cerebellum and the basal ganglia are both crucial for procedural learning. Another form of memory is *semantic memory*: contrast the memory of picking an apple when visiting an orchard during a memorable vacation, the skill of peeling an apple with a knife, and the knowledge that ripe apples are good to eat.

The most famous data point about the *human* hippocampus comes from the sad case of H.M. [5] Many papers were written about him, but his privacy was protected during his lifetime. It was only when he died in 2008 that we were told his name was Henry Gustav Molaison. As a young man he had massive epilepsy—electrical storms would rage through his brain. His neurosurgeon went overboard. Instead of seeking a small cut in the brain that might solve the problem, in 1953 he excised a huge region that included the hippocampus and much of the surrounding temporal lobe (Scoville & Milner, 1957; Figure 3.13).

---

5. We met the involvement of place cells in the *rat* hippocampus in "From schemas in the head to neurons and synapses" in §2.5.

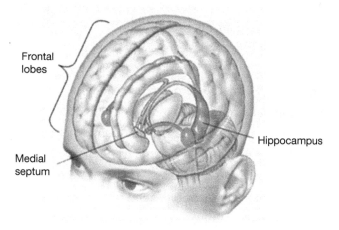

Figure 3.13 The brain region removed in surgery on H.M. (Henry Gustav Molaison) included most of the hippocampi on both sides and regions of nearby temporal lobe. It removed his ability to form new episodic memories, while preserving working memory and procedural memory. (https://pubs.niaaa.nih.gov/publications/arh27-2/IMAGES/Page191.gif. Public domain.)

While this cured the epilepsy, it had a tragic side-effect. H.M. lost the ability to form memories of new episodes. One colleague who went to do a study with him, back in the old days when people did not have mobile phones, was talking to H.M. but was called out of the room to take a phone call. When he came back, H.M. had no memory that they had met! If you were engaged in conversation with him, his *working memory* seemed to be functioning—he could keep the conversation going, or follow through on the current task. But once left alone, that working memory was no longer relevant and was discarded, leaving no trace in *episodic memory*. He could, however, recall episodes from before the operation, so that we now believe that hippocampus is necessary for the formation of episodic memories (episodic learning) but that, at least for more significant episodes, these memories can in due course be consolidated in cerebral cortex.

But there was a surprise. You could introduce H.M. to a game, and play it with him, and he would pick up something of the rules as play proceeded. However, if you came back the next day with the same game, he had no memory of playing it before. And so it would be, day after day. But over the days, even though he never remembered having played the game before, he became more and more skillful. He could not form episodic memories, but he could form new *procedural memories*.

The movie *Memento*[6] presented a fictional drama inspired by the clinical facts concerning H.M. The hero, having lost episodic memory, developed two new compensatory skills—one was to take photos of significant events, and the other was to have himself tattooed with useful aphorisms. The genius of the movie was that we, too, were placed in the position of having no memory of past episodes—the scenes were presented in the movie in reverse temporal order. In the end (when we reached the beginning!), we discovered that the external memory system he had devised was unreliable and the memories distorted. The movie is worth seeing, both in its own right, and to challenge you to think more about the human brain's orchestration of diverse processes, and what happens when they are disrupted.

Such data help us understand that the brain supports different memory systems. In this section, we have mentioned

- *working memory*, keeping track of what is currently relevant,

and three long-term memory systems:

- *procedural memory*, of how to perform diverse skills,
- *episodic memory*, of particular episodes in one's life, and
- *semantic memory*, of particular facts.

The last two types of memory are called "declarative" in that we can explicitly "declare" them, whereas procedural memory is non-declarative in that the fine tuning of neurons that let us, for example, walk swiftly on uneven ground are not open to our introspection. Figure 3.14 gives a classic and more comprehensive taxonomy of long-term memory systems together with neural correlates, but most of the details are outside our scope (see

6. https://en.wikipedia.org/wiki/Memento_(film)

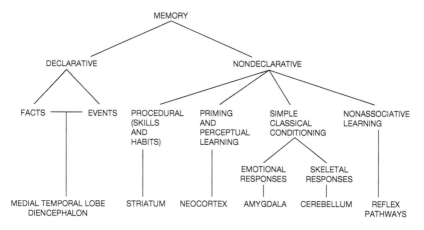

Figure 3.14 A classic taxonomy of mammalian long-term memory systems. The taxonomy offers one account of the brain structures thought to be especially important for each form of declarative and nondeclarative memory. (Reprinted from Squire, L. R. [2004]. Memory systems of the brain: A brief history and current perspective. *Neurobiology of Learning and Memory*, 82(3), 171–177, with permission from Elsevier.)

Squire & Wixted, 2011, for a more recent perspective). However, I would stress that the striatum and cerebellum work together with cerebral cortex in procedural learning, and that emotional responses are more complex than simple classical conditioning and are not restricted to the amygdala. We will return to the role of the hippocampus and the adjacent medial temporal lobe in semantic (facts) and episodic (events) memory in §10.3. One important family of neural mechanisms for memory involves changes in synaptic strengths (§5.3)—these reflect experience and change future computations of the neural networks and thus future behavior and experience.

3.4. VISIONS: SCENE PERCEPTION AS A FORM OF CONSTRUCTION

Magritte and Escher show us ways that visual perception can be fooled, but we now turn to a schema-based model of how our perception of a "normal" static visual scene may proceed. Although the VISIONS system model, created by my colleagues Ed Riseman and Al Hanson at the University of Massachusetts at Amherst (Hanson & Riseman, 1978; Riseman & Hanson, 1987), was implemented on a serial computer, I see its underlying logic of competition and cooperation as conceptually exemplifying "the style of the brain."

To understand their approach, consider a two-level analysis of a picture of a typical suburban scene near Amherst (Figure 3.15).

Segmentation/lower-level vision: As described in §3.2, competition and cooperation between local image features grows edges and regions to yield a first-pass subdivision of the image to ground semantic analysis. These processes populate the *intermediate representation* (*center*; region features not shown) as one of two *working memories* (WMs), which will change as perception proceeds.

Recognition/high-level vision: Data from the intermediate database on color, shape, location, and more for regions can initiate high-level vision, bringing perceptual schemas into play. *Schema instances* compete and cooperate in Visual WM, a second working memory, to interpret different regions to in time yield an interpretation (*right*).

But what are schema *instances*?

A *perceptual schema* for a type of object X provides processes sophisticated enough to recognize a viewed object as an X despite variations of size, location, and orientation, so long as the present X is not too atypical.

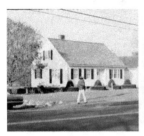 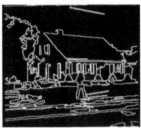 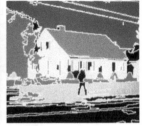

Figure 3.15 (*Left*) A suburban scene in Massachusetts. (*Center*) An initial segmentation of the scene into candidates for interpretation. (*Right*) An interpretation of parts of the scene provided by the VISIONS system. (Images courtesy of Allen Hanson.)

We postulate that each person's brain has a *long-term memory* (a *semantic memory*) that encodes a host of schemas, including how the schemas may be activated by bottom-up cues (certain cues of color and texture may increase confidence that a region is covered in grass) and top-down cues (relations between schemas that mediate competition [a cube in the middle of a fire is less likely to be ice] and cooperation [the region below a roof is likely to contain windows]).

However, if we are making sense of (a picture of) a room, there may be several chairs, and in understanding the scene one may want to keep track of the shape, style, and location of more than one of them. We use the term *schema instance* for the separate items in the working memory that keep track of the different regions that have been associated with each schema—not only the associated schemas but also their *activation levels*. These last are the confidence levels (does the schema really represent the object in that region?) that can increase through cooperation and decrease through competition. Each schema instance may also encode parameters such as shape, color, texture, depth, and more. *Visual WM* then holds the current state of interpretation of the scene as an assemblage of schema instances (Figure 3.16).

To further probe the dynamics of VISIONS, note that, in the middle panel of Figure 3.15, a crucial edge is missing at the left end of the roof, while edges due to a highlight or a shadow may fool the lower level processes. For all its imperfections, this is enough for visual schemas to start spawning instances to check whether various segments match their activation criteria. Putting this in anthropomorphic terms:

- The sky schema finds a region at the top of the image that has the right color and the right extent to create an instance with a confidence level of 0.9. This is a *bottom-up* process, driven purely by local data from the image.
- Just below the putative sky, there is a region of a similar color, fairly large, but lower in the image, and this might create an instance of the sky schema with a confidence level of 0.4.

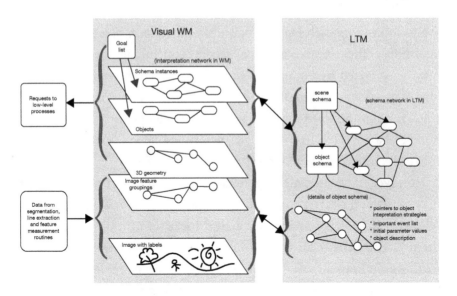

Figure 3.16 The logic of cooperative computation in VISIONS. Preprocessed visual data from the intermediate database (its input is at *lower left*) provides bottom-up cues that recruit schemas from long-term memory (LTM) to associate instances in the visual working memory (Visual WM). There, information about schema relationships in LTM can combine with top-down influence from previously active schema instances and bottom-up data from the intermediate database both to activate new schema instances and modulate the competition and cooperation of currently active instances. Instances with low activation levels may eventually cease to influence the process, but at some moment the more active instances may have their activation levels pass a critical threshold so that they and certain of their parameters may provide the perception of the scene. The *arrow* at *top left* indicates that processing may request updating of the intermediate representation. The goal list may include top-down influences based on partial interpretations seeking confirmation of hypotheses. (From Arbib, M. A. [2012]. *How the brain got language: The mirror system hypothesis*. New York and Oxford: Oxford University Press.)

The high initial confidence level for interpreting the top region as sky provides what is called an *island of reliability*. This is "part of the pattern" that will remain stable long enough for other elements to fall into place in relation to it. This may yield a larger part of the pattern that itself becomes a new island of reliability—or may be greatly modified before it can re-enter the process, if indeed it can. Even though an island may later be discarded, processing for now proceeds as if this interpretation were reliable so that context (*top-down influences*) begins to work, as schema instances have their confidence levels raised by cooperation with other schema instances, and decreased by competition.

- The roof schema can also assess the second region and find that it is not only the right shape for a roof but also in the right spatial relation with a region confidently assessed as sky, to give a roof schema instance for this region a 0.7. Note the combination of bottom-up and top-down influences (and recall that "up" and "down" refer to the processing stream, not to location in the image).

As VISIONS begins to interpret one part of a scene, this may guide attention to related parts of the scene in service of our interpretation. Then this roof schema instance will say (to continue with our anthropomorphism), "Well, if I'm a roof, then, unless this is a disaster scene, there should be a house underneath me, and so schemas should be able to detect windows or shutters in that region."

- Because wall-related cues are located, confidence in the roof hypothesis goes up and the region below it becomes linked to an instance of the wall schema.
- But that missing edge now causes problems—a large region has been confidently assessed as both wall and roof. However, this draws attention to the likely boundary, and a query to the intermediate database triggers further low-level processing of that part of the image. The boundary is indeed found, the large region is divided in two, and the top part is now unequivocally interpreted as sky and the bottom part as wall.
- And so interpretation goes to completion.

Given that the missing edge caused problems, one might ask, "Why didn't we just make it easier to find edges? Then we wouldn't have missed that edge." The answer is that this would yield so many little patches of shadow and highlight that it would have been nearly impossible to find regions that could reliably activate schemas.

In the right panel of Figure 3.15, we see the final interpretation of the image by that system of 40-plus years ago. It was able to correctly recognize foliage versus grass. It recognized the roof. It recognized the shutters and the walls fairly well, but it had not been programmed with schemas for "person" or "road" or "telephone wires," and so these could not be part of its interpretation. As humans, we are not "programmed" to recognize different objects and domains of interaction. Rather, it takes years of experience, with and without explicit education, to build up the repertoire of tens of thousands (or many more?) of perceptual schemas we each possess.

When we view VISIONS as an account of human vision, I reiterate that in many cases there will be no conscious awareness of the neural processes whereby you construct your perception of the scene. In other cases, conscious attention may be required to search out details that allow you to make sense of the overall scene, as in completing the different tasks assigned by Yarbus.

Taking stock

What is important about VISIONS for us in this book is not the neuroscience challenge of updating it in view of decades of research in visual neuroscience, but rather the fact that it provides a set of key concepts for our A↔N conversation concerning the experience and design of architecture. It thus seems valuable here to summarize those key points and give a sense of how they will be built upon later in the book.

Our understanding of a visual scene is a process of **construction**: we do not experience the "total reality" (an implausible idea in itself). Rather, current stimuli are "made sense of" on the basis of our brain's ability to construct an assemblage of instances of schemas. And these schemas encode aspects of our knowledge/long-term memory/prior experience of the world relevant to our current situation, tasks, and motivation.

Perception proceeds both *bottom-up* (extracting patterns from the sensory input) and *top-down* (with interpretation of portions of the scene conditioned by context and "islands of reliability" established by ongoing perception).

VISIONS models how visual perception can exploit *semantic memory* (the stock of interrelated perceptual schemas) to create *working memory* that is adequate to support current experience and behavior. What it does not model is (i) how salient features of an episode can be extracted from the dynamics of this working memory to support *episodic memory* (a major concern of Chapter 10), and (ii) how learning processes can exploit *working memory* patterns, coupled with ongoing feedback or reinforcement from behavior, to update *semantic memory* (some open to conscious analysis, some not) for both the specifically visual knowledge (the bottom-up cues that can evoke an instance of a schema) and the more general world knowledge (the lateral and top-down cues that can encode the knowledge that certain spatial relations between certain types of objects are more likely than others, and thus mediate the competition and cooperation of schema instances).

In Chapter 4, we will build on our understanding of VISIONS to consider the role of imagination in drawings and paintings as "inverting vision." I will argue that in imagining a scene, we may begin to mentally assemble visual schemas but with at best a vague specification of the details. Here, the visual working memory of the VISIONS model is extended to accommodate "top-down" imagination. The key carryover for design (Chapter 10) is that competition and cooperation between diverse hypotheses will give some more weight than others, until many are discarded and others remain as part of the final interpretation of a scene or design that meets varied criteria. Moreover, the design may converge on "what" to place, and *approximately* where, but may require fine-tuning to determine "how" to place the various elements to achieve a harmonious balance—transferring to the design side the perceptual capabilities of the "what" and "how" visual pathways in the guidance of hand movement.

VISIONS analyzes the perception of objects in static relationship, but in building upon it, a fuller account would have to infuse the scene with a perception of agency, actions, and emotions. In many cases, recognizing properties of an object and its present relation to us can offer affordances for our possible actions, whose parameters could be passed to the motor schemas that guide those actions, supporting ongoing processes within the action–perception cycle. These considerations certainly apply as well to multimodal perception in linkage with action, as I will spell out in §3.6 in offering a conceptual generalization I call MULTIMODES that exploits sensory cues from multiple modalities in developing a coherent understanding of dynamic episodes embedded within three-dimensional (3D) space. Here, we may interpret regions of the scene not simply in terms of "what" they are but also in terms of "how" we might interact with them, their affordances. Rather than having a single intermediate database restricted to vision, we have a separate intermediate database for each sensory modality, and these can be linked so that, for example, spatial layout cues can be coordinated between vision, audition, and touch—but they all contribute to the interpretation of the environment.

3.5. AESTHETIC JUDGMENT OF VISUAL FORM

We now turn to two proposals that link neural circuitry to aesthetic judgment of visual form, one based on the mechanisms supporting *general-purpose vision* exemplified in the study of initial stages of processing in monkey visual cortex by Hubel and Wiesel, and the other based on mechanisms for *action-oriented vision* exemplified in the study of "prey detectors" in the frog retina by Lettvin et al. Note that, of course, the general-purpose mechanisms in the human brain, akin to those of the monkey, evolved to work with diverse other brain regions to serve action and much more, including the elaboration of novel schemas as new types of environment become familiar. However, specifics of the more direct linkage of vision and action in the frog will prove relevant to thinking through one aspect of visual aesthetics.

Aesthetics and general-purpose vision

Tom Albright is among those vision neuroscientists who have combined analysis of the detailed neural circuitry of early visual cortex in the style of Hubel and Wiesel, with broad consideration of higher level vision to offer hypotheses on the neural basis of the experience of visual beauty. This section presents and assesses the approach to visual aesthetics in "Neuroscience for Architecture" (Albright, 2015b).[7] The key idea is that visual patterns can tap into intrinsic features of visual system organization to elicit "aesthetic responses." The emphasis here is on "pure vision" rather than the linkage of action and perception.

Albright's first example is based on the observation (§3.2) that the mammalian brain can take data from the Hubel-Wiesel edge detectors and use competition and cooperation to assess which of these can be aggregated to support our perception of contours. He argues that it is this brain operating principle that makes us appreciate patterns like those exhibited in Figure 3.17.

The catch is that every scene we encounter, whether beautiful or not, involves extensive contour extraction—for example, to separate figure from ground and assess the shape of a region. So, what distinguishes the three scenes in Figure 3.17 from most other scenes? If we are to seek principles of brain organization that privileges these examples, it cannot be that they contain distinctive contours. Perhaps we are "one level up," where the near parallelism of contours (whether straight or curved) offers a pleasing impression. In the Fay Jones Chapel, we might add symmetry as another higher level principle. Indeed, symmetry does seem to be a basic (but nonlocal) principle of visual organization, and the rating of symmetric human faces as being more attractive than asymmetric faces seems to be a culture-free preference (Zaidel & Hessamian, 2010; their

---

7. Background for Albright's approach comes from research on the visual system of monkey and human cerebral cortex as reviewed in his article, "On the Perception of Probable Things: Neural Substrates of Associative Memory, Imagery, and Perception" (Albright, 2012); further material on aesthetics may be gleaned from his unpublished lecture on "Contextual Influences on Visual Processing" (Albright, 2015a).

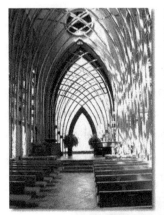
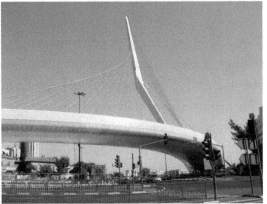
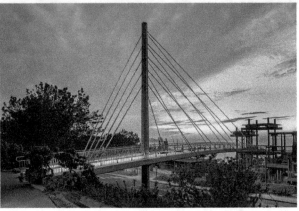

Figure 3.17 A chapel and two bridges: (*Top left*) The Mildred B. Cooper Memorial Chapel in Bella Vista, Arkansas, designed by Arkansas architect Euine Fay Jones. (*Top right*) The Jerusalem Chords Bridge. (*Bottom*) Scripps Crossing Pedestrian Bridge, La Jolla, California, by Safdie Rabines Architects (1993). (*Top left*: (http://beautifulbellavista.com/chapel.htm, Photo © Dustie Meads, reproduced with permission. *Top right*: https://upload.wikimedia.org/wikipedia/commons/e/e3/Jerusalem_Chords_Bridge_5.JPG. Public domain. *Bottom*: Photo © Pablo Mason, reproduced with permission.)

article belongs to a Special Issue on "Symmetry and Beauty"). However, neither of the bridges is symmetric—can it be that the "hint" of symmetry is more attractive to the sophisticated aesthete than symmetry itself? If so, this may be an example of the discrepancy principle of §3.2. In any case, I ask the reader: Which of the two bridges do you find more attractive? To what extent does the scene in which the bridge is embedded affect your judgment? And, since we have here a single photograph of each, would that judgment change if indeed you were able to walk around or across the actual bridges, experiencing how your view was modulated by your own dynamics? These are the sort of questions that might provoke architects and neuroscientists to embark on focused studies related to the visual aesthetics of buildings.

Albright is inspired by a book by E. H. Gombrich (1979), *The Sense of Order: A Study in the Psychology of Decorative Art*. He quotes from Gombrich's reply (Gombrich & Zerner, 1979) to a review by Henri Zerner (1979):

> I claim that the formal characteristics of most human products, from tools to buildings and from clothing to ornaments, can be seen as manifestations of that sense of order which is deeply rooted in man's biological heritage. [*Albright omits these sentences*: Organic life is governed by hierarchical structures which not only secure the interaction of internal functions (e.g. heartbeat and breathing), but also assist adjustment to the environment. Here the role of the "sense of order" is complementary to the perception of meaning, because the detection of food, of mates, or of danger first requires orientation in space and anticipation in time.] Those ordered events in our environment which exhibit rhythmical or other regular features (the waves of the sea or the uniform texture of a cornfield) easily "lock in" with our tentative projections of orders and thereby sink below the threshold of our attention while any change in these regularities leads to an arousal of attention. Hence the artificial environment man has created for himself satisfies this dual demand for easy adjustment and easy arousal.

Albright wraps this into his account of aesthetics by interpreting it as follows:

Easy adjustment: Albright links this to the ordered events in our environment that exhibit rhythmical or other regular features, which he identifies with familiarity. He sees simple, regular, repeating forms as activating specialized neuronal systems that have evolved because they facilitate detection of natural stimuli that confer selective advantage for survival and reproduction.

Easy arousal: Albright associates this with novelty, involving complex forms with irregular statistics. Here, there are no specialized neuronal system for detection, and indeed detection of novelty as such confers little *direct* value for survival and reproduction. Making sense of novelty, however, can be an important aspect both of survival and of human culture.

Contra to Albright's take on "easy arousal," I do not see the presence of irregular statistics as being contrary to "detection of natural stimuli that confer selective advantage for survival and reproduction." Rather, if an animal is exploring its environment, then its brain must exploit regularities in the overall field of view *and* have the capacity to respond appropriately to local irregularities that may, for example, support detection of prey or predator, and generation of the appropriate response. Such mechanisms may be relatively hardwired as in the frog, or based significantly on learning—in either case, the issue is to be able, on detecting irregularities in local statistics against a spatiotemporal background, to determine which course of action has the greatest likelihood of being beneficial. In either case, the animal or human performs as in some sense a probabilistic machine.

I think Gombrich was looking at a different dichotomy than that offered by Albright, one that we established in our discussion of lateral inhibition: the nervous system has evolved, in part, to detect changes in both space and time. It thus extracts a stronger "attention-catching" signal when and where change occurs. This is emphasized in one of the sentences that Albright omitted: "Here the role of the 'sense of order' is complementary to the perception of meaning, because the detection of food, of mates, or of danger first requires orientation in space and anticipation in time." This leads to my suggestion that for Gombrich,

- *easy adjustment* is the capacity of our brains to relegate certain aspects to the background or status quo, while
- *easy arousal* is the capacity of our brains to rapidly direct attention to unexpected changes so that they can be examined for relevance to our ongoing behavior.

But let's set this aside for now, and instead focus on how Albright employs *his* definitions of these terms in his approach to visual aesthetics. Although I will not be convinced by his argument, it will help us better understand the challenge of relating brain mechanisms to our ideas of beauty.

Figure 3.18 shows two examples of what Albright, in a talk on "Contextual Influences on Visual Processing" at NewSchool of Architecture and Design, San Diego, suggested were attractive because they exemplify what he sees as easy adjustment, based on a sense of familiarity engendered by simple, regular, repeating forms. However, if "simple, regular, repeating

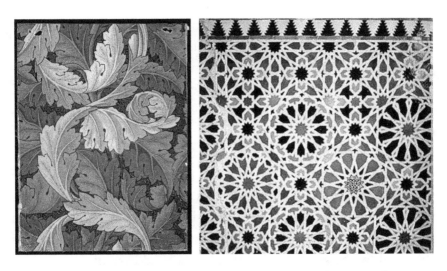

Figure 3.18 Two examples chosen by Tom Albright to exemplify his notion of easy adjustment, based on repeating forms. (*Left*) A design by William Morris for his Acanthus wallpaper, 1875. (*Right*) A tessellation (Nasrid Palace Mosaic, Alhambra, 10th century). (*Left*: Given by Morris & Co to Victoria and Albert Museum, London, reproduced with permission. *Right*: Public domain.)

forms" were the key to aesthetic appreciation, then a piece of graph paper would be even more appealing. Moreover, these two examples are unfamiliar, go far beyond mere repetition to gain their effect, and, it seems to me, are appealing in different ways.

For the William Morris wallpaper, the basic block combines two linked but different leaf patterns, and these blocks are arranged into an overall repetition that can be perceived in two ways—the repetition of the blocks, and (perhaps more strikingly) the alternating columns of lighter "foreground" leaves and darker "background" leaves. Perhaps, indeed, perception of the easy adjustment apparent in those columns gains aesthetic impact only as it unfolds into a deeper structural pattern while also revealing the aesthetic quality of the pattern within each block.

In the tessellation, the first impression is one of regularity, but here one discovers that there are at least three blocks that are repeated within the sample shown here, and two that are not, though each would, presumably, be repeated in a larger sample (and this does not exhaust further variations we can discover). The subtlety of local pattern combines with a scheme of repetition that eludes us at first glance to provide the possibility of aesthetic charge here. So, yes, we have evolved to recognize repetition—but whether that recedes into a negligible background or continues to engage our interest depends on higher level strategies of perception.[8]

In these two examples, we detect variation in the array and have some aesthetic appreciation for the elements that are repeated. We come to appreciate the pattern at different scales and need this interplay to elevate the overall aesthetic effect. Consider, too, the beauty of Persian rugs, where we see the pattern and interplay of defined geometries enhanced by the subtle choice of colors that adds another parameter to the geometry beyond the choices that would be captured in a line

---

8. Wikipedia has an excellent article on Islamic geometric patterns, https://en.wikipedia.org/wiki/Islamic_geometric_patterns, with insights into their design, as well as a photo gallery of impressive examples, some 2D, others 3D.

drawing alone. And, of course, the visual appearance of such a rug is enhanced by the feel and texture of the weaving and complemented by the way it is placed in the room. Moreover, for many people, this experience can be enriched by an appreciation of its role in Persian culture across the centuries.

Albright classified the Sydney Opera House as an example of easy adjustment (familiarity based on repetition, in this case repetition of the shell structure), but this analysis becomes less tenable as one sees the Opera House from diverse viewpoints on land, on the harbor, and from the Sydney Harbour Bridge, and moves in and around it (Figure 3.19). There is no reduction here to "specialized neuronal systems," but rather one expression of the experience of an exceptionally skilled architect, as we will see in §9.2.

In advancing neuroaesthetics, Albright's ideas have helped us see the interplay of diverse "forces" that yields an aesthetically successful visual

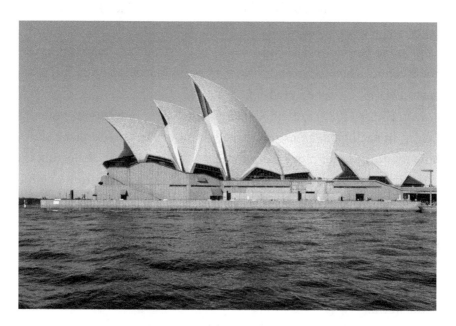

Figure 3.19 A side view of the Sydney Opera House. (https://upload.wikimedia.org/wikipedia/commons/3/38/Sydney_opera_house_side_view.jpg. Photo by Matthew Field. Permission granted under the terms of the GNU Free Documentation license.)

pattern—and this interplay exemplifies the competition and cooperation that I have offered as "the style of the brain." For example, in the William Morris wallpaper—or, indeed, in the Villa Savoye and the Parthenon—it is the blend of rhythm and novelty that best carries that aesthetic charge. But why one blend works, or why a nonrhythmic display may capture our appreciation, is beyond our (current?) objective analysis. What neuroscience can help us understand is some of the mechanisms that must be mobilized if that blend is to be achieved.

Aesthetics and action-oriented vision

A recurring theme of this book is that success of a building (as distinct from a painting) goes far beyond visual impact alone. Success must be registered in the action–perception cycles of those who use it. Frog visuomotor behavior offers a surprising insight here. Going beyond the Lettvin et al. study, my group developed computational brain models that included far more than retina and tectum to address the question, "What does the frog's eye tell the frog?" One particular challenge was to understand how neural networks could control *detour behavior*, where the frog must avoid an obstacle if it is to get to a worm or escape a predator.

Don House (1989) explained the frog's behavior in terms of "potential fields." In each field, an arrow at each point of the ground plane shows how the frog would move from that point (Figure 3.20). Following the arrows yields a trajectory the frog would follow, starting from any initial point.

- The *worm* creates *a field of attraction*. If nothing else were there, the perception of the worm would establish the field shown at top left, and the frog would come up with a trajectory straight toward the worm.
- But the *obstacle* creates a *field of repulsion*, which is much more local. The frog would go a long way to get to food, but an obstacle does not matter unless the frog is close to it.

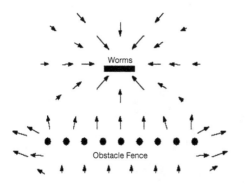 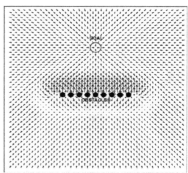

Figure 3.20 (*Left*) The worm and the obstacle are represented by "potential fields." If only a worm were present, the *arrows* would direct the frog to approach the worm no matter where it started, a long-range attractive field. By contrast, an obstacle has no effect unless the frog is close, and so is characterized by a short-range repulsive field. (*Right*) Combining the two fields, we get a new field of *arrows* that urges the frog on one side of the barrier to a worm on the other side, but via a trajectory that detours around the barrier.

- Integrating these two fields yields a new field, which supports a trajectory that will carry the frog around the obstacle to get to the worm.[9]

The relevance for architecture is that the notion of combining fields of attraction and repulsion has also entered the realm of aesthetics, as explored in Rudolf Arnheim's (1977) book on *The Dynamics of Architectural Form*. Arnheim was a distinguished art critic who had studied Gestalt psychology with Max Wertheimer and Wolfgang Köhler at the University of Berlin and then applied it to art, as masterfully presented in his earlier book, *Art and Visual Perception: A Psychology of the Creative Eye* (Arnheim, 1974). In the newer book, he explored what would carry over from this analysis of art to architectural form. However, despite the word "dynamics" in the title, his view is not action-oriented.

9. Combining attraction and repulsion to control behavior in the external world was not only important in our model of frog behavior but was also extended to analyze a range of behaviors in other animals, including humans. Our model of the frog was applied in the control of mobile robots (Arkin, 1989).

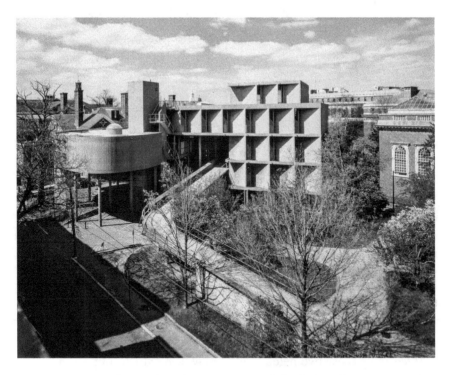

Figure 3.21 A view of Le Corbusier's Carpenter Center for the Visual Arts at Harvard University. (Photograph by Steve Rosenthal © Historic New England, from the Steve Rosenthal Collection of Commissioned Work at Historic New England.)

Discussing Le Corbusier's Carpenter Center for the Visual Arts at Harvard University (Figure 3.21),[10] Arnheim says:

> It was realized that the horizontal protrusion of the large curved North Studio on the second floor would lose much of its outward thrust unless a larger space beneath it rendered it more independent of the *attraction* exerted by the ground. For this reason, an essentially unfunctional pit was dug beneath the studio area, which, resting on relatively slim pilotis, acquired thereby the necessary *dynamic freedom*. [My italics.]

10. Strangely, Arnheim chose a view of the Center that does not match his text. I hope that the view I have chosen is more appropriate!

Notice the talk about attraction and dynamic freedom—not an actual dynamics of parts of the building moving, but rather the idea that close elements "attract" in that they may look closer together than they are, and distant elements "repel" in that they may look farther apart than they are. The challenge, then, was to balance the proportions to achieve a desired effect—an "equilibrium" between attraction and repulsion as "dynamics of form" rather than actual movement in the finished building.

The frog finding its way to its prey while avoiding a barrier balances the attraction and repulsion of various parts of the environment in finding its trajectory. The architect tries to create an aesthetic or visual balance in the appearance of a building, and Arnheim uses the language of dynamic fields to assess this judgment. I do wonder whether there is some evolutionary relationship between the sensorimotor dynamics of attraction and repulsion and the "static dynamics" of aesthetic judgment. Note that the frog midbrain bauplan is built upon in the dramatic process of corticalization (Figure 3.3) and that in many cases corticalization both preserves basic brain operating principles and opens them up to the impact of both our cultural milieu and our individual experience.

Our behavior rests not only on perceiving what objects (and people) are around us, but on *judging the spatial relations between them* in determining what to do and how to do it. Thus, our aesthetic judgment of spatial relations between parts of a visual display may well be rooted in ancient mechanisms that serve the action–perception cycle. The present analysis of the frog–Arnheim parallel provides my somewhat idiosyncratic stepping stone from the "it's just vision" account of the previous subsection to my emphasis in Chapter 5 on the role of the motor system in aesthetics.

3.6. SCHEMAS WITHIN AND BEYOND VISION

Art, illusion, and schemas

Albright was inspired by the Gombrich of *The Sense of Order* but, for us, Gombrich's more relevant volume may be *Art and Illusion: A study in the*

Psychology of Pictorial Representation (Gombrich, 1960). Gombrich was not simply interested in art as such, but wanted to understand the relevant psychological principles. In this, he was abetted by a partnership with Richard Gregory, the British psychologist of vision.[11] Together, they edited the book, *Illusion in Nature and Art* (Gregory & Gombrich, 1973), that brought together neuroscientists and psychologists along with those who studied pictorial art. Of especial relevance, Gregory (1967) had earlier written the paper "Will Seeing Machines Have Illusions?" with the unequivocal answer "Yes"—in the sense that any approach to recognition must be based on a limited sample, perhaps further limited by computational efficiency, that ensures that there will always be patterns that are misclassified or whose properties are misrepresented—as is indeed true for humans, as exemplified by the Muller-Lyer illusion (Figure 3.22).

Back to Gombrich's *Art and Illusion*. After quoting Oliver Zangwill's (1937) statement that "Reproducing the simplest figures, constitutes a process itself by no means psychologically simple," Gombrich invokes a certain notion of *schema* relevant to *pictorial representation*.

> [I]t is certainly possible to look at a portrait as a schema of a head modified by the distinctive features about which we wish to convey information. The American police sometimes employ draughtsmen to aid witnesses in the identification of criminals. They may draw any vague face, a random schema, and let witnesses guide their

11. Richard Gregory is best known for his book on *Eye and Brain* (Gregory, 1966 and many subsequent editions), a profusely illustrated book that I strongly recommend to anyone who wishes to get a deep, and highly readable, appreciation of the psychology and neuroscience of vision. His talk, "How the Brain Works Cognitively," (https://www.youtube.com/watch?v=BxtvvYb9FWA) gives a sense of his work and, most importantly, his personality. I first met Richard in 1961 and greatly valued his friendship and his sense of play. When I visited his home in 1986, he greeted me with an enthusiastic demonstration of his new book, *Odd Perceptions*. I made the obvious pun: "Ah, Richard, now you will have to write a sequel, *Even Perceptions*." But Richard went one (or several) better: "No, Michael, it will be called *Even Odder Perceptions*." Richard's sense of fun was captured by Colin Blakemore (2010), whose obituary for Richard concluded: "The only thing that mattered to him was enthusiasm, and his own was highly infectious. On 30 May [2010], his friends and family gathered in Bristol to celebrate his life. The event was fittingly entitled a FUNeral. Richard would have shaken with laughter."

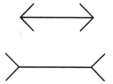

Figure 3.22 The Muller-Lyer illusion. It is hard to tell from visual inspection that the two lines are of the same length. There are diverse explanations based on possible occurrences of similar visual patterns on objects with which we might interact. One example: the bottom pattern might be seen in the far edge inside a box, while the top pattern might be seen in the near upper edge of the box, and we have learned to compensate for the smaller retinal projection of the further of two lines of equal length.

modifications of selected features simply by saying "yes" or "no" to various suggested standard alterations until the face is sufficiently individualized for a search in the files to be profitable. . . . [A]s a parable . . . [this] reminds us that the starting point of a visual record is not knowledge but a guess conditioned by habit and tradition. (Gombrich, 1960, p. 72)

In our schema theory of vision, a visual schema is a *general* process in the head for recognizing a certain type of object, and the brain sets parameters to yield a *schema instance* that accommodates particularities of a currently observed object. It seems, then, that Gombrich uses the term "schema" where we would use "schema instance," as when he says that the witness may "draw any vague face, a random schema." In some sense, the draughtsman or the (representational) artist is *inverting* vision—given the parameters, "run the schema backward" to achieve a sketch or drawing or painting or sculpture that can be recognized as the repository of these imaginings. They use the witness's binary choices, rather than direct visual experience, to set the parameters of the person, and the result is a drawing that may guide identification of the person seen by the witness by people who had not seen that person before. Where Gombrich says that

the starting point of a visual record is not knowledge but a guess conditioned by habit and tradition

I emphasize a sense of *a schema as a parametrizable process linked within a network of long-term memory to other schemas* and argue that the starting point of a visual experience is not direct knowledge but an initial assemblage of schema instances (the schemas themselves being active processes shaped by habit and tradition). The full experience emerges through a process (often subconscious) of competition and cooperation that melds both bottom-up processes driven by sensory stimuli and top-down processes driven by our current tasks and motivation and our accumulated knowledge.

Gombrich quotes an example from Bartlett's (1932) book *Remembering*, whose importance I noted in the history of schemas:

> Where such a pre-existing category is lacking, distortion sets in. Its effects become particularly amusing when the psychologist imitates the parlour game of "drawing consequences." Thus F. C. Bartlett had an Egyptian hieroglyph copied and recopied till it gradually assumed the familiar shape and formula of a pussycat. (Gombrich, 1960, p. 61)

We see in Figure 3.23 successive attempts to remember and reproduce the spatial relation of a pattern of lines (without recourse to a label) until Reproduction 9, which has achieved a shape that serves to activate the schema (in our sense) for "pussycat," and that, rather than the memory of how lines are disposed, influences the form of Reproduction 10. Bartlett shows that in the continuation of the sequence, Reproduction 11 onward, the sketches become simplified through appeal to the general cat schema (Bartlett, 1932, p. 181), with each reproduction providing input for the working memory that will drive the next action of drawing. However, for architecture, our concern is not for one drawing (noun) as a stimulus for further drawing (verb) but rather for designing the way in which a building can provide a frame for the ongoing action–perception cycles of its users (Chapter 10).

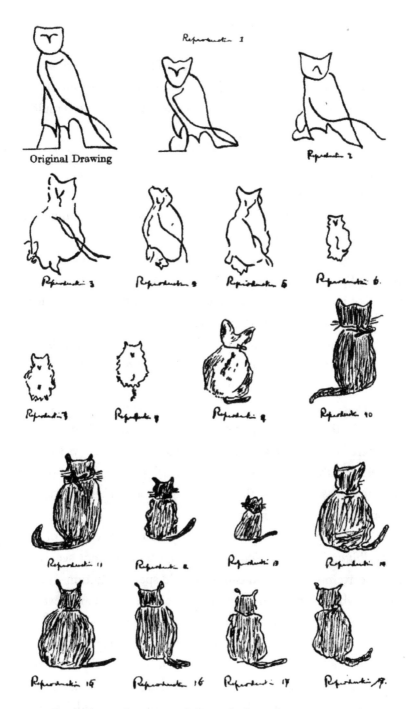

Figure 3.23 Bartlett's transformations of a hieroglyphic owl into a pussycat. (From Bartlett, F. C. [1932]. *Remembering: A study in experimental and social psychology.* Cambridge, UK: Cambridge University Press, pp. 180–181, with permission.)

Art and architecture of and for the blind

But vision is not enough for our approach to architecture, not even when coupled to drawing. For Gombrich, the focus is on vision and its relation to pictorial representation. Here, however, we must reiterate a multimodal view of schemas instantiated within the action–perception cycle. As one example of many, a visit to a cathedral will certainly involve visual experience, but this changes with our actions as we enter and walk through the church; as we sit in a pew, the feel of the seat beneath us relates to our contemplation of the form of the church and the light streaming through its stained-glassed windows. If we join in the singing of hymns, then the acoustics will affect how we sing and how we immerse ourselves in the sounds and actions of those around us. Moreover, perhaps subliminally, the smell of incense in the air may affect the quality of our overall experience. To probe these intuitions, this section will emphasize the nonvisual with a brief detour to consider art and architecture of and for the blind.

The blind architect Chris Downey was formerly sighted, but now employs an assistive technology that lets him sketch in terms of raised lines on a surface (Anderson, 2014). The sound within a space, such as the echoes of footfalls, may vary as one walks through it, not only adding to atmosphere but also helping the blind judge their trajectory. The foot-feel of carpet versus wood flooring can distinguish paths for locomotion from other floor areas. A table with straight edges and corners provides better positional cues than a round table. And so on.

Kennedy (1993) offers an intriguing psychological account of *Drawing and the Blind: Pictures to Touch*. While the blind cannot see 3D space, they can certainly hear it and can thus build spatial intuition—just as, for example, sighted people can recognize a train in the distance even if they cannot see it. Audition can determine the direction; memory of (for example) having walked to the train tracks can aid the estimate of distance. And don't forget the Doppler effect. However, in terms of the specifics of drawing, the linkage of tracing objects with our hands to both pantomime and drawing (more on this in §8.4) helps prepare us for Kennedy's studies. For most of us, drawing requires a technology for making enduring marks for later visual inspection. The blind can draw when a technology is available for making contours for later tactile inspection, such as that employed by Downey.

Perhaps more surprising is the case of a Turkish artist, Esref Armagan, who can paint, using appropriate colors (Figure 3.24). An fMRI study (Amedi et al., 2008) suggested that the occipital (visual) cortex played a key role in supporting mental representations even without prior visual experience. The key point here, I suggest, is that the brain evolved to link visual cortex with "higher" regions in both a top-down and bottom-up fashion. This fits in with our discussion of VISIONS—the visual working memory is constantly seeking to coordinate bottom-up signals based on retinal input and top-down signals that create expectations of what the scene contains, guide attention to seek out objects relevant to the current task, and so on. Consider, further, what happens when you take an object out of your pocket—your hand has already constructed a rough tactile image in 3D—and so when you look at the object, you are matching what you see with what you felt. Thus, top-down influences on visual cortex

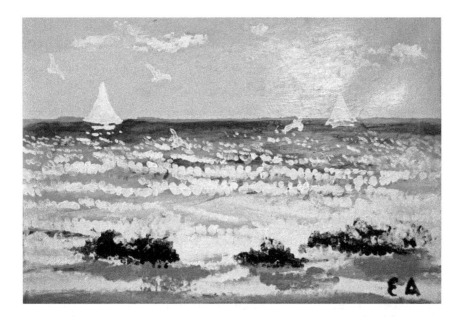

Figure 3.24 A painting by the blind Turkish artist Esref Armagan. (Alamy Stock Photo.)

in sighted people can come from other sensory systems (audition, touch, small) as well as task demands and other expectations.

Now consider a person who is blind because their retina is damaged or absent, but who still has the visual cortex intact. The regions in this cortex lack visual input but can still receive diverse signals from other regions. The rules of synaptic plasticity ensure that these regions will learn to seek out correlates with patterned activity from elsewhere, including signals from areas involved in current actions. So, how could such a brain fail to exploit all the computing capacity available in the neural networks of what would normally be the visual system? It's a bit like reading—train a sighted person to read, and the brain can restructure to accommodate it (Dehaene et al., 2010), adapting circuits that evolved to serve face recognition to also recognize the visual form of words.

Thus, spatial imagination can populate "higher" regions via hapsis (touch) to create pseudo-visual (contour relational) representations—so that even some of the features from what VISIONS models as the intermediate database can be accessed, such as edge information, tactile (not visual) texture, and so on. Again, we need to remember how strongly linked are the multiple regions in the brain—if we see the fur of a pet, for example, we not only see it, we also activate the expectation of the feel of it and even the urge (which we may or may not suppress) to stroke the pet and reinforce the integration of vision, touch, and action.

For the blind artist, perspective-dependent contours may be learned from exploring the raised contours of prior tactile-friendly drawings along with their interpretation. The "knitting together" required for extended objects or scenes is supplied by "prior art" and by interaction with a sighted person. Remember, a blind person understands perfectly well a sentence like "There is a yacht sailing 300 yards away across the water" and can learn how to "draw" waves, and how the size of an object in the drawing diminishes with distance. What about color? Again, although the blind person does not *see* color, they know *about* color— ripe apples are red, their driver stops when the traffic light turns red. Thus, after they learn the layout of a paint box, and can trust a sighted person to tell them what color pigment is located where, a blind artist can indeed learn to choose appropriate colors for different parts of a painting.

Turning from painting to everyday locomotion, a blind person can certainly build cognitive maps based on locomotor distance to get around their house and neighborhood. Claudia Folska (2012), herself blind, had blind participants sketch maps of their route from public transportation to the Colorado Center for the Blind. All participants exhibited a preference for relying on touch rather than audition for extracting environmental information. Passini and Proulx (1988) found that the blind made more decisions in navigating complex spaces and required more informational access points than those who navigated sighted, but were still able to navigate novel, complex spaces. This suggests the need to provide diverse tactile cues in designing for the blind. However, we also know the importance of auditory cues, as in telling a blind person when it is safe to cross the street in a certain direction. Similar considerations apply to aiding memory formation and recall, both providing means to help blind newcomers to the building orient themselves and supplementing the resident's working memory of where objects are to be found. The unavailability of visual affordances to guide navigation, and the related lack of visual cues about whether there is smooth terrain and an unobstructed path to the next "via point," requires a greater density of nonvisual via points if navigation is to be conducted efficiently.[12]

MULTIMODES: From vision to action and episodes

To conclude this chapter, I want to introduce a conceptual model—well, not so much a model as a set of discussion points—to remind us that schema theory is far more than a framework for the study of vision. I call it MULTIMODES to suggest its relation to VISIONS while linking

12. *Mobility of Visually Impaired People: Fundamentals and ICT Assistive Technologies* (Pissaloux & Velazquez, 2017) includes discussions of "Lived Space as an Interconnected Set (Network) of Places" and "Neuro-cognitive Basis of Space Perception for Mobility."

it to multimodal perception and action, and moving from static scenes to dynamic episodes. What I offer here is a preliminary sketch that will be extended in the approach to a cognitive neuroscience of design in Chapter 10.

- Figure 3.16 showed the logic of cooperative computation in VISIONS. Data from the intermediate database provided bottom-up cues that recruit schemas from long-term memory (LTM) to associate schema instances in the visual working memory (WM) with regions in the spatial environment. In MULTIMODES, rather than having a single intermediate database restricted to vision, we can have a separate database for each sensory modality, and these can be linked so that, for example, spatial layout cues can be coordinated between vision, audition, and touch—but they all contribute to the interpretation of the environment.
- The original VISIONS model accesses a static visual scene as input. However, in assessing its implications, we factored in the way in which visual attention can be directed to cumulatively enrich the intermediate-level input to mediate the competition and cooperation of schema instances. In MULTIMODES, it could be the sound of its meow that attracted our attention to a cat, and we could then enrich visual recognition of the cat by stroking it, thus integrating the visual and tactile representation of its fur and the flexibility of its body. A purr might then reward us by enriching the dynamic auditory component of the experience. The point of our discussion of Barlow remains—the high-level assemblage of schema instances can be enriched by lower level features, whether consciously or unconsciously, but now in multiple modalities.
- Our concern with aesthetics reminds us that the appreciation of an object or, more important, a scene, is not limited to identifying what the object is. It can be enriched by the appreciation of aesthetic qualities. In Chapter 4, we will extend our appreciation of the emotional impact of a scene in relation to our current

disposition, and exemplify this by exploring the notion of the "atmosphere" of a building.

- More generally, MULTIMODES must support the action–perception cycle: although perception may serve to recognize and analyze a static scene (whether in preparation for action, or for purposes of contemplation), we generally make sense of a dynamic scene as our behavior changes our immediate environment and/or our relationship to the environment, possibly to satisfy our current goals or to learn more about the current situation.

- Our concern with the thinking hand and its schemas demonstrated that perceptual schemas not only support recognition of objects but also may serve to pass the parameters of affordances to the motor schemas that implement the corresponding effectivities. We also saw the transition from visual to tactile guidance of action.

- The coordinated control program for the reach-to-grasp (§2.4) provides a basic example of a script that introduces a way of ordering actions to achieve some goal, but with the timing of the actions and the passing of control from one to another dependent on the current relation of the person to the relevant parts of the environment.

- The concern with the thinking hand and its brain (§2.6), as well as with the body schema, reminded us that affordances can serve both for planning (ventral) and for parameter-setting (dorsal). We can say that schemas in the ventral stream are semantic (what is this object good for?) but also procedural at the level of planning an overall course of action, while schemas in the dorsal stream are more directly procedural, given their role in passing parameters to motor schemas.

Such a list, reminding us of how VISIONS relates to lessons learned so far about the brain, invites the reader to reflect on these first three chapters and then take an active role when reading subsequent chapters in seeing how the list can be extended. The final payoff will come in Chapter 10 when we base IBSEN, our conceptual model of *Imagination in Brain Systems for Episodes and Navigation*, on investigations of how the user experiences the built environment, and then extend them to offer a preliminary account of the cognitive neuroscience of the design of architecture.

REFERENCES

Albright, T. D. (2012). On the perception of probable things: Neural substrates of associative memory, imagery, and perception. *Neuron*, 74(2), 227–245. doi:10.1016/j.neuron.2012.04.001

Albright, T. D. (2015a). *Contextual influences on visual processing.* PowerPoint Presentation, NewSchool of Architecture and Design, San Diego.

Albright, T. D. (2015b). Neuroscience for architecture. In S. Robinson & J. Pallasmaa (Eds.), *Mind in architecture: Neuroscience, embodiment, and the future of design* (pp. 197–217). Cambridge, MA: MIT Press.

Amedi, A., Merabet, L. B., Camprodon, J., Bermpohl, F., Fox, S., Ronen, I., . . . Pascual-Leone, A. (2008). Neural and behavioral correlates of drawing in an early blind painter: A case study. *Brain Research*, 1242, 252–262. doi:10.1016/j.brainres.2008.07.088

Anderson, L. (2014). How a San Francisco architect reframes design for the blind. *curbed.com.* https://www.curbed.com/2014/2018/2016/10064320/how-a-san-francisco-architect-reframed-design-for-the-blind

Arbib, M. A. (1987). Levels of modelling of visually guided behavior (with peer commentary and author's response). *Behavioral and Brain Sciences*, 10, 407–465.

Arbib, M. A. (2019). Poetics and more in performative architecture: Towards a neuroscience of dynamic experience and design. In K. Mitra (Ed.), *The Routledge companion to paradigms of performativity in design and architecture: Using time to craft an enduring, resilient and relevant architecture* (pp. 105–116). New York and Abingdon: Routledge.

Arkin, R. C. (1989). Neuroscience in motion: The application of schema theory to mobile robotics. In J.-P. Ewert & M. A. Arbib (Eds.), *Visuomotor coordination: Amphibians, comparisons, models, and robots* (pp. 649–671). New York: Plenum Press.

Arkin, R. C. (1998). *Behavior-based robotics.* Cambridge, MA: MIT Press.

Arnheim, R. (1974). *Art and visual perception.* Berkeley: University of California Press.

Arnheim, R. (1977). *The dynamics of architectural form.* Berkeley and Los Angeles: University of California Press.

Attneave, F. (1954). Informational aspects of visual perception. *Psychological Review*, 61, 183–193.

Barlow, H. B. (1959). Sensory mechanisms, the reduction of redundancy, and intelligence. In *Symposium on mechanization of thought processes* (pp. 535–539). London: Her Majesty's Stationery Office.

Bartlett, F. C. (1932). *Remembering. A study in experimental and social psychology.* Cambridge, UK: Cambridge University Press.

Blakemore, C. (2010). Obituary: Richard Langton Gregory (1923–2010). *Nature*, 466(7302), 45.

Chatterjee, A. (2014). *The aesthetic brain: How we evolved to desire beauty and enjoy art*. Oxford and New York: Oxford University Press.

Christensen, J. F., & Gomila, A. (2018). *The arts and the brain: Psychology and physiology beyond pleasure*. Cambridge, MA: Academic Press.

Cobas, A., & Arbib, M. (1992). Prey-catching and predator-avoidance in frog and toad: defining the schemas. *Journal of Theoretical Biology*, 157(3), 271–304.

Curtis, W. J. R. (2011, September 21). The classical ideals of Le Corbusier. *Architectural Review*.

Dean, P., Redgrave, P., & Westby, G. W. M. (1989). Event or emergency? Two response systems in the mammalian superior colliculus. *Trends in Neurosciences*, 12(4), 137–147. doi:10.1016/0166-2236(89)90052-0

Dehaene, S., Pegado, F., Braga, L. W., Ventura, P., Filho, G. N., Jobert, A., . . . Cohen, L. (2010). How learning to read changes the cortical networks for vision and language. *Science*, 330(6009), 1359–1364. doi:10.1126/science.1194140

Didday, R. L. (1976). A model of visuomotor mechanisms in the frog optic tectum. *Mathematical Biosciences*, 30, 169–180.

Dutton, D. (2009). *The art instinct: Beauty, pleasure, and human evolution*. New York: Oxford University Press.

Ewert, J.-P. (1987). Neuroethology of releasing mechanisms: Prey catching in toads. *Behavioral and Brain Sciences*, 10, 337–405.

Felleman, D. J., & Van Essen, D. C. (1991). Distributed hierarchical processing in the primate cerebral cortex. *Cerebral Cortex*, 1, 1–47.

Folska, C. L. (2012). *In blind sight: Wayfinding in the absence of vision*. PhD Thesis, University of Colorado at Denver.

Gombrich, E. H. (1960). *Art and Illusion: A study in the psychology of pictorial representation*. London: Phaidon Press.

Gombrich, E. H. (1979). *The sense of order: A study in the psychology of decorative art*. Ithaca, NY: Cornell University Press.

Gombrich, E. H., & Zerner, H. (1979, September 17). The sense of order: An exchange. *New York Review of Books*.

Gregory, R. L. (1966). *Eye and brain*. New York: McGraw-Hill.

Gregory, R. L. (1967). Will seeing machines have illusions? In N. L. Collins & D. Michie (Eds.), *Machine intelligence 1* (pp. 169–180). Edinburgh: Oliver & Boyd.

Gregory, R. L., & Gombrich, E. H. J. (Eds.). (1973). *Illusion in nature and art*. New York: Scribner.

Hanson, A. R., & Riseman, E. M. (1978). VISIONS: A computer system for interpreting scenes. In A. R. Hanson & E. M. Riseman (Eds.), *Computer vision systems* (pp. 129–163). New York: Academic Press.

Hewitt, C. (1977). Viewing control structures as patterns of passing messages. *Artificial Intelligence*, 8(3), 323–364. doi:10.1016/0004-3702(77)90033-9

House, D. H. (1989). *Depth perception in frogs and toads: A study in neural computing*. Berlin and Heidelberg: Springer-Verlag.

Hubel, D. H., & Wiesel, T. N. (1959). Receptive fields of single neurones in the cat's striate cortex. *Journal of Physiology*, 148(3), 574–591.

Hubel, D. H., & Wiesel, T. N. (1977). Ferrier lecture: Functional architecture of macaque monkey visual cortex. *Proceedings of the Royal Society of London. Series B, Biological Sciences*, 198(1130), 1–59.

Humphrey, N. K. (1970). What the frog's eye tells the monkey's brain. *Brain Behavior and Evolution*, 3, 324–337.

Huston, J. P., Nadal, M., Mora, F., Agnati, L. F., & Conde, C. J. C. (2015). *Art, aesthetics, and the brain*. Oxford: Oxford University Press.

Ingle, D. J. (1968). Visual releasers of prey catching behaviour in frogs and toads. *Brain, Behavior and Evolution*, 1, 500–518.

Ingle, D. J. (1983). Visual mechanisms of optic tectum and pretectum related to stimulus localization in frogs and toads. In J.-P. Ewert, R. R. Capranica, & D. J. Ingle (Eds.), *Advances in vertebrate neuroethology* (pp. 177–226). New York: Plenum Press.

Ingle, D. J., Schneider, G. E., Trevarthen, C. B., & Held, R. (1967). Locating and identifying: Two modes of visual processing (a symposium). *Psychologishe Forschung*, 31(1 and 4).

Kaas, J. (Ed.). (2017). *Evolution of nervous systems* (2nd ed.; in 4 volumes). Elsevier.

Kagan, J. (1970). Attention and psychological change in the young child. *Science*, 170(3960), 826–832.

Kennedy, J. M. (1993). *Drawing and the blind: Pictures to touch*. New Haven, CT: Yale University Press.

Kirk, U., Skov, M., Christensen, M. S., & Nygaard, N. (2009). Brain correlates of aesthetic expertise: A parametric fMRI study. *Brain and Cognition*, 69(2), 306–315. doi:10.1016/j.bandc.2008.08.004

Kolarevic, B., & Malkawi, A. M. (2005). *Performative architecture: Beyond instrumentality*. Routledge.

Kuffler, S. W. (1953). Discharge patterns and functional organization of mammalian retina. *Journal of Neurophysiology*, 16, 37–68.

Le Corbusier. (1927). *Towards a new architecture* (Translated from the 13th French edition with an introduction by Frederick Etchells). New York: Brewer, Warren & Putnam.

Le Corbusier. (2007). *Toward an architecture* (Translated from the French by John Goodman). Los Angeles: Getty Research Institute Publications Program.

Lettvin, J. Y., Maturana, H., McCulloch, W. S., & Pitts, W. H. (1959). What the frog's eye tells the frog brain. *Proceedings of the IRE*, 47, 1940–1951.

Li, L., Zhu, H., Zhao, S., Ding, G., & Lin, W. (2020). Personality-assisted multi-task learning for generic and personalized image aesthetics assessment. *IEEE Transactions on Image Processing*, 29, 3898–3910. doi:10.1109/TIP.2020.2968285

Passini, R., & Proulx, G. (1988). Wayfinding without vision: An experiment with congenitally totally blind people. *Environment and Behavior*, 20(2), 227–252.

Pissaloux, E., & Velazquez, R. (Eds.). (2017). *Mobility of visually impaired people: Fundamentals and ICT assistive technologies*. Springer.

Pitts, W. H., & McCulloch, W. S. (1947). How we know universals, the perception of auditory and visual forms. *Bulletin of Mathematical Biophysics*, 9, 127–147.

Prescott, T. J., Lepora, N., & Verschure, P. F. J. (2018). *Living machines: A handbook of research in biomimetics and biohybrid systems*. Oxford: Oxford University Press.

Ratliff, F. (1965). *Mach bands: Quantitative studies on neural networks in the retina*. San Francisco: Holden-Day.

Reisner, Y. (2019). *Beauty matters: Human judgement and the pursuit of new beauties in post-digital architecture*. New York: John Wiley & Sons.

Reisner, Y., & Watson, F. (2010). *Architecture and beauty: conversations with architects about a troubled relationship*. New York: John Wiley and Sons.

Rifkind, D. (2011). Misprision of precedent: Design as creative misreading. *Journal of Architectural Education*, 64(2), 66–75.

Riseman, E. M., & Hanson, A. R. (1987). A methodology for the development of general knowledge-based vision systems. In M. A. Arbib & A. R. Hanson (Eds.), *Vision, brain and cooperative computation* (pp. 285–328). Cambridge, MA: Bradford Book/ MIT Press.

Rowland, I. D., & Howe, T. N. (Eds.). (1999). *Vitruvius: Ten books on architecture* (I. Rowland, Trans.). New York and Cambridge: Cambridge University Press.

Saint, A. (2007). *Architect and engineer: A study in sibling rivalry*. New Haven, CT: Yale University Press.

Schneider, G. E. (2014). *Brain structure and its origins: In development and in evolution of behavior and the mind*. Cambridge, MA: MIT Press.

Scoville, W. B., & Milner, B. (1957). Loss of recent memory after bilateral hippocampal lesions *Journal of Neurology, Neurosurgery, and Psychiatry*, 20, 11–21. (Reprinted in *Journal of Neuropsychiatry and Clinical Neurosciences*, 12, 103–113, 2000.)

Shannon, C. E. (1948). A mathematical theory of communication (parts I and II). *Bell System Technical Journal*, 27, 379–423, 623–656.

Shannon, C. E., & Weaver, W. (1949). *The mathematical theory of communication*. Urbana: University of Illinois Press.

Shimamura, A. P., & Palmer, S. E. (2012). *Aesthetic science: Connecting minds, brains, and experience*. New York: Oxford University Press.

Simon, H. A. (1969). *The sciences of the artificial*. Cambridge, MA: MIT Press (2nd ed., 1981).

Skov, M., Vartanian, O., Martindale, C., & Berleant, A. (2018). *Neuroaesthetics*. Routledge.

Squire, L. R., & Wixted, J. T. (2011). The cognitive neuroscience of human memory since H.M. *Annual Review of Neuroscience*, 34(1), 259–288. doi:10.1146/ annurev-neuro-061010-113720

Starr, G. G. (2013). *Feeling beauty: The neuroscience of aesthetic experience*. Cambridge, MA: MIT Press.

von Békésy, G. (1967). *Sensory inhibition*. Princeton, NJ: Princeton University Press.

Wang, Z., & Quan, H. (2019, July 14–19). *Fashion outfit composition combining sequential learning and deep aesthetic network*. Paper presented at the 2019 International Joint Conference on Neural Networks (IJCNN).

Weiskrantz, L. (1974). The interaction between occipital and temporal cortex in vision: An overview. In F. O. Schmitt & F. G. Worden (Eds.), *The neurosciences third study program* (pp. 189–204). Cambridge, MA: MIT Press.

Wiener, N. (1948). *Cybernetics: Or control and communication in the animal and the machine*. New York: Technology Press and John Wiley & Sons.

Yarbus, A. L. (1967). *Eye movements and vision*. New York: Plenum.

Zaidel, D. W., & Hessamian, M. (2010). Asymmetry and symmetry in the beauty of human faces. *Symmetry*, 2(1), 136–149.

Zangwill, O. L. (1937). An investigation of the relationship between the processes of reproducing and recognizing simple figures, with special reference to Koffka's trace theory. *British Journal of Psychology, General Section*, 27(3), 250.

Zerner, H. (1979, June 28). The sense of sense (Review of The Sense of Order: A Study in the Psychology of Decorative Art). *New York Review of Books*.

Atmosphere, affordances, and emotion

The colloquial sense of the word "atmosphere" may refer to the air around us, but its use in architecture invokes its figurative sense of the pervading tone or mood. When we encounter a building or a landscape, it may have an immediate impact upon us. Is it calming or forbidding? Does it inspire humility or invite us to act in a masterful way? The experience of atmosphere may frame our appreciation of details of the building that invite contemplation or that invite action, but as we register those details, our perception of the atmosphere may change. A welcoming atmosphere may rapidly dissipate if we subsequently observe armed guards blocking our entry; a sense of nervous tension in a strange environment may ease as we come to see accessible affordances for the actions that we came to the building to perform. And, of course, we may register unexpected affordances that allow us to appreciate and use the building in unanticipated ways.

The serenity of a Japanese temple garden, the hustle and bustle of a city street that may be energizing or frustrating, the welcoming aura of one house but not of another—all these demonstrate the idea of atmosphere as the general "feeling" you get from a space, as well as reminding us that in this book, *architecture* may at times serve as shorthand for *the design and experience of rooms, buildings, and larger ensembles*, whether or not they succeed functionally or aesthetically. Thus, when we consider atmosphere or the relation between the utilitarian and the aesthetic, I ask you to keep calibrating the ideas developed here against the buildings you encounter in your daily life—your home, your workplace, the shops and restaurants you frequent, and so on—and continue to ponder for each example what "better" might mean to you.

Our concern with the mood evoked by a building will lead us to look at brain mechanisms for emotion, and so we explore motivation and emotion and their relation to the limbic system and other parts of the brain. Motivation can include such basic drives as hunger, thirst, and fear, as well as the demands of familial affection. Emotion builds on this set of primordial emotions, but in humans an amalgam with cognitive states and memories adds subtlety and long-term components, as in envy and jealousy as well as in aesthetic emotions.

Earlier, we introduced J. J. Gibson's notion of an affordance as a perceptual cue that could invite and guide a specific type of action. Here, we explore the notion that in some sense the atmosphere of a building can provide a *non-Gibsonian* affordance that provides cues for moods and emotion to set, perhaps, a general disposition toward certain courses of action rather than others, though not offering cues for specific actions.

We take a detour from architecture to explore paintings by Turner and Constable to gain some insight into how they develop atmosphere in their paintings. Of particular interest is Turner's *The Slave Ship*, in which we find that the initial atmosphere evoked by viewing a sunset on a stormy sea changes dramatically as we pay attention to details of the scene, or if we know the tragic story that provided the inspiration for the painting. Moreover, the discussion takes us beyond the phenomenology of atmosphere to explore the idea that the artist "inverts" vision. The VISIONS model gave us some sense of how the brain may transform a visual image into an assemblage of schema instances that come laden with a range of parameters that can express details of the objects seen in different parts of the scene. The challenge for *inverting* vision, then, is to start with some sort of mental image in the form of a schema assemblage that may be precise in some ways yet completely vague in others and find a way of transforming it into motions of the hand holding a paintbrush or pencil or moving a computer mouse to create patterns that in some sense "realize" the mental image. This involves a process linking the visual pathway (from visual pattern to mental image) with an inverse pathway (from mental image to visual pattern). The first judges the emerging sketch—assessing the extent to which the interpretation of the current sketch matches the imagined scene—and the other seeks to update the sketch. In the process, not only will the sketch or drawing or painting change, but so too will the mental image as what was vaguely conceived at first becomes more and more precise, or ideas that had seemed appealing become rejected in favor of others. Understanding how equilibrium is achieved in this process sets the stage for our exploration of the extent to which the design of architecture may similarly be seen as "inverting" the experience of architecture (a theme to be explored in much detail in Chapter 10).

With this, we will turn to an extended analysis of one specific study in which brain imaging (using functional magnetic resonance imaging [fMRI]) was used to assess what regions of architects' brains became activated when they observed a sequence of images corresponding to a "contemplative" building as distinct from images of a noncontemplative building. We will not only discuss what the study achieved but also offer an extended critique that suggests challenges for designing further experiments. Our A↔N conversation can only prove fruitful if we recognize that our understanding is imperfect, welcoming the way in which each partial understanding can provide a basis for future insights into how brains meet buildings. A crucial obstacle to our conversation is the distance between cog/neuroscience experiments that seek to isolate the influence of a few key variables and the whole-person experience of using and contemplating a building in all its varied complexity.

Finally, we turn from contemplation to "varieties of religious experience" or, more generally, "experiences of ultimacy," those oceanic feelings that may be interpreted by some in religious terms but in others as a feeling of emotional totality. To focus this discussion we leave the domain of architecture to examine a hypothesis that, just as religious experience may be seen as a highly enculturated form of underlying experiences of ultimacy, so may the prayers of believers instantiate a more general feeling of trust that is essential to family life and to social relations. This discussion is underwritten by the comparison of two differently focused brain imaging studies. A major challenge for the A↔N conversation implied here is to further develop an integrative view of cog/neuroscience that inform the designing of buildings that offer an atmosphere of trust that can support social belonging rather than the isolation of the individual.

4.1. ATMOSPHERE EXEMPLIFIED

Although we are concerned with the totality of being in a space, and although our impression of a building or a room may depend on sound and touch and even smell, not merely its visual impact, I will nonetheless use a few photos to offer examples of atmosphere.

In this temple garden in Kyoto (Figure 4.1), the atmosphere is, for me and many others, immediately one of tranquility and relaxation. If you are a Buddhist, steeped in certain types of practice, the atmosphere would have further dimensions than those I experienced. However, some Western observers find the atmosphere created by the compositions of Japanese gardens to be unsettling. Thus, here and elsewhere, we see that evocation of the "atmosphere" involves a relationship between observer and building (or, in this case, garden). Nonetheless, atmosphere will be one of the targets of the architects' design process, and so they may speak of the atmosphere of the building itself as shorthand for "the atmosphere that I expect this building to evoke in many of the people for whose use it is intended." The reader should be alert to this two-fold use of the term.

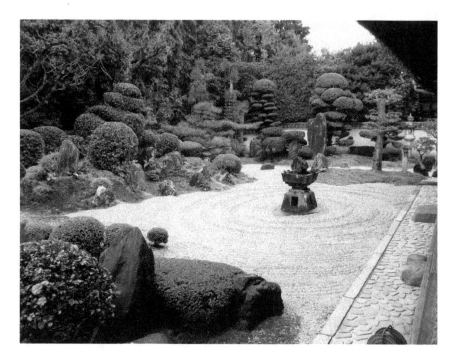

Figure 4.1 A temple garden in Kyoto. (Author's photo.)

Back to the temple garden. After we get our initial sense of the overall atmosphere, it can be reinforced as we begin to look at the way the
sand has been raked or at the disposition of the stones and the bushes.
We may then wonder about that wall at the back. Is it there as part of setting the atmosphere, or is it there just to separate this garden from the
temple next door? We get a very strong sense of both how the details have
come together to give us the atmosphere of tranquility and how, when
established, this atmosphere then frames our appreciation of the details.
In this case, the atmosphere gained on first impression may endure as we
continue to experience the setting.

Remaining in Kyoto, consider the very different atmosphere of Hiroshi
Hara's addition to Kyoto Train Station. If instead of looking down as we
did in Figure 1.8 at the hustle and bustle of people buying tickets, hurrying
to and from trains, buying snacks, and so on, we look across the vestibule,
we are greeted with a very different scene (Figure 4.2)—the surprisingly

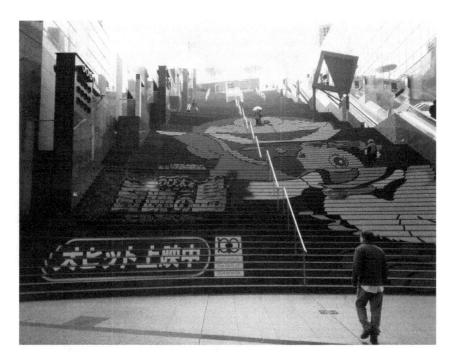

Figure 4.2 The ascending stairs of the Kyoto Station extension. (Author's photo.)

broad, little-populated expanse of the stairs (and escalators) linking stores at each level.

Let's travel from Japan to Scotland. Edinburgh castle (Figure 4.3) was built both as a fort and as a royal palace. As such, it may be said to symbolize fortitude as well as power. As a castle on a hilltop, it was at certain stages of history configured for battle. If you approached it at such a time as one of the invading troops, you would be very much aware of the fortifications that you would have to attack and the threat of counterattack that they pose. If you come at a time of peace and tourism, you get a different set of affordances, both atmospheric (historical grandeur?) and Gibsonian—the large door at right may afford you a chance to enter and tour the castle. You might initially be struck by the castle's foreboding aspect, and then the sight of that door might shift the atmosphere to one of being welcomed as a tourist for a historical adventure. We thus see that a first impression not only may be highly personal (but also dependent

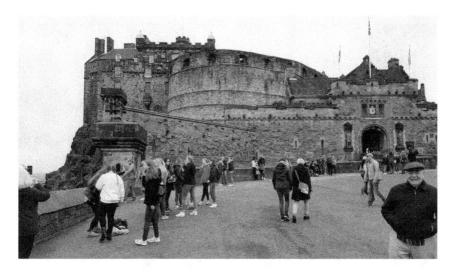

Figure 4.3 The approach to Edinburgh Castle. (Author's photo.)

on social role and historical period), but also may change for us as we assess the details of the building before us, and may change further as we act upon those initial impressions. Note, too, how the atmosphere offered here depends not only on the Castle as we see it (an impression strengthened by the changing perspectives during the strenuous walk up the Royal Mile toward the Castle) but also by the sight of people casually milling around the courtyard.[1]

Descending the Royal Mile from the Castle, one looks down a side street (Figure 4.4) to encounter a totally different atmosphere. This street's descent with a curve invites one to walk down it. There is an overall atmosphere offered by the general style of the architecture, and yet there is a real delight in visually exploring the diverse shapes of the towers and windows and chimneys. In addition, of course, each shopfront offers affordances to enter and temptations to buy. The architecture provides not only an overall atmosphere but also further details, both aesthetic and

1. Further notions relevant to analysis of atmosphere are the notions *mystery* and *complexity* as explored in environmental psychology. See, for example, the studies of "Mystery, Complexity, Legibility and Coherence" (Stamps, 2004) and "Complexity and Mystery as Predictors of Interior Preferences" (Scott, 1993).

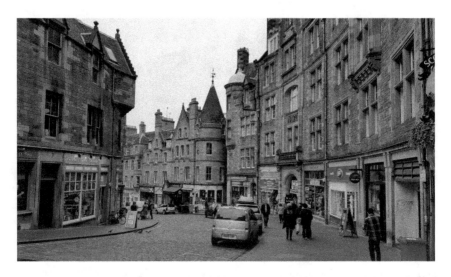

Figure 4.4 The Royal Mile descends from Edinburgh Castle to Holyrood Palace. Here is a side street. (Author's photo.)

practical. Even though all the storefronts have the same function, urging you to come in and spend your money, each one is nonetheless distinctive. Complementing this, as we visually explore the rooftops, we experience a certain joy in form rather than functionality.

Alvar Aalto, perhaps the greatest of Finnish architects, wrote:

> I am led to believe that most people, but especially artists, principally grasp the emotional content in a work of art. This is especially manifest in the case of old architecture. We encounter there a mood so intense and downright intoxicating that in most cases we don't pay a great deal of attention to individual parts and details, if we notice them at all. (Aalto, 1978, p. 1)

But is the emotional content of the earlier examples so "downright intoxicating" that we are unaware of the details?

To further make this point, consider Boa Nova (Figure 4.5), originally a tea house and now a restaurant, on the coast near Porto in Portugal, designed by the architect Alvaro Siza. Each view offers a somewhat different atmosphere,

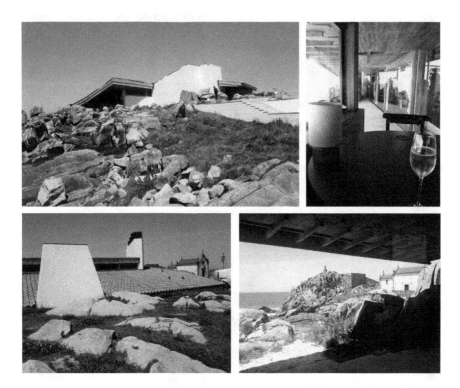

Figure 4.5 Four views of Alvaro Siza's Boa Nova, near Porto, Portugal. (Author's photos.)

and each atmosphere enhances one's appreciation of the organic embedding of the building among the rocks and the hillock rising above the beach. The white walls and terracotta roof echo the chapel (*bottom left*), yet in a completely different architectural style; while the interior offers an atmosphere of its own (*top right*), and affords views (*bottom right*) that enrich the appreciation of the building as explored from the outside.

Let's next contrast sacred places of two very different religions to assess what their atmospheres hold in common and what differs. The first is Todai-Ji Temple in Nara, Japan (Figure 4.6). The temple complex was first built in the eighth century and has been replaced twice after fires. The current building was completed in 1709, and until very recently was the largest wooden building in the world. The view of the interior is dominated by two immense statues of the Buddha. The second is one of the great Christian cathedrals of Europe, Notre-Dame de Paris (Figure 4.7).

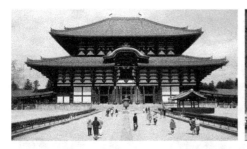
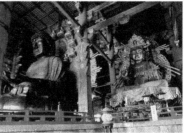

Figure 4.6 Todai-Ji Temple, Nara, Japan. (Creative Commons Attribution-Share Alike 2.0 Generic; https://www.justonecookbook.com/nara-guide-todaiji/#.)

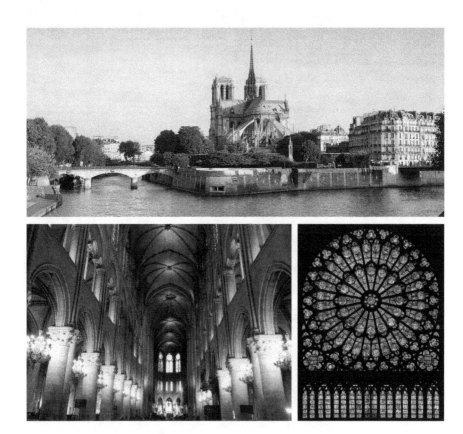

Figure 4.7 Notre-Dame de Paris. (*Top*: https://www.france.fr/en/paris/list/notre-dame-de-paris-in-6-secrets. © Paris Tourist Office—Photograph: Daniel Thierry*Bottom left*: https://upload.wikimedia.org/wikipedia/commons/e/e4/Notre_Dame_de_Paris_interior_looking_east_2012-11-5180_straight.JPG, Creative Commons. *Bottom right*: https://upload.wikimedia.org/wikipedia/commons/d/d8/North_rose_window_of_Notre-Dame_de_Paris%2C_Aug_2010.jpg, Creative Commons.)

Ironically, since this section was first written, it too has been consumed by fire.

Let's consider the interior atmospheres. In Todai-Ji, the eyes rise up to the dark space above the heads of the Buddhas, whereas in the cathedral, one lifts one's eyes to light flooding in through the stained glass windows. "Height" is also about feelings of superiority and power and may thus combine different influences—tapping into a primeval awe in looking up at great mountains, but also the relation of child looking up to the parent both literally and metaphorically, so that Christians may pray "Our Father, which art in Heaven."

In Gothic Cathedrals, God was believed to be "present" in the light of the soaring space. However, there is no heaven in Japanese Buddhism, and certainly not one like that in Christianity. The point of Buddhism is not to look up, or even out . . . it is to look within. Whatever the shared biological substrate here, note the strong cultural overlay. Each space induces something of religious awe, but the faithful of that religion will have their feeling of awe enriched by the signs and symbols of their own faith.

A building may support multiple atmospheres—such as those outside the building and within an interior sppace. This can be enhanced by the contrast between the space that one has been in, and the space that one now enters. Here is an example from Le Corbusier:

> In Broussa in Asia Minor, at the Green Mosque, you enter by a little doorway of normal human height; a quite small vestibule produces in you the necessary change of scale so that you may appreciate, as against the dimensions of the street and the spot you come from, the dimensions with which [the mosque's interior] is intended to impress you. Then you can feel the noble size of the Mosque and your eyes can take its measure. (1927, p. 181)

He offers this as evidence for the claim that a "[p]lan proceeds from within to without; the exterior is the result of an interior," but I suggest that it shows only the drama of transitions (whether from inside to outside or vice versa, or from room to room), rather than showing the primacy of interior to exterior in planning. Indeed, in a mosque, the minarets form a key external element that is (almost) unrelated to the interior, and in Utzon's Sydney Opera House, the design of the shells was only loosely constrained by his (unrealized) design of the auditoriums. The transition may be such that the outside gives only a limited sense of the inside or foreshadows it. The architect must choose whether the exterior tightly embraces that inner form or, by leaving certain inner spaces unfilled, expands to meet other criteria than such an embrace.

4.2. MOTIVATION, EMOTION, AND BRAINS

Given the previous discussion, we might redefine architectural atmosphere as that which, when a person encounters a building or an architected space, establishes an overall emotional response or mood. Our ongoing conversation thus demands that we now look in more detail at the cognitive science and neuroscience of motivation and emotion.

The touchstone for the study of emotion is the range and subtlety of human emotions as we experience them ourselves, as we observe them in others, and as we extend our understanding vicariously through art and literature. Motivation and emotion play crucial roles in both the utilitarian and the aesthetic dimensions of architecture. As people act within buildings, they are motivated to meet various needs, from basic drives like finding food or a toilet or place to sleep all the way to a desire to view great works of art in a gallery or find religious inspiration. Thus, architects seek to understand (among so much else) how buildings affect the emotions of their users, while cog/neuroscientists or ethologists deepen our understanding of human emotion by detailed study of humans as well as comparative study of the brains and behaviors of other animals.

In this section, I sketch a path from the study of basic motivation to varied "everyday" emotions like love, anger, and fear and on to aesthetic emotions, including those of awe. For the last, consider the difference in emotion if we visit Notre-Dame de Paris or Todai-Ji as a tourist or—as the builders intended—as devotees of the religion for which either was built.

Motivation and emotion are the engines that drive the action-perception cycle. We have all had days when we have wanted to stay in bed, but eventually got up and started the day. This might have been because of basic motivational systems—the insistent pressure on the bladder, or the hunger demanding that you break your fast—or perhaps fear of a very abstract kind, the fear of losing your pay or even your job if you do not get to work on time. The motivating emotion may also be a social one—the love for your children, and the consequent desire to spend time with them before they leave for school. Nonetheless, in many cases the emotional pressure is (almost?) absent—one starts the day because one has developed ingrained habits, scripts, for how the day begins. Perhaps only on weekends does the anticipated enjoyment of leisure allow you to override those weekday habits. In other words, where most animals may act primarily in response to the state of basic systems for motivated behavior, humans have developed elaborate systems for recalling the past and planning the future, and our current behavior may depend on knowledge acquired through past experiences, including those charged with emotion, as much as on present emotion—which may, indeed, be the anticipation of future emotion based on those experiences. Note, however, that the most basic behaviors that we share with other creatures are also based on expectation—hunger may drive complex behaviors directed to finding food and then enjoying the pleasure of eating it; the drive to reproduce may invoke lengthy and energy-consuming courtship rituals before the intense reward of mating, an innate reward that evolved to support the continuation of the species.

Internal and external roles of emotion

Emotions have both internal roles and external, social roles. For example, anger may mobilize the body's resources in preparation for a fight, while the expression of anger warns others that a fight may be imminent, so they should prepare to fight, to submit, or to flee—or, in terms of a behavior more specifically human, to conciliate. More formally, then, as we consider people acting and interacting, we distinguish the following:

- *Emotion for the organization of behavior.* These *internal aspects* affect prioritization, action selection, attention, and learning and thus contribute to successful behavior (yet sometimes have a downside).
- *Emotional expression for communication.* These *external aspects* support social coordination, communicating clues as to one's possible course of behavior, and allowing others to adjust their behavior accordingly.

These internal and external aspects of emotion have co-evolved in animals. Animals need to survive and perform efficiently within their "ecological niche." Patterns of coordination will greatly influence the suite of relevant emotions and the means whereby they are communicated. A full analysis of motivated behavior and the emotional behavior that builds upon it must certainly include somatomotor behavior (bodily movement)—as in feeding and fleeing, and orofacial expression—but even more important may be autonomic effects (as in the regulation of heart rate and blood pressure) and viscero-endocrine effects (cortisol, adrenaline, release of sex hormones). I will not dwell on these effects in this book, but their measurement already provides key data for researchers seeking objective measures of how variations in the built environment affect the stress and emotional state of people they observe. Gathering and analysis of such data rest on detailed study of the *autonomic* nervous system, combining the *sympathetic* and the *parasympathetic* nervous systems. However, the focus here will continue to be on the *central* nervous system.

Charles Darwin's (1872) concern with relating facial expressions of certain animals to human emotional expression placed the *external role* of emotion within a comparative, and thus implicitly evolutionary, framework. This in turn set the stage for the notion that the internal role of emotions in affecting behavior has an evolutionary base with a strong social component. With this, let's introduce some related neuroanatomy, offer a few ideas on the evolution and roles of emotion, and consider various mechanisms of the central nervous system.

An anatomy of emotion

The anatomical core of our emotional system is the so-called *limbic system*. It has nothing to do with our limbs. It gets its name because early neuroanatomists noted how it "throws its arms" (metaphorically speaking) around the *thalamus*, the set of key waystations through which all sensory systems except olfaction pass signals from the periphery to their primary sensory cortex. Figure 4.8 shows the relative position of key components—the amygdala, hippocampus, and cingulate gyrus—in the human brain. Of course, emotions affect and are affected by so many of our mental processes that it comes as no surprise that the limbic system is linked to many other areas of the brain—the figure shows orbital and medial prefrontal cortex, and the temporal lobe as areas with especially tight interactions.

Paul MacLean, one of the foremost contributors to our understanding of the limbic system, put forward a famous theory of brain evolution, that of the *triune brain* (MacLean, 1990). It is still suggestive, but we now know it was too simplistic. In his account, the human brain combines three "brains" that were established successively in response to evolutionary needs. The usual caution: We are not descended from present-day species of reptiles, though primates (and mammals more generally) are descended from ancient reptile-like creatures.[2]

---

2. For a quick tour, see http://www.bobpickett.org/evolution_of_mammals.htm. Mammals evolved from a group of reptiles called the *synapsids* that arose during the Pennsylvanian Period (310 to 275 million years ago). A branch of the synapsids called the *therapsids* appeared by the middle of the Permian Period (275 to 225 million years ago). Over millions of years, some of these therapsids would evolve many features that would later be associated with mammals. It's impossible to know from which of the reptiles the first mammals evolved since hair, warm blood, and milk-producing glands do not fossilize.

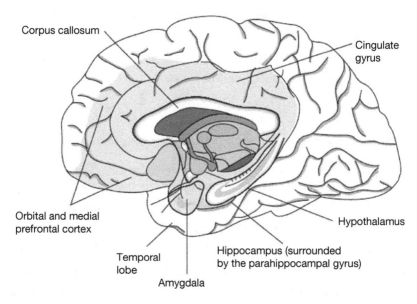

Corpus callosum

Cingulate gyrus

Orbital and medial prefrontal cortex

Hypothalamus

Temporal lobe

Hippocampus (surrounded by the parahippocampal gyrus)

Amygdala

Figure 4.8 A medial view of the human limbic system, showing relative placement of amygdala, hippocampus, cingulate gyrus, orbital and medial prefrontal cortex, and temporal lobe in the human brain. (From Arbib, M. A. [2012]. *How the brain got language: The mirror system hypothesis.* New York and Oxford: Oxford University Press. Adapted from Williams, S. M., White, L. E., & Mace, A. C. [2007]. *Sylvius 4: An interactive atlas and visual glossary of human neuroanatomy.* Sunderland, MA: Sinauer Associates, Inc., Publishers, in association with Pyramis Studios.)

For MacLean, the core is the so-called **"reptilian" brain** and includes the hypothalamus, brainstem, cerebellum, and basal ganglia. Its purpose is closely related to actual physical survival and maintenance of the body. The cerebellum and basal ganglia orchestrate movement, while other subsystems regulate reproduction, circulation, breathing, and the execution of the "fight or flight" response in stress.

Next comes the **limbic system,** including the amygdala and the hippocampus. The amygdala comes into play in situations that arouse feelings such as fear, anger, or outrage. The hippocampus may assess "emotion markers" to bias what events are more likely to be remembered. The limbic system may inhibit the "reptilian" brain's responses. It also supports activities related to expression and mediation of emotions and feelings, including emotions linked to attachment.

The neocortex, or cerebral cortex, makes long-term planning, language, and formal thinking possible.

However, although reptiles (as well as amphibians, like frogs) have a great proportion of the brain in what we now call the midbrain, and little in the way of a forebrain, the human midbrain is *not* just like a reptile brain. Not only has the cortex evolved, but so have the cerebellum and basal ganglia, with new regions working in concert with the neocortex. Substructures involved with more basic functions may be more similar to those in reptiles. For example, the head movements of reptiles become supplemented by eye movements in humans. Moreover, when neocortex evokes voluntary actions, it may well inhibit the automatic "reptilian" responses that would otherwise occur.

Such inhibition may itself depend on one's current emotional state. When relaxing in one's living room with an engrossing book, all but the strongest external stimuli may be ignored, but if one is afraid, as when walking in strange woods on a moonless night, cortex will be "on full alert" to signals from the midbrain system as you react to every movement seen "out of the corner of your eye," and every sound but your own footsteps, even the wind soughing in the trees.

With increasing *encephalization* (MacLean's third stage, wherein the neocortex occupies a larger and larger proportion of the nervous system) comes the ability to integrate one's immediate wants, needs, and desires into a longer term perspective. To use vocabulary introduced in discussing vision, our behavior is not a simple "bottom-up" realization of our instinctual patterns; rather, it combines these with "top-down" influences reflective of our personal experiences and the culture that partially shaped them. I offer a somewhat different perspective on the evolution of emotion in the later subsection, "From motivation to emotion."

Let's focus for now on one limbic area, the *amygdala* (whose name, Latin for *almond*, evokes its shape as discerned by early neuroanatomists), a crucial part of the brain's emotion system. It has been linked to how mammals learn that certain objects or places are to be feared (LeDoux, 2000) and in humans is related to the recognition of facial expressions that tell one that someone is to be feared or distrusted (Adolphs, Tranel, & Damasio, 1998). People with lesions to the amygdala can still recognize other people on seeing their faces, but can no longer make sound judgments as to the likelihood that a stranger should be mistrusted. Thus, our social interactions with others involve gaining a reliable impression of their general character as well their current emotions and intentions. The amygdala can influence cortical areas by way of feedback from proprioceptive or visceral signals or hormones and via projections to various "arousal" networks, while cognitive functions organized in prefrontal regions can in turn regulate the amygdala and its fear reactions.

This exemplifies a major principle for organization in the human brain: the limbic system can be somewhat controlled by cortical systems, but it also projects *back* massively to the voluntary control systems of cerebral cortex. Our behavior does not toggle back and forth between emotion and cognition, but involves a constant interaction between the two (indeed, they are not truly separated)—which is not to deny that one or the other can predominate in different situations.

We cannot understand what brains contribute to our humanity unless we understand how emotion interacts with basic behaviors all the way up to higher cognition. Further, the contribution of any one brain area must be seen in the context of larger networks of which it is part. Each part of the brain is a context for other brain regions, and these evolve in conversation with each other as they help contribute to survival—just as our own development has meaning only within a social context of interpersonal interaction.

Neuromodulation

In §2.5, we saw that the effect of a spike arriving at a synapse may be *excitatory*, making the postsynaptic neuron more likely to fire or, conversely, *inhibitory*, tending to make it less likely to fire, and we noted that *synaptic plasticity*—differential changes in the weights of the input synapses of a neuron—can greatly affect the set of input patterns that will cause a neuron to fire. This is why such plasticity plays a central role in many theories of the neural mechanisms of learning and memory. However, I also noted that some synaptic inputs emit a chemical substance called a neuromodulator that can modulate the way the postsynaptic neuron behaves in diverse ways other than excitation or inhibition.

Neuromodulators are released by neurons of a few specialized brain nuclei with diffuse projections (i.e., widespread distribution of their axons to allow transmission of the neuromodulators at their synaptic endbulbs). These nuclei receive inputs from brain areas at all levels of behavior. Each neuromodulator typically activates specific families of macromolecules called "receptors" that are inserted in postsynaptic membranes. The receipt of its neuromodulator by a receptor yields specific effects on the neuron at various time scales from a few milliseconds to minutes and hours. Each class of neuron has its own mix of receptors. Neuromodulation thus provides a high impact signal that can fundamentally change the way anything from single neurons and synapses to large neural systems "computes."

In Chapter 3 we talked about how notions of what is beautiful differ from person to person. This chapter offers a similar perspective on atmosphere. How can shared biology support such differences, yet also support widespread human responses? I invite you to read the following guided tour of neuromodulators with these questions in mind. Intriguingly, the same neuromodulator can play different roles in the nervous systems of different creatures.

Ann Kelley (2005) offered a thoughtful review of three great neuromodulatory systems. Here are some key points from her richly detailed survey, "Neurochemical Networks Encoding Emotion and Motivation: An Evolutionary Perspective":

Dopamine: reward and plasticity: In mammals, dopamine plays a major role in motor activation, appetitive motivation, reward processing, and cellular plasticity, and may well play a major role in emotion. *Dopaminergic* neurons are those that release dopamine at their synapses to modulate activity in postsynaptic neurons. In the mammalian brain, a major dopamine pathway ascends from the midbrain to innervate the striatum (part of the basal ganglia). Studies in the awake, behaving monkey show dopamine neurons that fire to predicted rewards, and track expected and unexpected environmental events. Moreover, dopamine plays essential roles all the way from "basic" motivational systems to the working memory systems in prefrontal networks that are essential to linking emotion and consciousness. In §5.3, we will see that neural mechanisms for "reinforcement learning" are strongly linked to the dopaminergic system.

Here are two comments focused on the role of dopamine in mediating reward:

EvoDevo: At the more or less innate level, normal development will distribute the dopamine signals to specific brain regions and to specific neuron types with possibly distinctive receptors. Thus, the very distinctiveness of the circuitry in these regions will lead to very different effects of reward signals—there is no reason to expect a visual stimulus to be rewarding in the same way as a muscular effort.

Socio: One of the best known studies of learning is the classical conditioning study by Ivan Pavlov (1927) in which, after repeated ringing of a bell just before a dog was given food, the ringing of the bell alone was enough to make the dog salivate. The point is that learning can make a stimulus pleasurable if the environment (whether natural or in the laboratory) is such that the stimulus is associated often enough with a pleasurable outcome. Similarly, conditioning can create aversion to something that previously elicited neutral affect. The dog's salivation is a long way from appreciating the beauty of a symphony, but one can imagine that the soothing tones of a mother about to feed her infant may create a disposition to enjoy hearing the mother's voice, and hearing similar tones may then serve as a reward for further development of an aesthetic sense. In humans, such cumulative experiential impact on reward systems can be immensely modified by the use of language—so that social dynamics can enter as we take pleasure in experiences that others tell us are pleasurable. And so it goes.

Serotonin: aggression and depression: Serotonin has been implicated in many functions, including behavioral state regulation and arousal, motor pattern generation, sleep, learning and plasticity, food intake, mood, and social behavior. The cell bodies of serotonergic neurons are found in midbrain and other regions in the mammalian brain and have extensive descending and ascending projections. Serotonin plays a critical role in the modulation of aggression and agonistic social interactions in many animals. Even in crayfish, serotonin plays a specific role in social status and aggression (Edwards & Spitzer, 2006)—showing how far back in the evolutionary tree these neuromodulatory systems must have emerged. In primates, with the system's expansive development and innervation of the cerebral cortex, serotonin has come to play an even broader role in cognitive and emotional regulation than in other creatures, particularly control of negative mood or affect.

Opioid peptides: pain and pleasure: Opioids, which include the endorphins, enkephalins, and dynorphins, are found particularly within regions involved in emotional regulation, responses to pain and stress, endocrine regulation, and food intake. Increased opioid function is clearly associated with positive affective states such as relief of pain, and with feelings of euphoria, well-being, or relaxation. Activation of opioid receptors promotes maternal behavior in mothers and attachment behavior and social play in juveniles. Separation distress, exhibited by archetypal behaviors and calls in most mammals and birds, is reduced by opiate agonists (i.e., substances that work with opioids) and increased by opiate antagonists (substances that work against opioids) in many species (Panksepp, 1998). Opiates can also reduce or eliminate the physical sensation induced by a painful stimulus as well as the negative emotional state it induces.

Much of the investigation of central opioids has been fueled by an interest in understanding the nature of addiction—these drugs and the neuromodulatory systems they stimulate may have great adaptive value in certain contexts yet may be maladaptive in others. We now know all too well that opioids developed to reduce pain can be abused to produce pleasure in a way that comes to dominate other motivations, and lead to an addiction so powerful that it can ruin the lives of addicts and those around them. The lesson here is that the modern world can build on our basic motivational and neuromodulatory systems in beneficial ways, or can develop technologies that overstimulate one or more of these systems to an extent that proves destructive.

What is striking here is the way in which these three great neuromodulatory systems seem to be distinct from each other in their overall functionalities, while each exhibits immense diversity of behavioral consequences. The different effects depend both on molecular details (the receptors that determine how a cell will respond to the presence of the neuromodulator) and global arrangements (the circuitry within the modulated brain region, and the connections of that region within the brain). However, exploring how relevant such details are to the A↔N conversation is a challenge outside the scope of this book.

From motivation to emotion

The animal (including the human) comes with a set of basic *drives*—for hunger, thirst, sex, self-preservation, social behaviors, and more—and these provide the basic "motor," motivation, for behavior. These drives, which Derek Denton calls *primordial emotions* (Denton, McKinley, Farrell, & Egan, 2009), yield animal behaviors that we may want to label as akin to those of humans. However, there is much debate as to the extent to which other animals have feelings in the way humans do. Presumably, the human neocortex supports emotional experiences that are unavailable to other animals, or are akin to human experiences only in diluted form. There is a danger of *anthropomorphism*, blurring the distinction, but there is also a danger of ignoring essential commonalities.

Drives correspond to the genetically programmed behavior patterns that aid *homeostasis*, balancing the milieu interieur—such as thirst, various hungers (e.g., for air, food, specific minerals), and avoidance of pain—as well as those that contribute to other aspects of survival, such as fear to help avoid predators, the sex drive to move on to reproduction, and so on—but also maternal behavior and hierarchies of social dominance. Karl Pribram (1960) quipped that the limbic system is responsible for the four Fs: feeding, fighting, fleeing, and reproduction. Interestingly, three of the four have a strong social component—and we may add a fifth F, Family, to his list.

The *hypothalamus* has specialized nuclei (subregions) whose circuitry organizes basic motor behaviors appropriate for such drives. Stimulate one nucleus and the animal is compelled to drink; stimulate another and the animal flies into a sham rage—real in behavioral terms, sham only in that there is no environmental or social reason for the animal to be enraged. It requires other parts of the brain to determine which motor routines the hypothalamus needs to activate at any particular time. The limbic system provides basic systems to mobilize them.

In nonhumans, "knowing" when to eat or drink (related in part to the day–night cycle) or to mate (related in most nonhumans to a mating season) is handled for the most part by bodily systems and innate, specialized neural systems closely coupled to them. A crucial aspect of mammalian evolution that may be intimately linked to distinguishing motivation from emotion is the ability to plan behaviors on the basis of future possibilities rather than only in terms of present contingencies. A frog lives in the present, with very little predictive ability. As we compare frog to rat to cat to monkey, the ability to link current decisions to past experiences and future possibilities becomes more explicit and more diverse as the role of cortex expands to form increasingly complex associations, time evaluation, and so on. For example, hunger may stimulate behaviors that engage (through evolution and/or learning) an increasingly complex cognitive map to reach sites that support hunting or foraging, and increasingly subtle and longer term strategies to guide the behaviors that locate and capture the food. This may support in turn the development of the ability to make preparations for hunger even when one is not experiencing it, as in the caching of food by blue jays and squirrels. Within the EvoDevoSocio framework and the perspective of biocultural evolution, we may see architecture as expressing, after eons of evolution, a highly encephalized extension of such foresight—of making efforts to provide shelter or other spaces in advance of the needs they will assuage.

When the emotional state of one individual induces a matching or closely related state in another, we speak of *emotional contagion* (Hatfield, Cacioppo, & Rapson, 1994), extending the familiar effects of yawning and smiling to emotion—for example, contagion of sadness or joy. Going beyond this simple spread of undirected feeling, emotional and motivational states often manifest themselves in behavior specifically directed at a partner. If you recognize that someone else is angry, then your general behavior is probably framed within some overarching emotion such as *fear* (in which case you may try to avoid this person), *sympathy* (in which case you may seek to understand and soothe the other's anger), or your own *anger* (perhaps trying to get in the first punch). We shall have more to say on this topic in our discussion of empathy and the aesthetics of architecture in Chapter 5.

Emotions serve not only to regulate our current behavior and immediate social interaction. The more emotionally charged our current state, the more likely are we to remember aspects of the current situation. Memories too may be emotionally charged, or we may simply remember that the experience was emotional yet not feel the emotion itself. We may speak of the *heat* of the emotion; others would speak of the visceral sensations that provide the true intensity of an emotion, invoking the autonomic nervous system. On one occasion, you may recall somebody's reprehensible behavior and feel the heat of anger in doing so; on another occasion, you may coolly recall that, yes, his behavior really was quite deplorable. In one case, you are reviving that heat, those bodily feelings of anger; in the other case, you just recall your cognitive appraisal of the other's behavior.

A primordial emotion can, using Denton's phrase, have "plenipotentiary power" over behavior. Hunger, for example, is accompanied by specific sensations that when severe may compel one to seek gratification by a consummatory act—seeking food and then eating it. Fear and pain can lead to extreme patterns of avoidance. This is a far cry from the quiet contemplation of a wide range of courses of action. It may be an important part of what makes us human—that these two faces of emotion can at times be separated even though normally they coexist.

Antonio Damasio (1994) takes a somewhat benign and overemphatic view of the emotions:

> Rather than being the antithesis of rationality, emotions aid human reasoning. People can reason and deliberate as much as they want, but, as neuroscientists have found, if there are no emotions attached to the various options in front of them, they will never reach a decision or conviction.

Certainly, as in our example of getting started in the morning, motivation and emotion may shape our overall plans. But if you decide to visit Todai-Ji and start checking the airline schedules for flights to Osaka, it seems that the long-term planning involved is far removed from the eventual gratification of an aesthetic or religious motivation perhaps weeks later. Or, again, consider a teenager assiduously studying mathematics in the hope of becoming, many years later, an aeronautical engineer. Yes, emotions (or, more basically, drives) can provide a necessary impetus for action and a beneficent modulation of our perception, but as the neocortex becomes more and more important in the evolving brain, so do we go from the obligatory linkage of appetitive to consummatory behavior—if we are hungry we must find a way to get food—to an increasingly long-term view of our priorities, in which a lengthening chain of goals and subgoals may temporarily override the almost-imperatives of the primordial emotions and of other emotions as well.

Both as individuals and social actors, we are able to take actions that are defined within a long-term timeframe, supported in part by our use of language to explicitly analyze alternative futures and to contemplate hypothetical as well as actual situations. This complexity in turn supports new emotions, of which perhaps the most human, though not the most worthy, is what the Germans call *Schadenfreude*, the taking of pleasure in the misfortunes of others—a long way from primordial emotions, yet able to color our behavior in many subtle ways. Indeed, emotions are not always beneficial—they can help or hinder our long-term efforts. Passions can override one's thoughtful control of behavior. In humans, an emotion may surge up and dominate the stream of consciousness (e.g., lust or rage), submerging any coherent rationality.

But what might this mean for the architect? To begin answering this, let's consider the aesthetic emotions.

Aesthetic emotions

Writing in the context of the relationship between music and language, Klaus Scherer (2013) refers to emotions such as anger, fear, joy, or disgust as *utilitarian emotions*—the ones that build fairly directly on the basic emotions shared across many species to help shape our practical behavior. However, biocultural evolution has led to other functions of emotional expression in humans, particularly in the domain of social empathy and bonding, where shame and guilt seem to depend on a certain richness of symbolic expression in which various social norms can be made explicit. Such a capacity for symbolism can also support magic/religious ritual and the tapping of the capacity for pain and pleasure in ways that go beyond the failure or success of consummation of basic drives. This in turn can lead to the pursuit of beauty, involving what Scherer calls *aesthetic emotions*, which are desired and sought out through engagement with cultural practices such as music, art, or literature.

Our EvoDevoSocio framework suggests that, rather than biological evolution yielding new genetic mechanisms to support the broad range of aesthetic emotions, the appreciation of beauty may have emerged as part of mechanisms for family bonding, for mate selection, for finding refuge, and for foraging. What further changed was that in human *cultural* evolution, the basic biological mechanisms became enmeshed with ever more complex social structures and practices made possible by neocortical circuitry. These in turn have made new technologies possible, as well as the resources to develop music, art, and literature—and even architecture. With this, the aesthetic emotions could become separate targets for individual development and cultural evolution with respect to these new bodies of social practice.

We might thus speak of an ancient endowment of protoaesthetic emotions that provided the basis for the cultural evolution of aesthetic emotions. The suggestion is that, while protoaesthetic emotions are part and parcel of utilitarian emotions, aesthetic emotions evolved (culturally) beyond the realm of the utilitarian—though there are no hard and fast boundaries here. Praxic goals and coping potential came to play a much less important role in aesthetic emotions than they do in utilitarian emotions. An aesthetic experience is one in which the appreciation of the intrinsic qualities of a piece of visual art or music or architecture is of paramount importance. This corresponds in many ways to the distinction made by William James (1890) between "coarse" and "subtle or refined" emotions. Frijda and Sundararajan (2007) suggest that refined emotions tend to occur in situations in which goals directly relevant to survival or fundamental well-being are not in the center of the individual's attention, proposing that such emotions are more felt than acted upon, and do not show strong physiological arousal. Note, though, that we can experience complex combinations of emotional response—in looking at a painting, for example, you may simultaneously admire its beauty, feel anger through empathy with what the painting portrays, and be surprised that its style is not what you have come to expect from that artist. Moreover, these emotions are socially instilled atop a biological basis of feeling, but with individual experience our aesthetic judgments may remain attuned to the local norm or may come to diverge considerably.

Another piece of the puzzle is offered by Koelsch et al. (2015, §2.3.3):

Once an organism has satisfied bodily needs and achieved homeostasis, the organism is satiated, and stimuli that were incentive before can become even aversive. . . . [But] a brain system for attachment-related affect that does not satiate is evolutionar[il]y adaptive, because feeling attached to a child, loving a child and feeling the joy of being together with the child are emotions that serve the continuous protection, and nurturing of the offspring.

Perhaps these emotions of childrearing (the fifth F) may be a surer basis than the primordial emotions of the four Fs for understanding aesthetic emotions. Yes, child care invokes primordial emotions in many (but by no means all) species, but its sense of prolonged attachment can provide the evolutionary core of a range of emotions that seem specifically human. Aesthetic emotions can produce physiological changes that may serve behavioral readiness or the specific, adaptive action tendencies for attention, sharpening of sensory perception, and regulation of arousal (Frijda, 1986). Bodily symptoms such as goosebumps, shivers, or moist eyes can be external markers of what the connoisseur would consider the essence of such emotions.

In architecture, as in other utilitarian arts, the aesthetic and the utilitarian are somehow intermixed, and there is no hard boundary between the two. Nonetheless, there is a distinction, and architectural design involves a tradeoff between them. Indeed, sophisticated architects can use an enlarged understanding of human experience—such as that the A↔N conversation is intended to provide—to find ways that the two can be developed together to serve each other. In a store that sells expensive jewelry, a spacious layout with the jewelry displayed in vitrine tables will be arranged to heighten the aesthetic appeal of the jewelry—but, of course, this is all to the utilitarian end of attracting wealthy customers and persuading them to buy. Contrast this with a convenience store where the accessibility of diverse products predominates over the aesthetics of their display.

Or consider, for example, walking in a city around lunchtime. One may be somewhat hungry, but one's hunger does not yet have "plenipotentiary power." Then one turns a corner and sees signs proclaiming a variety of restaurants. This incentive raises hunger to one's prime motivation. But where to eat? The signs may provide an initial screening, but one uses each attractive sign to locate a doorway—not, initially, as an affordance for entry but as an affordance for the process of searching for a menu. If the menu proves appetizing, then a glimpse through the door or window may establish whether the atmosphere is one of uncomfortable but fast eating, of conviviality, of elegant leisure, or of off-putting opulence. . . .

The deciding incentive may even come from the atmosphere in the literal sense: the odors of the cooking that may provide, or suppress, the incentive to eat.

Here, we see the ongoing interaction between motivation, incentives, atmosphere, and relevant Gibsonian affordances in driving the continuing action–perception cycle. Note that neither hunger, incentive, nor atmosphere is itself an affordance in the Gibsonian sense. Between them, they may motivate one, but satisfying that motivation rests on determining a series of actions—enter the restaurant, sit at a table, order food, use utensils to get the food, and so on—each of which requires the recognition of affordances for that specific action.

Even in a contemplative act like admiring a painting, one exploits Gibsonian affordances to position oneself in a good vantage point. The architect and curator of an art gallery have, hopefully, worked together to determine the likely number of visitors at any one time and then set the distribution of paintings to accommodate their viewing, as well as designing the lighting so that most visitors will be able to find a vantage point where enjoyment of the painting is not marred by highlights and reflections.

4.3. ATMOSPHERE AS A NON-GIBSONIAN AFFORDANCE

Gibson (1979, p. 140) wrote that "the perceiving of an affordance is not a process of perceiving a value-free physical object to which meaning is somehow added in a way that no one has been able to agree upon; it is a process of perceiving a value-rich ecological object." It is the word *ecological* that is crucial for Gibson—he is referring to the *action-value* of an object, its pragmatic affordance, the opportunities for action it provides. Clearly, the affordances we perceive in an object vary with our intentions—as in distinguishing affordances for menu location for the door of a restaurant and the "usual" affordance of a door for the action of movement from one space to another.

However, Tonino Griffero (2015) argues that we should also consider *atmosphere* as a form of affordance, what I shall call a "non-Gibsonian" affordance. He asserts that forms do not "merely" express causal relations and pragmatic affordances but also "sentimental and therefore atmospheric ones that permeate the space."[3] Our slogan is thus "Gibsonian affordances are for motion, for action; whereas atmospheric affordances are for emotion, for feeling, for overall impact." Some might view this as a difference between "effects" and "affects," respectively. Although there are no hard-and-fast distinctions, I think drive- and emotion-related incentives—think of the smell of freshly baked bread as both an invitation and an incentive to eat bread, while architectural atmosphere offers perceptual cues for experiencing a particular mood—are non-Gibsonian, rather than Gibsonian, affordances.

As a tantalizing parallel, we can relate this complementarity to our discussion (§3.5) of Arnheim's vector fields of "non-Gibsonian" attraction and repulsion that support aesthetic form, and the "Gibsonian" potential fields invoked in modeling frog visuomotor coordination. This comparison offers another area in which the neuroscientist might look for an evolutionary relationship between Gibsonian and non-Gibsonian affordances, and between utilitarian and aesthetic emotions.

Whether primary or not, symbolism may be an important part of the design of a building, and may serve as one aspect of atmosphere. Consider an impressive courthouse with a grand entrance and then, below it, a mean little door on the steps leading down to the prison beneath—symbolizing the majesty of the law and the crushing weight of justice bearing down on the guilty. An alternative symbolism—of prisoners being consigned to

---

3. A major source for this chapter section was a symposium on *Architecture and Atmosphere* (Tidwell, 2015) held in Helsinki under the auspices of Juhani Pallasmaa and his colleagues. There were three speakers. Gernot Böhme spoke on "Atmosphere: New Perspectives for Architecture and Design," Tonino Griffero on "Architectural Affordances: The Atmospheric Authority of Space," and Jean-Paul Thibaud on "Installing an Atmosphere." For more on the topic, see *Atmospheres* by Peter Zumthor (2006), and the collections *Building Atmosphere* (Havik, Teerds, & Tielens, 2013) and *Architectural Atmospheres: On the Experience and Politics of Architecture* (Borch, 2014), which contain further essays by Böhme, Pallasmaa, Zumthor, and others.

their fate—is afforded by the Bridge of Sighs in Venice, but note that this symbolism is not inherent in the bridge itself, which may appear rather attractive unless one knows the way in which it was employed. The relation between symbolism and atmosphere poses a continuing challenge.

Gernot Böhme (2015) urges us to think of the atmosphere of a building as "a kind of a spatially extended feeling, that it creates." He suggests that atmosphere is "the sort of smell of the nest, the 'air' that allows one to feel at home."[4] However, this is not very helpful for assessing buildings other than homes. Our lunchtime example provided another bridge to the colloquial use of the term "atmosphere"—the initial impression of a restaurant may be olfactory as well as visual. But the atmosphere of, for example, a bank or a hospital may be completely different from that of a nest or some place with happy associations. Indeed (back to Edinburgh Castle in time of war), the atmosphere may be highly negative, such as one of foreboding. Conversely, a modern hospital may be explicitly designed to attempt to counteract the unease and uncertainty associated with disease. More generally, then, atmosphere is both spatial and emotional at the same time. Zumthor (2012, p. 12) tells us,

> I do not think of (Architecture) primarily as either a message or a symbol, but as an envelope and background for life which goes on in and around it, a sensitive container for the rhythm of footsteps on the floor, for the concentration of work, for the silence of sleep.

Böhme offers an integrated view of "atmospheric affordances"—the stage-setting and the shifting mood—and the physical affordances for the range of actions the user will take within the action–perception cycle within the space:

> The architect . . . is . . . primarily concerned with . . . the structure and articulation of spaces. These spaces may be open or closed,

---

4. Compare the emphasis offered by Sarah Robinson (2011) in her choice of title, *Nesting: Body, Dwelling, Mind*, for her book on architecture.

narrow or wide, pressing or uplifting. They may have a center and thus a directional orientation; they may frame sights or open to the indefinite. . . . [T]he architect at the same time sets "suggestions for movement," actual movement as when the visitor steps around the space or virtual movement as when he follows lines and surfaces with his eyes. All these considerations mean that the architect when designing anticipates what sort of lived place he is constructing and how the future visitor or dweller will feel [and not just feel!] there. (Böhme, 2015, p. 13)

Here, Böhme shifts the emphasis from the structure of the building to the spaces that these buildings create, whether in providing affordances for behavior in the building or for creating atmosphere—the texture of a wall may be as important as the space it encloses. The visual impact is important and can have strong emotional correlates, but the true measure is how people use the space and how they live in it. Just as in vision there is the idea of a *gist*, a building makes a first impression that can then be integrated in various nuanced fashions. For Griffero, that impression *is* the atmosphere:

Architectural atmospheres are . . . responsible for "immediate understanding, immediate contact, immediate rejection," and are generated fundamentally by everything [sic!]: "things, people, air, noises, tone, colours, material presences, structures, also forms" . . . [B]y generating "orientations, kinetic suggestions, markings," buildings produce therefore a wide range of atmospheres and as authentic scripted spaces force the perceiver to immerse themselves in them.

For Jean-Paul Thibaud (2015), the atmosphere may change dynamically. My concern is that Griffero here ignores the temporal impact of the details. Moreover (as will be seen further later), though the spaces may be scripted to meet specific user needs, they are (often) places in which people can also write their own scripts rather than being "forced" into a particular form of immersion.

Let's now relate the comments of Böhme and Griffero to the observation that there are many "maps in the brain"—action-oriented spatial reference frames—that offer different perspectives on the external world as part of the brain's organization of sensory and motor data relevant to specific types of action (§2.2). There are representations that we can use when walking around, representations that guide the way we reach, and representations that shape our hand in anticipation of the object we reach for. Our conscious experience gives us the "illusion" of a unified experience of the world around us as our brain integrates visual maps with those for sound, touch, and other senses and then, as the action–perception cycle progresses, translates these data into the diverse maps that control the action of the arm, the shape of the hand, the movement of the eyes, locomotion, and much more.

When preparing construction drawings, the architect may employ the precise distances and angles of Euclidean space as the frame in which the building is located. However, our experience of the spaces the architect designs are, instead, in terms of how the surfaces are shaped that enclose or confront us, including those that we readily perceive from the current vantage point, and different neural systems will accept diverse invitations of the affordances for exploration and action, as well as the atmosphere that shapes our mood, or offers opportunities for aesthetic experience. There is a real value to architects if they think in terms of the "unfolding" and changing of all these varied affordances as we spend time within a building, acting, interacting, or contemplating.

Griffero (p. 30) suggests that the impressive entrance hall of a traditional bank will express an *atmosphere of power* for those who venture there in search of a loan but an *atmosphere of proud belonging* for an employee who has developed a strong *esprit de corps*. "What generates both atmospheres (uneasiness and pride) is still the same: the spatial-sentimental quality of solemn vastness." Griffero (p. 37) adds that in "designing buildings architects . . . should indeed contrive places that invite certain behaviors and so be aware of how to create affordances and how they are perceived," blending atmosphere with affordances in the Gibsonian sense.

The atmosphere of a hospital is, as hinted earlier, tense precisely because we anticipate the situation to follow (e.g., the visit, the diagnosis) and we remember earlier ones (e.g., further waits). "Am I going to get better or not? What's the operation going to be? What drugs am I going to be forced to take?" The architect, though, can find ways of creating an atmosphere that will, for many patients, reduce that sense of fear or foreboding and instill a measure of confidence. There is both a function of the hospital and an atmosphere of the hospital, and the architect can strive to defuse the "default" atmosphere by providing conditions that, at least to some extent, relax the tension, as in a children's hospital with murals of favorite story characters on the wall. Indeed, a soothing atmosphere can contribute to the functional goal of healing by its psychosomatic effects.[5]

Thus, not only is the atmosphere of a space defined by the relation between the person and the place, but also the person's perception differs greatly depending on their current tasks. A winding path that is delightful when one has time for a quiet stroll may be frustrating when one is running late for an appointment. This does not deny that the architect may seek to instill a place with a certain atmosphere for a certain range of users—but one that may vary for different types of user (the bank example) or for its inhabitants with time of day, as in a restaurant with a very different atmosphere at breakfast, lunch, and dinner that may be accompanied by changes in table setting and layout, lighting, and background music. Note, too, the different spaces that matter to staff and clients, and the very different affordances that each will exploit.

Nonetheless, despite these differing roles, and differences between individuals, architects have a program to meet, and so they must seek to ensure

---

5. This ties back to the main question addressed by the Academy of Neuroscience for Architecture (ANFA): "How do you take a particular typology of building and seek to understand the neural and mental processes of people, and adjust the building to improve its impact on humans? What sort of building will provide the right affordances and atmosphere?" The "menu" of needed affordances and appropriate atmosphere is different for each typology. We are back to Eberhard's original vision (§1.3).

that the building will serve the purposes suggested for its various groups of users. Here, they will rely on the notion that there is a dimension to atmospheres that is objective in at least statistical terms, otherwise the design could not be expected to achieve some commonality of responses. This, then, might define what comes to be considered as "the" atmosphere of a building, abstracted from the variation of individual experience. Indeed, the discussion of Todai-Ji and Notre-Dame suggests that there may be fundamental organic responses (with some evolutionary basis, as for awe) that may then be subject to various cultural and personal influences.

Stage-setting

We keep looking at photos in this book, but we must always be thinking back to our multisensory experience as we act within real buildings, real landscapes. It is that interaction that cumulatively provides both the overall (possibly dynamic) atmosphere and those details that are essential to the way we act. This requires cog/neuroscience to develop a neuroaesthetics for architecture, as distinct from paintings or music, that emphasizes how people act and react in architected spaces, and how this may have a lasting impact on individuals.

We have seen Griffero's comment that "buildings produce . . . a wide range of atmospheres and *as authentic scripted spaces* [my italics] force the perceiver to immerse themselves in them." Similarly, Wigley (1998) says that "architecture is but *a stage set* that produces a sensuous atmosphere."[6] What can we learn from this comparison?

In the theater, the stage designer has created an environment that contains the scenes that are meant to capture our whole attention as we become engaged with the emotions and experiences portrayed by the actors. We stop thinking about the rustling of the programs, or the noisy

---

6. In his cognitive history of architectural design, *Draw in Order to See*, Mark Alan Hewitt (2020) devotes Chapter 6 to a highly relevant historical account of "Scenography and Craft in the Baroque."

popcorn eaters, and instead are transported into that little world on the stage. The stage designer is given a script that already exists and establishes an environment for the behavior of the actors as set down in that script by the dialogue and stage directions, helping the actors engage the audience, drawing them into the experience of the characters in the play (who are not the same as the people on the stage). However, with architecture, we leave the line-by-line scripts of the playwright for scripts in the sense introduced in §2.1 of setting forth general rules for a particular kind of behavior. The architect creates a "stage" on which we become active participants. Its affordances may support diverse behaviors—as customers in a restaurant or a bank, say, we tend to follow a basic script with variations, while we have diverse scripts and variations for living at home.

Within these constraints, and the social schemas that both support and constrain behavior in different environments, people will vary the scripts, and the scripts will in some sense play out differently, depending on how the currently available affordances match their needs and goals—and depending on how the various incentives modify the needs and goals that were driving them before this encounter. In addition to the impact of Gibsonian affordances, though, these self-generated scripts will also play out differently depending on the general mood that the building engenders. Am I depressed when I am here, in an old hospital with dingy walls and the smell of disinfectant? Or am I exhilarated when I am here, as I was (long ago) in the central hall of Saarinen's TWA Terminal? The idea of architecture as providing a stage set is provocative, but a building does not just produce a sensuous atmosphere. It provides an environment in which we not only follow variations on scripts considered by the architect but also develop our own scripts within certain constraints of the typology of the building, as adjusted to our own needs.

But is it possible to design atmospheres? Böhme (p. 75) asserts:

Stage design succeeds in producing a certain climate, and so stage designers tacitly know how to do this. Moreover, their work proves the inter-subjectivity of atmospheres. If this were not the case, the whole project of stage design would be nothing at all.

However, the stage-setting itself does not determine the atmosphere. As the actors perform and the script unfolds, the atmosphere changes from scene to scene, and with dramatic turns changing the atmosphere within many scenes as well. We see how crucially the presence of other people can be vital to the creation of a mood. In the same spirit, when architects design, they don't (or should not!) think of an empty building—they envision it as a web of *inhabited spaces*, and so the atmosphere(s) they envision should include the users of those spaces. Indeed, Thibaud holds:

> We must consider atmosphere as the interaction between that space and people living in it. . . . I don't think that we can design an atmosphere, but *we can design the conditions for an atmosphere to appear*. We can design conditions that afford certain activities or actions of people in a place. The interaction between the space and the activity in that space has the potential to produce an atmosphere. [My italics.] (2015, p. 75)

He then returns to the dynamics of atmosphere:

> When we project a space we must also project a way that evolves in time. For that I believe we must have the presence of people immersed in that space or we are only considering a fixed image, which is not an atmosphere. (p. 76)

But Griffero (2015, p. 76) remains unconvinced:

> If an atmosphere changes over time, then which is the real atmosphere of a place? Is it always the last one? The first impression for me is important because it is the point of departure for every other experience. Every experience unfolds from this first impression. This

is for me the real atmosphere of a place. The others are part of a story of atmosphere that is developing with our perception.

Where the atmosphere is the first impression for Griffero, for Thibaud the atmosphere may change dynamically—and it is Thibaud's view that I share. Reverting to our discussion of the external expressions of people's emotions, we may note how differently we may interact with the same person as their mood or emotion shifts, as indeed our appreciation will shift with our own emotion—jolliness that would be welcome on one occasion would become off-putting when we are distressed. Perhaps we should speak of the *action–emotion–perception cycle*, with emotion part of our human dynamic that is open to the emotion of others and the atmospheres-as-we-experience-them of the spaces (whether inhabited or not) that we encounter.

In line with our earlier riffs on stage-setting, we have seen that Thibaud stresses that people (inhabitants, city dwellers, passersby) are part of the production of atmosphere, something exemplified in our view of the tourists outside Edinburgh Castle. People going about what they do creates an atmosphere. Imagine that you're walking down a street, and it has a lively atmosphere. But as you walk on for another block or two, you suddenly realize there's nobody else on the street, and even with no change in architectural style, the atmosphere may change for you from one of pleasure, happy relaxation, to one of, perhaps, fear. You wonder, "What is going on? Why have people gone? Why am I alone? What's going to happen to me?" As night falls, a place that looked friendly may become unfriendly. Or, alternatively, sparkling illuminations may suddenly come on in a place that had looked dull before, and the atmosphere may become joyous.

And what are we to make of the Nuremberg crowd (Figure 4.9), caught up in the Hitler mania of the day and place? For them, a thrilling atmosphere of national solidarity; for us, a chilling atmosphere of Nazi fanaticism. Here, atmosphere and our current understanding of the symbolism made explicit in the swastikas are intertwined. We experience it as enculturated biological beings, historically aware and with a wealth of personal experience and the attendant associations. The affordances the architect

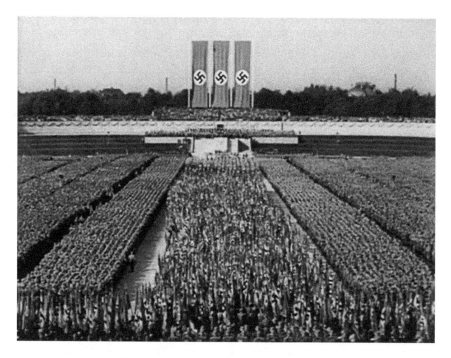

Figure 4.9 The Nuremberg rally. (Still from Leni Riefenstahl's 1935 propaganda film, *Triumph of the Will*, covering Hitler's 1935 Nuremberg Rally. Public domain.)

and the "stage-setting" provide may allow for a wide range of behaviors, or may regiment those behaviors as at the Nuremberg rally—a sinister version of Griffero's notion of "authentic scripted spaces [that] force the perceiver to immerse themselves in them." Here, the individual may become immersed in the psychology of the crowd (Canetti, 1978; Freud, 1959); and in large public arenas it is the psychology of the crowd, rather than the psychology of the individual or the specifics of the architecture that, for good or ill, may dominate the atmosphere.

4.4. THE EVOCATION OF ATMOSPHERE IN PAINTINGS

Despite my general emphasis on action and interaction in a person's response to architecture, consideration of paintings can enrich our encounter with atmosphere. I thus turn now to two paintings that demonstrate how shading, color, and texture can convey atmosphere as well as depicting objects and scenes. The resultant insights will offer a fresh perspective on how architecture may evoke different atmospheres that may vary not only for different observers but also over time for any one observer. Moreover, this section hints at some of the brain mechanisms that support the imagination of the artist—providing ideas that I will apply in charting the beginnings of a cognitive neuroscience of design in architecture in Chapter 10.

Two masterpieces

"Atmosphere is my style," a comment made by J. M. W. Turner to John Ruskin in 1844, provides the epigraph of *Atmospheres* (Zumthor, 2006). When we view Turner's *The Slave Ship* from 1840 (Figure 4.10), our first impression is indeed atmospheric, a bracing experience of beauty, a vivid sunset above a stormy sea. But as we begin to look more closely, the mood changes. There is a ship, and it is obviously in great distress—the storm is no longer merely bracing, there is an atmosphere of tragedy. As the details accumulate, the atmosphere becomes horrifying as we become aware of the manacled hands and legs rising from the water and the sea creatures closing in on them. The back story, which contemporary viewers would have known and which the title *The Slave Ship* suggests, is that the captain of the ship has thrown the slaves overboard to lighten the load and reduce the risk of sinking in the storm. The slaves were treated not as humans but as mere property. Now the atmosphere perhaps shifts again, as we recognize the beauty and the danger of the scene but also reflect with horror on the cruelty of the slave trade (whether from looking at the painting alone, or also through learning more of the back story).[7]

7. This analysis of Turner's *The Slave Ship* was informed in part by the article at https://en.wikipedia.org/wiki/The_Slave_Ship.

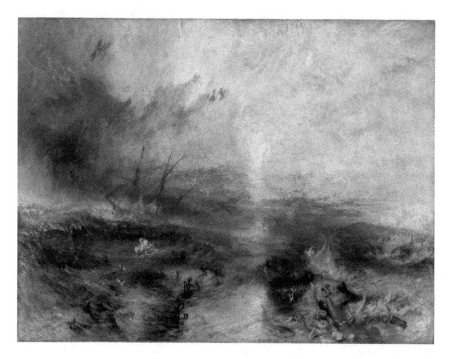

Figure 4.10 J. M. W. Turner, *The Slave Ship* (1840), Museum of Fine Arts, Boston. (https://commons.wikimedia.org/wiki/File:Slave-ship.jpg. Public domain.)

Turner's painting offers a strong social message, but the painting is atmospheric first, and only secondarily representational—but that representation then "installs" a new overall atmosphere of, perhaps, righteous horror, sympathy for suffering, and indignation. The appreciation of the atmosphere and construal of the "intended" meaning of a painting will be to a great extent subjective, but the same may be said of buildings if one compares (with a certain sense of irony) the views of different architectural critics writing about the same building.

When we turn to John Constable's *Salisbury Cathedral From the Meadows* of 1831 (Figure 4.11), we see a painting that is much more clearly delineated. We did not have to search to recognize Salisbury Cathedral and then see the horse drawing a cart across the stream. We clearly recognize the rainbow and the trees as such, and we appreciate

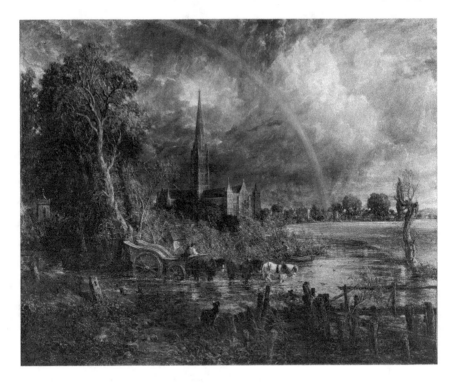

Figure 4.11 John Constable, *Salisbury Cathedral From the Meadows* (1831), Tate Britain, London. (https://commons.wikimedia.org/wiki/File:Constable_Salisbury_meadows.jpg. Public domain.)

the overall composition of these elements. And yet as we look longer at the massing of clouds (perhaps Constable's imaginative collage of multiple observations of cloudscapes near Salisbury) as counterbalanced by the foliage, and with light shining through in judiciously chosen places, we can see that Constable is as much a master of layered evocation of atmosphere through "nonobjects" as Turner. Here, again, creating and evoking atmosphere goes beyond the definition of clear spatial relationships through well-delineated contours to evoke feelings that do not rest on classification of what object appears in precisely which part of the image (or building, when we return to architecture). Saying that part of Constable's painting depicts a cloud does not go far toward giving us its evocative impact.

Inverting vision

The paintings by Turner and Constable are works of the imagination—combining and morphing familiar forms and impressions to create a new ensemble that is an end in itself, that can both inform the viewers and play on their emotions. The sketches prepared by the artist in preparation for the painting may be compared to the sketches and models produced by the architect as intermediary steps toward the detailed specifications that will guide the construction of a building.

How do these behaviors—sketching, drawing, painting, model-making—relate to our discussion of the neuroscience of vision that we met in Chapter 3? To get started, consider "drawing from life" or from memory of real scenes. For example, Albrecht Dürer's *Study of Three Hands* (c. 1490) is, presumably, based on Dürer's observation of his own left hand in three different poses (Figure 4.12). It is the other hand, coupled with eye and brain, that is crucial in transferring each pose to paper. We can see that this involves not only the tracing of contours but also the use of shading to suggest aspects of three-dimensional (3D) shape. Let's try, briefly, to understand something of the neurocognitive basis of Dürer's drawing—though with no attempt to explain Dürer's exceptional genius in drawing and in etching. §8.5 offers further analysis of the neuropsychology of drawing.

In seeking to understand visual perception, we used the VISIONS system (§3.4) to underwrite the way in which a visual scene might be understood by combining *low-level* processes (such as extracting the shape and color of a particular region) with *higher level* processes of competition and cooperation to converge on a set of instances of perceptual schemas as enriched by some of the lower level properties of the regions that emerge through the dynamics of visual processing. But even earlier, in "The thinking hand and its schemas" (§2.4), we had stressed that vision was to be considered within the action–perception cycle—so that, in many cases, recognizing properties of an object and its present relation to us could offer affordances for our possible actions whose parameters could

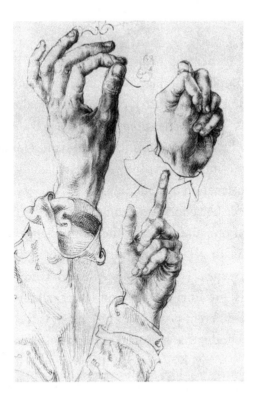

Figure 4.12 Drawing from life: Albrecht Dürer's *Study of Three Hands* (c. 1490), Albertina, Vienna. (https://uploads5.wikiart.org/images/albrecht-durer/study-of-three-hands.jpg. Public domain.)

be passed to the motor schemas that guide those actions. Seeing a hand extended toward us by someone with a welcoming smile, we might grasp the hand and shake it; seeing the hand of a beloved, we might caress it; seeing a hand shaped like a fist, we might move to avoid it and retaliate.

When we turn to drawing from life, the challenge is to use vision of a scene in the real world to create instances of perceptual schemas that can drive motor schemas that do something rather different. Instead of driving interaction with the objects, they drive the motion of the drawing hand to make marks on the paper that will—as exemplified by Dürer's *Study of Three Hands*—create a new visual stimulus that has the possibility to activate some schema instances similar to those evoked in the mind or brain of the artist viewing the original scene.

The primary skill of drawing from life assembles motor schemas that control the hand, using visual feedback all the while, to create on the page a semblance of the scene. But this is far from a photograph. The skilled artist knows what to exclude as much as what to include and knows how to "distort" the drawing in ways that better convey patterns and emotions than would an exact placement of the projection of the 3D scene on the page.

In summary, we see here that *drawing "inverts" vision*: Where vision runs in one direction,

- real-world object (observed scene) → schema assemblage ("mental image"),

drawing runs in the *inverse* direction:

- schema assemblage ("mental image") → real-world object (drawing).

This is the inverse (opposite) in effect, but requires different brain mechanisms for its success.

In the case of drawing from life, the two are combined:

- real-world object (observed scene) → schema assemblage ("mental image") → real-world object (drawing), with the special property that the drawing resembles, in some ways, the appearance of the observed scene.

With repeated practice, the artist becomes skilled in drawing diverse objects and highlighting certain relations between them. However, once this skill has been mastered, the artist can create a schema assemblage that does not emerge from direct observation, or episodic memory of earlier experience, but is new. Artists choose what they wish the viewer to attend to, both immediately and on closer inspection. The work may develop through multiple sketches as the artist not only places representations of objects on paper but also adjusts them and their relationships to achieve atmospheric as well as "semantic" effects—and, in the process, the original conception of the piece may change as the initial work reveals new possibilities and while, perhaps, some of the earlier ideas come to feel unsatisfactory.

In discussing Turner, we saw that as we paid attention to hitherto unobserved details (bottom-up), our understanding of the scene shifted dramatically—and as this occurred, our attention to the painting became more fully directed top-down. In creating *The Slave Ship*, Turner worked back from the horrific story of the event that inspired his painting, complementing his famous style of evocative abstraction of massed color with telling details to create an image that provides the viewer with the dynamic perceptual experience interweaving emerging atmosphere and telling details. Though his brush strokes and palette were judiciously chosen, few defined contours are apparent in the painting. Rather, objects are defined by patterns of color in the painting, and the most prominent colors are the red of the sunset that encroaches into the water and ship as well, and the maroon of the bodies and hands of the slaves.

In summary, then, the task of the artist is in some sense to "invert" vision—creating an artificial object whose visual impact may achieve some intended effect or may, at least, offer some opportunity for contemplative visual exploration. For the architect, the challenge goes further, "inverting the action–perception cycle," to create a new external environment in which people can act and interact (Chapter 10). Here, vision becomes but one of many senses—and, indeed, in designing for the blind, it drops out altogether in the desired effects, though the architects themselves may employ vision in their design practice.

4.5. SEEKING NEURAL CORRELATES OF ENVIRONMENTS INDUCING CONTEMPLATIVE STATES

How can we link a growing understanding of atmosphere in architecture to study of the brain and its emotion-related mechanisms? Some initial steps "in the right direction" are provided by an exploratory fMRI study of architects' responses to "contemplative" architecture (Bermudez et al., 2017). Bermudez et al. sought neural correlates for the way certain buildings may support contemplation for those so inclined. They stress that this is an exploratory study. I view it as a positive step but will offer a critical analysis in this section—not to be negative, but rather to show how their exploration may provide stepping stones to further investigation. But first I need to say something about the methodology of fMRI used in their study, extending the brief comments in §1.4.[8]

Imaging the human brain

In the 19th century, much was learned about the human brain by studying how brain damage, whether through a lesion or some neurological disease, could affect perception. In studying Penfield's homunculi, we saw that much could also be learned from electrical stimulation of the brains of people undergoing neurosurgery. However, a major problem with such studies is that they are based on damaged brains. *Electroencephalography* (EEG), the study of variations in electrical activity from scalp electrodes, has been an invaluable tool since its discovery in 1929 in detecting the timing of various "components" of brain functioning and is still widely employed today in neuroscience. However, while it can report *timing* of activity with millisecond precision, it cannot *localize* the source of that activity in the brain with any precision.

A breakthrough, from the 1970s onward, came with the development of scanning methods that could map the overall structure of a person's brain or pick up how levels of neural activity in the brain would vary as the intact, healthy human subject performed different tasks. We will be particularly concerned with two kinds of data obtained from magnetic resonance imaging (MRI):

8. My thanks to Julio Bermudez for his comments on this section, and on the chapter as a whole.

- *Structural* MRI charts the structure of the brain, essentially by differentiating the magnetic resonance (the explanation of which is outside our scope) of structures with high and low fat content. MRI can be applied to any part of the body, but our interest here is that the MRI view of the 3D structure of the brain allows us to better assess the spatial extent of brain structures as they vary from individual to individual. This permits assessing with which part of which structure a particular activity revealed by functional MRI is associated—the key to the localization that EEG cannot provide.

- *Functional* MRI (fMRI) looks at the changes in activity of different brain regions as the person carries out different tasks. When "activity" of an area of the brain increases, so does blood flow to that region. fMRI can make a 3D scan of the *blood-oxygen-level-dependent* (BOLD) signal (again, I won't go into the details). The technique can localize activity to within a *voxel* (compare the "pixels" that serve as the building blocks for a digital display of a picture), a volume element a few millimeters on a side, but with a time window of a second or so. The BOLD signal is noisy and varies minutely from task to task. It thus takes sophisticated analysis to determine the statistical significance of the claim that the blood flow through a voxel is greater for task A than for task B. Intense computation generates a 3D representation of this statistical significance. As Figure 4.13 shows, we may examine this by looking at *computed* slices of the brain color-coded for statistical significance. Other ways of viewing or analyzing the data are, of course, available. A connected region of high statistical significance is often referred to as a "blob."

The opposite of EEG, fMRI has *relatively* precise localization but poor precision in timing (seconds rather than milliseconds). Its precision is much finer than that of the Brodmann areas, but each voxel contains a few million neurons.

What is the neural activity that the BOLD signal correlates with? My favorite is integrated synaptic activity, the total activation of both excitatory and

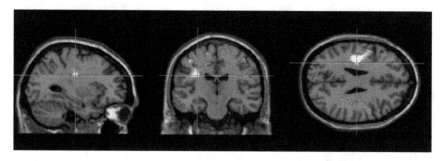

Figure 4.13 An example of functional magnetic resonance imaging (fMRI). The color code represents *statistical significance* that the various voxels have a greater blood-oxygen-level-dependent (BOLD) signal in some task A compared with some other task B—*not* the actual blood flow—over a time course of a few seconds in either task. The details of the study are irrelevant to the present exposition. While the expert can link the location of such "blobs" to the involvement of specific brain regions, the reader is not expected to develop this skill, but simply accept the labeling when offered in particular studies. Some, hopefully, will be motivated to develop this expertise for themselves as the basis for designing and interpreting new studies motivated by the work of Bermudez et al. reviewed later. (From Bermudez, J., Krizaj, D., Lipschitz, D. L., Bueler, C. E., Rogowska, J., Yurgelun-Todd, D., & Nakamura, Y. [2017]. Externally-induced meditative states: An exploratory fMRI study of architects' responses to contemplative architecture. *Frontiers of Architectural Research*, 6[2], 123–136; doi:10.1016/j.foar.2017.02.002. Open access.)

inhibitory synapses, and so I suggest we need the vampire model of neurons, which assesses not only how they compute but also how they suck blood.

Just as our faces vary, so does the anatomy of our brains. The precise 3D location within the head of a particular named brain structure like primary visual cortex will vary from individual to individual. And so, if we want to really understand where the blobs are, we must, in some sense, register them against the structure of the individual's brain. One can use structural MRI to locate anatomical features of the individual brain, and then morph the 3D significance map fonto a "standard" brain so that we can estimate which specific, named brain regions are more active in one task than another.

All this requires sophisticated use of MRI equipment and statistics, with specific decisions made in setting up experiments for each fMRI study. These details will be set forth in in the Methodology section of each fMRI paper. For example, the "technical stuff" on the fMRI image processing of each subject's scans is a major component of the Bermudez et al. (2017) report, but I will not review it there.

A cautionary note: We may find areas more active in task A than in task B, and vice versa. The problem is with interpretation. There is sometimes a tendency to say that a blob that is more active for task A than for task B is the site of the computations necessary for task A and not for B. However, this is misleading. In a system of systems, multiple systems may be engaged but differentially involved in both tasks.

Another brain imaging technique, called *diffusion tensor imaging*, can yield estimates of the strength of connections between two brain regions, and even reveal how this strength varies on different occasions. These brain imaging techniques provide vital cues to the "systems architecture" of the human brain, but can tell us nothing about the fine details of synaptic connections that determine the details of our memories or our performance and experience in different situations. This is where comparative studies linking behavior and neurophysiology in other species play a crucial role.[9]

An exploratory fMRI study of "contemplative" spaces

Bermudez et al. (2017) offered their study to "add to the growing evidence-based design movement in architecture and the construction industry that seeks to use empirical knowledge to better teach, plan, construct, and assess the built environment." In seeking neural correlates for the ability of some buildings to induce contemplative states, they used fMRI

---

9. Those of us working in computational cognitive neuroscience seek to use computational models, like the FARS model of Chapter 2, to get a handle on the actual computations in the (possibly overlapping) neural networks that support these different tasks. My group is among those who have developed methods to convert activity in simulated neural networks into predictions for fMRI studies and the related method of positron emission tomography (Arbib, Bischoff, Fagg, & Grafton, 1995; Bonaiuto & Arbib, 2014) and for EEG (Barrès, Simons, & Arbib, 2013). Griego, Cortes, Winder, and Tagamets (2016) offer a textbook exposition of "Synthetic Brain Imaging."

and self-reports to study the responses of 12 architects to photographs of "ordinary" and "contemplative" architectures. An important point: We can contemplate anything, even a building that is ugly, derelict, and no longer useful. What the authors are getting at is that some buildings are designed to "induce contemplative states," and others are not. They sought neural correlates for this distinction. I will assess strengths and weaknesses of their approach.[10]

The study used 10 image-sequences in an attempt to explore differences in brain activation for five "ordinary [buildings that are] typical of contemporary American urban life" (Figure 4.14)and five "contemplation-inducing" buildings (Figure 4.15). The authors sought photos that present the "phenomenological essence of the particular building" in a progression from outside to inside the building. This raises the question of whether a walk from outside to inside—let alone viewing a sequence of four images from such a walk—is the way to elicit a "contemplative" experience. Contrast sitting still or standing within the space, visually exploring the overall space, then fixing attention within it.

Let's concentrate here on the actual experimental design to evaluate the implications of its findings in themselves and in thinking through ideas for future studies. The first problem is that the five "contemplation-inducing" buildings were chosen from the 10 most cited buildings reported to provoke an Extraordinary Architectural Experience (EAE) in a previous survey (Bermudez, 2008, 2009). This raises the concern: In what sense does the study test neural correlates for "contemplative spaces" rather than for evocation of associations with famous works of architecture? And let's consider the five famous examples in more detail:

- The interiors of Chartres and Ronchamp were designed as "contemplative spaces"—and, more particularly, as sites for Christian worship.

10. I will relate the present section to a brief but broader review of studies in neuroaesthetics in §5.7, "Neuroaesthetics revisited, and more."

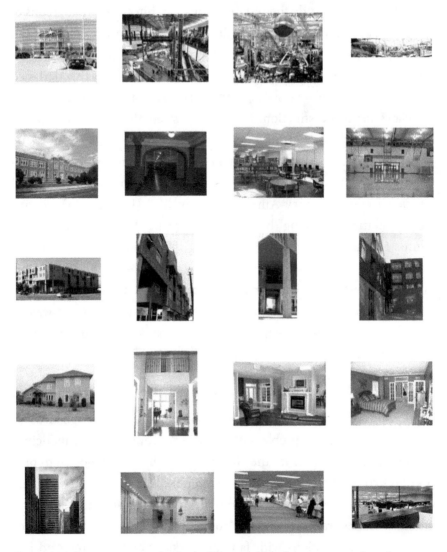

Figure 4.14 Image-sequences for five buildings typical of contemporary American urban life. Each building is represented by a progression of four images from outside to inside. From *top* to *bottom*: a shopping mall, a high school, an urban multiunit housing complex, a single-family suburban dwelling, and a downtown office building.

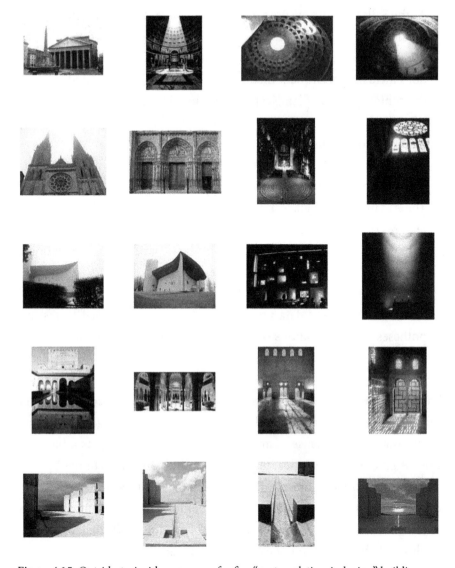

Figure 4.15 Outside-to-inside sequences for five "contemplation-inducing" buildings. From *top* to *bottom*: Pantheon (Rome), Chartres Cathedral (France), Ronchamp Chapel (France), Alhambra (Spain), and Salk Institute (California). (Images courtesy of Julio Bermudez.)

- At the Salk Institute, visitors may "contemplate" the space offered by the Salk courtyard, and all four Salk scenes are of the courtyard, not inside the buildings where scientists conduct research. What does inclusion of the Salk Institute say for components related to the contemplation of landscape rather than internal space, and what do these have to say about tapping into the experience of nature in some religious traditions?

- The Pantheon may now be used as a church, but for many visitors it is more evocative of the Roman Empire.

- The Alhambra is a palace, not a mosque, and for many it is the water features of the courtyard (a precursor of the Salk's?) that many find (when the crowd permits) to be the primary space for contemplation.

Note that my analysis of these five buildings is both brief and purely subjective. No specific data are available that might be used to test my hypotheses on what features of any of the buildings would contribute to one reaction rather than another. This points to the need for in-depth comparative analysis of how the experience of different observers varies with properties of the spaces—and this could be conducted with a large number of subjects and would be of value in itself (cognitive science rather than narrow-sense neuroscience) as well as serving as a basis for the design of more analytical feature-based brain imaging studies.

Returning to the Pantheon, the experience of visitors with various pre-occupations and backgrounds will differ, but for some, contemplation may take the form of reflection on the majesty of the dome or the light cast by the oculus as it changes during the day. Such considerations raise further questions for assessing the sequences used by Bermudez et al. for the "contemplation inducing" buildings. Each contains a shaft of light. Might this feature, rather than "contemplatability" or "architectural merit," be the key feature that distinguishes these images from those for the five "ordinary" buildings, none of which exhibits this feature? It would require a minor change in the selected images as the basis for a study to address this question.

We are here confronted with the general problem of "evidence-based" design, whether or not we seek neural correlates. If indeed we see an effect (as did Bermudez et al.), how do we decide which features were crucial in creating that effect? We must always be alert to competing interpretations of what are the "true" correlates of the observed differences in brain activity. For example, would we see the same effect if we contrasted the five "ordinary" buildings with architecturally exceptional buildings of the same five typologies? And then how would we determine whether the effect was due to contemplatability, architectural merit, or familiarity? Consider familiarity. The subjects in this study were all architects. If an architect sees a novel image-sequence, much brain activity may be required to fit the four images together into a plausible progression, while the progression can immediately be recognized in the case of a familiar building, quickly freeing the observer to contemplate prior experience of the building rather than the images themselves.

However, Julio Bermudez (personal communication) comments that figuring out the correlation of particular formal-spatial features in buildings with particular forms of experience is beyond the current state of the art in technology and, even more so, the funding of architectural research. Rather, his intention is to show that architecture, holistically, has a profound impact and begin to measure that impact neurophenomenologically. He further notes that whereas there are hundreds of architectural analyses of the Pantheon, the Salk Institute, and so on, there are distressingly few scientific studies of their impact on humans—although architects have at least tacit knowledge of what tends to produce certain effects.

With these caveats, let's look at the imaging paradigm. Each subject was scanned in two conditions—first the control block ("ordinary" buildings) and then the experiment block ("contemplative" buildings). Before the start of each block, subjects were read the following:

> We ask you to relax, be present, and try to imagine yourself being and experiencing the places you will be shown. We are interested in your perceptual, emotional, or intuitive response, not in your critical judgment. Therefore, imagine yourself transported to the buildings shown in the images. Just be present in that place and situation and let the experience be whatever it may be. Please, focus on the image and the image alone.

These instructions can be seen as an invitation to enter a state of contemplation, and as such might be disrupted if the sequence poses puzzles because of its unfamiliarity. In other words, perhaps the test was not, "Is the space contemplative?" but rather, "Will the shown images support or disrupt your attempt to enter a contemplative state?" In the latter case, it becomes unclear whether the experiment is about architecture or a more general sense of familiarity versus unfamiliarity.

The fMRI part of the study presented the subject with the sequence of four images for each building, each image presented for 20 seconds "to simulate a dynamic architectural experience." More precisely, each block lasted 10 minutes, comprising five 80-second sessions, each preceded by a 40-second neutral presentation (viewing a gray plane).

The initial analysis of the fMRI images just showed the difference between what, on the average, "lights up" more when people look at the control buildings versus what lights up more when people look at the experimental buildings. You may find Figures 4.16 and 4.17 and the descriptions of what they show to be overwhelming. However, the point here is to emphasize that while much of the conversation between architecture and neuroscience can be conducted at the level of this book, its full development will require detailed knowledge of both architecture *and* neuroscience. This does not mean that the architect must master neuroscience or vice versa, but it does mean that (as in any *meaningful* conversation) each

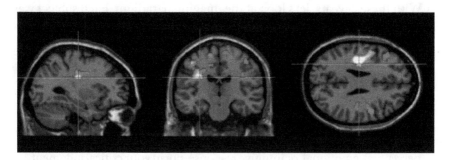

Figure 4.16 When activation was assessed using the inferior parietal lobe as the region of interest, analysis revealed significantly greater activation during the experimental condition compared to the control condition in the left and right inferior parietal lobule, Brodmann area (BA) 40. (From Bermudez, J., Krizaj, D., Lipschitz, D. L., Bueler, C. E., Rogowska, J., Yurgelun-Todd, D., & Nakamura, Y. [2017]. Externally-induced meditative states: An exploratory fMRI study of architects' responses to contemplative architecture. *Frontiers of Architectural Research*, 6[2], 123–136. Open access.)

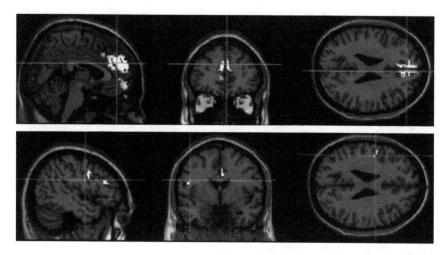

Figure 4.17 Using prefrontal cortex region (PFC) as the region of interest: there was significantly greater activation of PFC in control, *top*, compared with experimental, *bottom*, buildings. The *top panel* shows control > experimental activation in left and right medial frontal gyrus (BA 9), left middle frontal gyrus (BA 10), right superior frontal gyrus (BA 8), and left inferior frontal gyrus. The *bottom panel* displays Experimental > control activation in left inferior frontal gyrus (BA 9), left inferior frontal gyrus, left middle frontal gyrus (BA 46), and right precentral gyrus (BA 6). (From Bermudez, J., Krizaj, D., Lipschitz, D. L., Bueler, C. E., Rogowska, J., Yurgelun-Todd, D., & Nakamura, Y. [2017]. Externally-induced meditative states: An exploratory fMRI study of architects' responses to contemplative architecture. *Frontiers of Architectural Research*, 6[2], 123–136. Open access.)

partner must master enough of the other's vocabulary for the conversation to provide insights of interest or utility to each of them.

To reinforce this point, let's return to my earlier suggestion of the need for in-depth comparative analysis of how the experience of different observers varies with properties of the spaces. It is architects who could offer a subtle analysis to reveal such features, and these could be the basis for a purely cognitive analysis. The results of this analysis could then focus interest on a few key variables to be emphasized in the choice of spaces and key tasks to be given to the subjects of a brain imaging study. The results could be quite complex—and their interpretation would require detailed interaction between the architect and neuroscientist partners in the study. Each would leave many of the details of the other's specialty to their colleague, but each would have to know enough of the other's specialty for their conversation to reveal the full implication of the assembled data.

Back to the figures. The captions name the neuroanatomical regions that Bermudez et al. associate with the various blobs of high significance. The quick summary is that, for architects following the stated protocol, images of the five buildings classified as "contemplative," when compared to those classified as "ordinary," (i) induced attentive, receptive, and absorbing experiences and diminished internal dialogue; (ii) involved decreased engagement of prefrontal cortex; and (iii) activated the occipital lobe, precentral gyrus, and inferior parietal lobule.

A very nice feature of the Bermudez et al. study was that they did not confine data to those gathered from the scanner. After leaving the scanner, subjects filled out a written questionnaire and then had a face-to-face dialogue with a researcher—trying to bridge the two worlds of phenomenology and neural activity, the worlds of lived experience, of "what am I experiencing as I look at the images" versus "what do the scan comparisons reveal?" Most of the subjects said that they felt really engaged, drawn into, and relaxed when they were looking at the contemplative buildings and much less so when they were looking at the everyday buildings. However, as already noted, the issue here may not be "contemplation" so much as the contrast between "revisiting" something familiar and cherished (remember, all the subjects were architects) versus something novel, relatively mundane, and puzzling, as in, "How could these four images fit together in relation to a single building?"

Given these interviews, the researchers went back to the *individual* fMRIs, as distinct from the images obtained by averaging over the scans of a given condition for all subjects after registration of the scans to a common template. This allowed them to assess how the activity recorded with fMRI varied with that individual's "depth of experience" (not experience as an architect, but experience while viewing each sequence). Eleven of the 12 subjects were able to fully engage, enjoy, and relax while viewing the "contemplative" buildings. Nine said they were emotionally moved, transported, and connected to the settings, and described the experience as intense. Two participants went one step further and reported that they experienced a loss of the sense of self, attaining a state of "oneness" with the images of the buildings presented. Only one subject reported that he could not fully engage in the tasks, as required by the study instructions. The researchers concluded that as subjects became more immersed in the experience of the images rather than worrying about other "outside" events, certain brain areas would damp down. This finding fits evidence from elsewhere showing that, as people become more engaged or more skilled in some behavior, the brain can reduce the activity of extraneous areas so that most brain activity is focused in a few regions that can handle the bulk of the necessary processing for that task.

These results yield no immediate lessons for those who design contemplative spaces—or for the more general challenge of how we can design the atmospheres of buildings. Nonetheless, we have gained two important insights. One is that not only can the same architectural stimuli (though here limited to the presentation of a few static images) have different "atmospheric depth" for different subjects, but also that these difference have neural correlates that can be revealed by fMRI. The other is that big questions require the cumulative analysis of many experiments—with interpretation of both insights and shortcomings of any one study raising issues that demand the design of new experiments. The conversation between architects and neuroscientists is an ongoing one that should lead to the enrichment of both groups—new awareness of how the built environment may affect experience and behavior and action–perception–emotion cycles of users for the former; and new inspiration to take back to the laboratory for new experiments and modeling of brain mechanisms for the latter.

Let's celebrate, then, what the authors openly label an exploratory study. It is an attempt to move into the area that can address the concerns of those who question the relevance of neuroscience to architecture by exploring how we can get some new insights into the phenomena, in this case depth-of-experience, by understanding that different parts of the brain are differentially engaged in different architectural experiences.[11]

---

11. If you have somebody in a scanner, there's not much you can do about experience in actual buildings, so in the future we will have to turn to studies making use of portable EEG helmets to monitor brain signals as people experience the actual spaces. Indeed, in 2020, Bermudez received a grant from the Templeton Religious Trust for a focused study of this kind. His group will acquire and analyze data on ambulatory EEGs to test the power of architecture on laypeople (in this case, Catholic believers) in relation to a detailed assessment of the atmospheres of Union Station and the Catholic Basilica, both in Washington, DC.

4.6. EXPERIENCES OF ULTIMACY

In the Bermudez et al. study, some of the contemplative buildings are associated with religious practice; others are not. To complement their study, then, I briefly consider religious experience and a more general class of "experience of ultimacy," and briefly examine fMRI studies that suggest that one root of religious experience may be the experience of trust as a key ingredient of social cohesion.

Religious views not only are social schemas that were developed as answers to great questions about human existence but also arise from so-called religious experiences, whether experienced directly or indirectly. The classic charting of such experiences was provided by the Harvard psychologist William James—brother of the American novelist Henry James—in his classic, *The Varieties of Religious Experience: A Study in Human Nature* (James, 1902).[12] However, following the ideas of Wesley Wildman and Leslie Brothers (1999), I think it useful to see religious experiences as examples of a broader class of what they call *experiences of ultimacy*.

I had such an experience when I stood on the rocks of Cape Leeuwin at the southwest corner of Western Australia where the Southern Ocean meets the Indian Ocean. The sun was setting, the clouds were piled up gorgeously in the sky, the wind was blowing strongly, and the waves were pounding against the rocks below. These sights and sounds and the feeling of the wind conspired to give me an experience captured by the colloquialism of being "blown away," feeling part of the natural scene rather than a separate ego. (Figure 4.18 approximates the visual component of that experience, although the photo was taken at another place [the southwest corner of South Africa] in another time.)

For someone imbued with a theistic religious faith, this might have become a religious experience of connection with God, but in my case it did not. It was a feeling of *ultimacy* in the sense of feeling part of a greater whole of Nature without in any way feeling that that whole is God's creation. Perhaps the architect

---

12. James's book was based on his Gifford Lectures on Natural Theology delivered at the University of Edinburgh in 1901–1902. Mary Hesse and I delivered our Gifford Lectures there, the basis for our book on *The Construction of Reality*, in 1983.

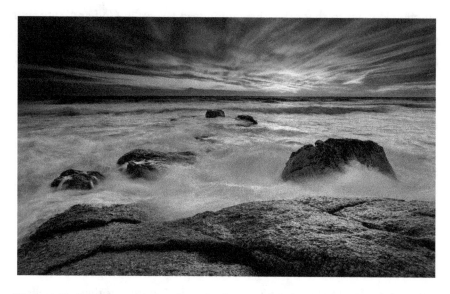

Figure 4.18 Consider nature in relation to the natural underpinnings of the architectural experience. An experience of ultimacy—the wind whipping a stormy sea at sunset. (Photo © Lee Slabber, with permission. https://leeslabber.com/product/stormy-waters/)

in creating an atmosphere of transcendence is tapping into innate ways that we evolved in interaction with nature that long predated architecture itself.

Recent decades have seen the rise of a new field called *neurotheology* (not to be confused with *neuroethology*, the study of brain mechanisms underlying animal behavior), based in large part on the results of conducting brain imaging of people meditating, engaging in religious practice, or reliving a religious experience. Some researchers approach the task in terms of how it is that God gave us brains that would allow us to have religious experiences, whereas others (myself included) would ask what it is about biological and cultural evolution that allows human brains to let people have experiences of ultimacy that some, immersed in a particular cultural milieu, make sense of in a religious framework.

Here, I offer one example. Schjødt et al. (2008) conducted an fMRI study that relates trust in God to interpersonal trust, arguing that their results support the hypothesis that religious prayer as a form of frequently recurring behavior is capable of stimulating the dopaminergic reward system (see §4.2) in practicing individuals. They studied a group of religious Christians in Denmark, having questioned them to check that they did indeed believe in God and not Santa Claus. The researchers then imaged their subjects' brains while they performed four tasks: making a wish to Santa Claus, reciting a rhyme that was not religious, offering a personal prayer, and reciting the Lord's Prayer. They hypothesize that, for a devout Christian, reciting this prayer is not the rote recitation of a formula, but instead a heartfelt affirmation of an intense relation with a Heavenly Father.

Schjødt et al. focused attention on the right caudate nucleus of the basal ganglia, a key target for neuromodulation by dopamine, and a key area in processing reward signals. The study revealed that activity in the caudate nucleus is below the baseline for the nonreligious tasks (making a wish to Santa Claus or reciting a nonreligious rhyme), was somewhat above baseline for personal prayer, and was activated even more for reciting the Lord's Prayer (Figure 4.19). Schjødt et al. argue that this highest activation during recital of the Lord's Prayer supports the hypothesis that this behavior stimulates the dopaminergic reward system in practicing individuals. This is clearly a big leap from a rather limited set of data. Why would this particular form of rote repetition invoke the reward system?

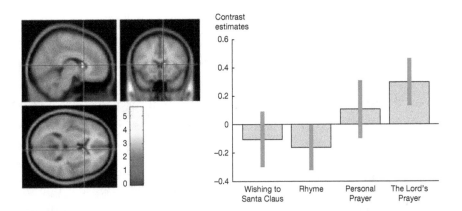

Figure 4.19 At *left*, we see three cuts through the brain to show the location of the caudate nucleus. At *right*, we see the BOLD response (the measure of blood flow that fMRI employs as a correlate with neural activity) in the caudate nucleus in a group of Danish Christians. Of the four conditions tested, the response was greatest during recitation of the Lord's Prayer. The *red bars* show the considerable deviation in individual response for each condition. (Reprinted from Schjødt, U., Stødkilde-Jørgensen, H., Geertz, A. W., & Roepstorff, A. [2008]. Rewarding prayers. *Neuroscience Letters*, 443, 165–168, with permission from Elsevier.)

To address this, Schjødt et al. cited a study in which people were scanned while playing a game with another person. The key point of the kind of game studied was that how you play the game depends on whether or not you believe that you can trust the other player. King-Casas et al. (2005) found that, in such games, participants learned about their partner's trustworthiness through trial and error, which made them able to optimize and predict monetary reward. This learning to trust partners was predicted and reflected in activation of the dorsal striatum, an area that includes the caudate nucleus and the putamen. This suggests that the caudate nucleus is also actively involved in evaluating future rewards dependent on interpersonal reciprocity.

This led Schjødt et al. (2008) to argue that the activation of the caudate nucleus in their study may reflect that, in reinforcing the relationship of the believer to God, prayer builds on general mechanisms for building trust through the evaluation of future rewards depending on interpersonal reciprocity. This relation of prayer to expectation for future rewards or reciprocity holds in some non-Christian religions as well—and may also relate to achieving a sense of security, protection, balance, submission, and tranquility. This is an example of where seeing the overlap in brain activation data between different studies suggests relationships that the neuro-data render more plausible. The challenge for architecture is to build environments, and not just faith-related environments, whose atmosphere can help address the needs of individuals who feel lonely, unprotected, and desperate—but in many ways this is, more importantly, a challenge for health care and the political will to build a social safety net.[13]

Our look at the Bermudez et al. study has set us off on a complex path, both by having us develop a sense of the pluses and minuses of fMRI as a tool for finding neural correlates of human experience, and by taking us from the action–perception cycle of moving through and acting within

13. This sentence was written long before the Covid-19 pandemic, but when read during that period of self-quarantine, unemployment, and social distance, it had an especial poignancy. I am reminded of the fiction, "Pierre Menard, Author of the Quixote" by the Argentine author Jorge Luis Borges. Menard prepared himself so that when he wrote his novel (he did not copy the earlier book), the text was identical to that of Cervantes. However, Borges judges the book by Menard to be far superior to that of Cervantes (!!) because sentences that were mere rhetorical flourishes for Quixote were possessed of great depth when written by someone who had experienced the cataclysms of the 20th century.

the (built) environment to the realm of contemplation. Fruitfully, this has tied in to the notion of atmosphere with its general link to mood and emotion, and in particular with the aesthetic emotions. We have thus started to get some sense of how the evolutionary journey from needs and motivation toward human emotions in general, and to the aesthetic emotions in particular, may provide pointers for much future effort in developing the A↔N conversation between architecture and neuroscience.

The challenge is to further develop an integrative view of cog/neuroscience that can span the many criteria that architects must address in balancing utility and aesthetics in designing a building. The discussion of ultimacy points us to the way in which highly developed cultural systems may co-opt far more ancient brain mechanisms. It has further shown that these mechanisms go beyond systems for perception and action and their linkage through memory to include systems that are essential to social interaction. Our discussion of how the external expression of the emotions serves social coordination provided one example of this; the discussion of mirror systems and empathy in the next chapter provides another.

REFERENCES

Aalto, A. (1978). Motifs from times past. In G. Schildt (Ed.), *Alvar Aalto: Sketches* (S. Wrede, Trans.). Cambridge, MA and London: MIT Press.

Adolphs, R., Tranel, D., & Damasio, A. R. (1998). The human amygdala in social judgment. *Nature*, 393(6684), 470–474.

Arbib, M. A., Bischoff, A., Fagg, A. H., & Grafton, S. T. (1995). Synthetic PET: Analyzing large-scale properties of neural networks. *Human Brain Mapping*, 2(4), 225–233.

Barrès, V., Simons, A., & Arbib, M. A. (2013). Synthetic event-related potentials: A computational bridge between neurolinguistic models and experiments. *Neural Networks*, 37, 66–92. doi:10.1016/j.neunet.2012.09.021

Bermudez, J. (2008). *Mapping the phenomenological territory of profound architectural atmospheres: Results of a large survey.* Paper presented at the Electronic Proceedings of the International Symposium "Creating an Atmosphere," Ecole Nationale Supériure d'Architecture de Grenoble, France.

Bermudez, J. (2009). Amazing grace: New research into "extraordinary architectural experiences" reveals the central role of sacred places. *Faith & Form*, 42(2), 8–13.

Bermudez, J., Krizaj, D., Lipschitz, D. L., Bueler, C. E., Rogowska, J., Yurgelun-Todd, D., & Nakamura, Y. (2017). Externally-induced meditative states: An exploratory fMRI study of architects' responses to contemplative architecture. *Frontiers of Architectural Research*, 6(2), 123–136. doi: 10.1016/j.foar.2017.02.002

Böhme, G. (2015). Atmosphere: New perspectives for architecture and design. In P. Tidwell (Ed.), *Architecture and atmosphere* (pp. 7–14). Espoo, Finland: Tapio Wirkkala–Rut Bryk Foundation.

Bonaiuto, J. J., & Arbib, M. A. (2014). Modeling the BOLD correlates of competitive neural dynamics. *Neural Networks*, 49, 1–10.

Borch, C. (Ed.). (2014). *Architectural atmospheres: On the experience and politics of architecture*. Basel: Birkhäuser Verlag.

Canetti, E. (1978). *Crowds and power* (C. Stewart, Trans.). New York: Seabury Press.

Damasio, A. (1994). *Descartes' error: Emotion, reason, and the human brain*. New York: Putnam.

Darwin, C. (1872). *The expression of the emotions in man and animals* (republished in 1965). Chicago: University of Chicago Press.

Denton, D. A., McKinley, M. J., Farrell, M., & Egan, G. F. (2009). The role of primordial emotions in the evolutionary origin of consciousness. *Consciousness and Cognition*, 18(2), 500–514.

Edwards, D. H., & Spitzer, N. (2006). Social dominance and serotonin receptor genes in crayfish. *Current Topics in Developmental Biology*, 74, 177–199.

Freud, S. (1959). *Group psychology and the analysis of the ego* (J. Strachey, Trans. 1992 ed.). New York: W. W. Norton.

Frijda, N. H. (1986). *The emotions*. Cambridge, UK: Cambridge University Press.

Frijda, N. H., & Sundararajan, L. (2007). Emotion refinement. *Perspectives on Psychological Science*, 2, 227–241.

Gibson, J. J. (1979). *The ecological approach to visual perception*. Boston: Houghton Mifflin.

Griego, J. A., Cortes, C. R., Winder, R., & Tagamets, M. A. (2016). Synthetic brain imaging. In M. A. Arbib & J. J. Bonaiuto (Eds.), *From neuron to cognition via computational neuroscience* (pp. 457–482). Cambridge, MA: MIT Press.

Griffero, T. (2015). Architectural affordances: The atmospheric authority of space. In P. Tidwell (Ed.), *Architecture and atmosphere* (pp. 15–47). Espoo, Finland: Tapio Wirkkala–Rut Bryk Foundation.

Hatfield, E., Cacioppo, J. T., & Rapson, R. L. (1994). *Emotional contagion*. New York: Cambridge University Press.

Havik, K., Teerds, H., & Tielens, G. (Eds.). (2013). *Building atmosphere: Journal for Architecture/Tijdschrift voor Architectuur #91*. Rotterdam: nai010 publishers.

Hewitt, M. A. (2020). *Draw in order to see: A cognitive history of architectural design*. ORO Editions.

James, W. (1890). *Principles of psychology*. New York: Holt.

James, W. (1902). *The varieties of religious experience: A study in human nature*. New York and London: Longmans, Green.

Kelley, A. E. (2005). Neurochemical networks encoding emotion and motivation: An evolutionary perspective. In J.-M. Fellous & M. A. Arbib (Eds.), *Who needs emotions: The brain meets the robot* (pp. 29–77). Oxford and New York: Oxford University Press.

King-Casas, B., Tomlin, D., Anen, C., Camerer, C. F., Quartz, S. R., & Montague, P. R. (2005). Getting to know you: Reputation and trust in a two-person economic exchange. *Science*, 308(5718), 78–83.

Koelsch, S., Jacobs, A. M., Menninghaus, W., Liebal, K., Klann-Delius, G., von Scheve, C., & Gebauer, G. (2015). The quartet theory of human emotions: An integrative and neurofunctional model. *Physics of Life Reviews*, 13, 1–27. doi:10.1016/j.plrev.2015.03.001

LeDoux, J. E. (2000). Emotion circuits in the brain. *Annual Review of Neuroscience*, 23, 155–184.

MacLean, P. D. (1990). *The triune brain in evolution: Role in paleocerebral functions.* Springer Science & Business Media.

Panksepp, J. (1998). *Affective neuroscience.* New York: Oxford University Press.

Pavlov, I. P. (1927). *Conditioned reflexes: An investigation of the physiological activity of the cerebral cortex* (G. V. Anrep, Trans.). Oxford: Oxford University Press.

Pribram, K. H. (1960). A review of theory in physiological psychology. *Annual Review of Psychology*, 11(1–40).

Robinson, S. (2011). *Nesting: Body, dwelling, mind.* Richmond, CA: William Stout Publishers.

Scherer, K. R. (2013). Emotion in action, interaction, music, and speech. In M. A. Arbib (Ed.), *Language, music, and the brain: A mysterious relationship, Strüngmann Forum Reports* (Vol. 10, pp. 107–139). Cambridge, MA: MIT Press.

Schjødt, U., Stødkilde-Jørgensen, H., Geertz, A. W., & Roepstorff, A. (2008). Rewarding prayers. *Neuroscience Letters*, 443, 165–168.

Scott, S. C. (1993). Complexity and mystery as predictors of interior preferences. *Journal of Interior Design*, 19(1), 25–33. doi:10.1111/j.1939-1668.1993.tb00149.x

Stamps, A. E. (2004). Mystery, complexity, legibility and coherence: A meta-analysis. *Journal of Environmental Psychology*, 24(1), 1–16. doi:10.1016/S0272-4944(03)00023-9

Thibaud, J.-P. (2015). Installing an atmosphere. In P. Tidwell (Ed.), *Architecture and atmosphere* (pp. 49–66). Espoo, Finland: Tapio Wirkkala–Rut Bryk Foundation.

Tidwell, P. (Ed.). (2015). *Architecture and atmosphere: A Tapio Wirkkala–Rut Bryk design reader* (with contributions by Gernot Böhme, Tonino Griffero, Jean-Paul Thibaud, and Juhani Pallasmaa). Espoo, Finland: Tapio Wirkkala–Rut Bryk Foundation.

Wigley, M. (1998). The architecture of atmosphere. *Daidalos*, 68, 20–27.

Wildman, W., & Brothers, L. (1999). A neuropsychological-semiotic model of religious experiences. In R. Russell, N. Murphy, T. Meyering, & M. A. Arbib (Eds.), *Neuroscience and the person: Scientific perspectives on divine action* (pp. 347–416). Berkeley, CA/Vatican: Center for Theology and the Natural Sciences/Vatican Observatory.

Zumthor, P. (2006). *Atmospheres.* Basel: Birkhäuser Verlag.

Zumthor, P. (2012). *Thinking architecture* (3rd, expanded ed.). Basel: Birkhauser.

From empathy to mirror neurons and back to aesthetics

5.1. Empathy and Einfühlung in life, architecture, and art
5.2. Mirror neurons and their larger setting
5.3. How neural nets enable us to learn and remember
5.4. Modeling how mirror neurons learn and function
5.5. Empathy and the brain
5.6. Einfühlung and the motor component of contemplation
5.7. Neuroaesthetics revisited, and more

If there are two "facts" that have been broadly shared between architects about brains, they are that mirror neurons support a resonance between people as well as between people and works of art and architecture, and that the hippocampus provides a GPS for navigation and wayfinding. In each case, there is a grain of truth, but the claim is simplistic, and to proceed further we need a deeper understanding of the neuroscience to ground a deeper understanding of its implications. This chapter undertakes the task for mirror neurons, the next chapter for the hippocampus.

My struggle in discussing aesthetics is to bridge the distance between the basic idea of the action–perception cycle and the aesthetic judgment of an art object or a building. My concern with "aesthetics" continues to be with "aesthetic judgment," the appreciation of the *value* along a range of aesthetic criteria for a work of art or architecture—or, indeed, for many of the elements of everyday life. Such judgment of a given object or experience may vary greatly from individual to individual. Our aesthetic response is rooted in both basic brain + body emotional systems and their refinement through our individual development in a specific physical and cultural milieu—and encompasses many more aspects of "evaluative feeling" than our (possibly idiosyncratic) appreciation of beauty. Even though vision often dominates our aesthetic sense of a building or a room, it is our integrated experience within the action–perception cycle that informs much of our appreciation of architecture. Since there are so many sources of pleasure—as well as sources of pain, fear, discomfort, and disgust—there is no "one size fits all" here. What makes this chapter distinctive is that it emphasizes roles the motor system may play in aesthetic judgment—judgment that ranges from the preconscious reaction to conscious evaluation, in some cases fusing sensorimotor integration and the recognition of actions.

We examine the general idea of empathy in human relations and explore the extent to which it does and does not correspond to the 19th-century notion of *Einfühlung* as the process whereby we "feel ourselves into" objects of artistic (or architectural) contemplation. We then turn to some key data on *mirror neurons*, noting that these were discovered in the monkey brain as neurons that were active both when the monkey performed a particular kind of manual action and when it observed another performing a similar action. This discovery provided a major impetus to social cognitive neuroscience, complementing the study of emotional reactions to conspecifics with new insights into the linkage in the brain of neural encoding of the execution of one's own actions and the recognition of the similar actions of others.

The discoveries in the monkey inspired new studies of humans using brain imaging. The search was on for brain regions that are more active compared to controls both for the execution and for the observations of the same class of actions. In this way, various *mirror systems* have been discovered in the human brain. However, as we probe the way in which mirror systems operate, we come to realize that this is possible only because of their linkage with other regions of the brain. Thus, the understanding of mirror neurons or mirror systems is incomplete without a study of brain regions *Beyond the Mirror*. Much of what has been attributed to mirror neurons alone is in fact a property of the interaction of multiple brain regions.

While the initial studies on monkeys focused on the ability to, for example, distinguish between precision pinches and power grasps, later studies showed mirror neurons specific to both the sight and sound of the breaking of peanuts, and others attuned to tearing paper. This made clear that the wiring of mirror neurons must be learned rather than being innately specified in detail. My group was the first to provide a computational model of how such learning might occur. To understand it, we need some background on how neural networks enable us to learn and remember, and so we briefly explore three ways in which the synaptic connections between neurons may change as a function of experience. *Unsupervised learning* is based on capturing statistical regularities in the input to the network. In *supervised learning*, a "teacher" (which may be another network) specifies exactly what output is required of the network in response to each input pattern within a training set. By contrast, *reinforcement learning* does not require specific details of what each neuron should or should not do. Rather, synapses are adjusted on the basis of positive or negative reinforcement, supplied by a "critic," of the overall behavior that the neural network controls. We will also discuss, very briefly, how these rules have been exploited to develop the "deep learning" that has been the driver of the immense upsurge in successful application of artificial intelligence (AI) in recent years.

With this background, we can turn to brain modeling. We first consider the MNS model of how mirror neurons may be formed by learning to associate the observed trajectory of one's own performance in a specific type of action with the activity of dedicated neurons, and then being able to exploit that to activate the same neurons when similar trajectories are observed in the performance of others. Providing cues to the similarity of those actions of self and others may provide a useful basis for social interaction and learning by imitation. Since most of the discussion of mirror neurons focuses on such social interaction, it will be important to stress that the original value of mirror neurons, in evolutionary terms, may have been to assist in observing one's own behavior as a basis for acquiring new skills. This will be demonstrated by the augmented competitive queuing (ACQ) model, which looks at how adaptive sequences of behavior may be mastered through learning the *desirability* and *executability* of actions within some particular task domain. The contrast between ACQ and scripts in the control of action exemplifies how the brain may achieve similar ends by different means. In the first account, diverse actions actively compete to be executed; in the latter, there is chaining in which the successful completion of one action triggers the next, though with the ability to recognize when one can start partway along the chain. The script could have been learned either through repeated flexible scheduling of a novel chain or through explicit training to perform the actions in the given order.

With this enriched understanding of mirror neurons and systems beyond the mirror, we can finally return to the issues that motivated the interest of mirror neurons within the A↔N conversation. Specifically, we look at data linking empathy to mirror systems before looking at a particular study that showed some evidence for a mirror system for the experience of disgust. However, we will offer an "experiment" that shows how our behavior goes far beyond the simple re-expression of observed behavior to vary in subtle ways that depend strongly on the influence of those systems beyond the mirror.

All this prepares us to explore a motor component for the aesthetics of art and architecture, in that we may enrich our appreciation of a piece by recognizing the actions and agonies of the protagonists in a representational sculpture or painting, or by gaining some feeling for the actions of the artist or sculptor or architect in creating the work. Of course, we have already seen how early visual processing may enter into our appreciation of art and architecture. Thus, the claim here must not be that the mirror system alone underlies aesthetic appreciation, but rather that it adds a crucial dimension that may be overlooked (literally) when the focus is on vision alone. In any case, the action-oriented use of a building enriches experience in a way that goes beyond the mere contemplation of art works.

Finally, we return to the earlier discussion of neuroaesthetics, offering a small sample of focused case studies that seek neural correlates for aspects of aesthetic appreciation and examining an approach to environmental psychology that exploits new instrumentation to take urban psychology "out of the laboratory and onto the street." Such studies share the general problem noted before that scientific studies focused on a few key variables cannot readily be linked to the richness of experience afforded by a building. Nonetheless, such work can contribute to the steady accumulation of a tool kit of new ways of assessing the experience of buildings to enrich future design.

5.1. EMPATHY AND EINFÜHLUNG IN LIFE, ARCHITECTURE, AND ART

The *Oxford English Dictionary* (OED) defines *empathy* as "The power of projecting one's personality into (and so fully comprehending) the object of contemplation," and notes that this term was apparently introduced into English in 1909 by E. B. Titchener in his *Lectures in the Experimental Psychology of Thought-Processes.* He wrote, "Not only do I see gravity and modesty and pride . . . but I feel or act them in the mind's muscles. This is, I suppose, a simple case of empathy, if we may coin that term as a rendering of *Einfühlung*." Today, we do not think of the mind as being the product of even a metaphorical set of muscles—we link it to the dynamic activity and plasticity of networks of neurons in the brain, a brain in the body of a creature engaged with the physical and social environment. But for now, let's leave neural mechanisms aside, and move beyond these basic definitions.

First, rather than seeing empathy as encompassing "personality" as a whole, we normally relate it to the current mental state of another person—though this may be framed by one's overall judgment (conscious and/or subconscious) of the other. Adding to this our general understanding that perception is dependent on our own prior experience and current state, let's first edit the OED definition to view *empathy* as "[t]he power of projecting one's personality into (and *to some extent* comprehending) the current state of the object of contemplation." However, I need to stress that there are many ways to comprehend an object of contemplation that involve no "projection of one's personality." If I see an apple and decide to eat it, I in no way treat it as a person (unless I have bizarre cannibalistic tendencies, which is not the case). Empathy is but one of many paths to understanding.

Much confusion has arisen because many people (including myself, on occasion) treat *empathy* and *sympathy* as synonyms. Let me try to disentangle them. The OED defines *sympathy* as "[t]he quality or state of being affected by the condition of another with a feeling similar or corresponding to that of the other." *Sympathy* may in some sense be the opposite of *antipathy*, a contrariety of feeling, disposition, or nature; people may feel antipathy for things as well as other people.

In empathy, one represents the state of the other as possibly distinct from one's own, and this neither implies nor disallows that to some extent one's observation of the other leads one to experience some of the feelings of the other. Sympathy is that special case of empathy that involves a partial conflation of the two states—"this is what the other is feeling, and now this is what I feel too" as the basis for further behavior.

Here is a possible scenario to try and get a handle on these three concepts:

> You are walking through a public square when you are confronted by a beggar who asks you for money. Your reaction may be one of antipathy with no empathy involved—you simply categorize the creature as a *beggar*, and your disposition is to never give money to beggars. I used the word "creature" in the previous sentence to highlight the fact that in this case, you do not really consider the beggar as a person, let alone project your personality into them.
> But let's consider two cases where empathy is involved. You may indeed stop awhile and "project your personality into (and so to some extend comprehend) the object of contemplation." But this comprehension may take different forms. You may judge the person

as genuinely needy and imagine yourself in such need; you feel *sympathy*. Then you may either press a dollar or two into the beggar's hand and walk on with, perhaps, a certain glow of self-approval, or walk on without this act of charity and, perhaps, feel somewhat guilty. Conversely, your empathy may lead you to conclude that the beggar is not needy but simply after your money, you feel *antipathy*, and you walk on, perhaps feeling a touch of anger at the beggar's apparent dishonesty.

Note a problem here. *When you project a personality into another, and so to some extent comprehend their mental state*, the projected personality may not be your own! In the case of sympathy for the beggar, you may imagine yourself in a situation where you have been hungry and without money. In the case of antipathy, you may indeed recall some occasion on which you acted dishonestly, and the tinge of shame involved in this exercise of empathy may indeed contribute to your antipathy. Or, thanks to reading the papers or watching videos, you may be able to imagine what it would be like to be dishonest, even though you find such behavior abhorrent. Through your many personal interactions and through your reading of stories and absorption of movies, you have met and imagined diverse personalities, some very different from your own. For example, if you are meek you may know all too well the type of person who is aggressive. Comprehending that someone you meet for the first time may be aggressive, then, is not projecting *your* personality, but rather projecting an understanding of diverse personalities, only some of which may share more than a few features with your own.

Back to *Einfühlung* and on to architecture. Harry Mallgrave, author of *The Architect's Brain*, has done much to bring the work of 19th century scholars in architecture to our attention—see, for example, *Empathy, Form, and Space: Problems in German Aesthetics, 1873–1893*, which collects essays by Robert Vischer and others (Mallgrave & Ikonomou, 1994). Vischer (1873) used *Einfühlung* to connote the active process by which we "feel ourselves into" objects of artistic contemplation. He stated:

Every work of art reveals itself to us as a person harmoniously feeling himself into a kindred object, or as humanity objectifying itself in harmonious forms. (Translation from Mallgrave & Ikonomou, 1994, p. 117)

Here, I must confess I have trouble with Vischer's talk of "every work of art reveals itself to us as a person harmoniously feeling himself into a kindred object." First, I wonder if adding the term "harmoniously" moves us from empathy to sympathy? Second, even if one were to offer the alternative, "When we experience a work of art, we are in some sense gaining a measure of harmony with it, much as we would in feeling empathy [or sympathy?] for another person," this would still raise the question: "Does *Einfühlung* for *objects of artistic contemplation* use the same brain mechanisms as *empathy for other humans*?" I will argue that this identity only holds in some cases. Gallese and Gattara (2015, p. 167) observe:

Vischer described *Einfühlung*, literally "feeling-in," as the physical response generated by the observation of forms within paintings. Particular visual forms arouse particular responsive feelings, depending on the conformity of those forms to the design and function of the muscles in the body, from our eyes to our limbs and to our bodily posture as a whole. Vischer clearly distinguished a passive notion of vision – *seeing* – from the active one of – *looking*. According to Vischer, looking best characterizes our aesthetic experience when perceiving images, in general, and works of art, in particular.

However, our discussion of Yarbus's study of diverse strategies for eye movements in visual attention, as in the distinct strategies for judging the ages of people versus assessing the clothes they are wearing (§3.2), makes clear the active process of looking need not invoke "feelings [that conform] to the design and function of the muscles in the body . . . and to our bodily posture as a whole." Thus, we may emphasize perception of images (and of works of architecture; more on this later) as an active process, and agree that in some cases it evokes patterns of bodily movement, and yet deny that this is the key aspect of looking.

Einfühlung implies a projection of the *dynamically embodied self* on the work of art or architecture. Nonetheless, we can often experience beauty—for example, a beautiful sunset—without sensorimotor correlates. Alternatively, the motor correlate may be very different from "feeling into" the object of contemplation—when I tap my foot or even dance as I appreciate a piece of music, I am following the overall rhythms of the piece whether the music itself conveys sadness or joy. Perhaps in such cases music does "arouse particular responsive feelings, depending on the conformity of those forms to the design and function of the muscles in the body," and experiences like singing hymns or dancing with others do indeed involve positive feedback between the experience of ourselves and of the others around us in heightening our emotions.[1] Of course, sharing an overall emotional state and detailed pattern of movement is a limited aspect of entering the "personalities" of those around us—the brain mechanisms that support people-centered empathy may overlap at most partially with those that support building-centered Einfühlung.

Geoffrey Scott in his 1914 book *The Architecture of Humanism: A Study in the History of Taste*[2] gives a satisfying account of how empathy may affect our response to a building, but in emphasizing appearances, he says nothing about how we act and interact around and within the building:

> The spaces, masses and lines of architecture, as perceived [visually], are appearances. We may infer from them further facts about a building which are not perceived; facts about construction, facts

---

1. This and many other issues are explored in Arbib, M. A. (Ed.). 2013. Language, music and the brain, a mysterious relationship. *Strüngmann Forum Reports*, 10. Cambridge, MA: MIT Press, based on diverse contributions to a Strüngmann Forum held in Frankfurt in 2011.

2. My thanks to Robert Lamb Hart for drawing Scott's book to my attention. On the occasion of a reprinting of the book, Witold Rybczynski wrote an essay ("The Triumph of a Distinguished Failure," *New York Review of Books*, 2004) that summarized key observations of Scott's complementing those quoted here and offered an extended biographical sketch.

about history or society. But the art of architecture is concerned with their immediate aspect; it is concerned with them as appearances. . . .

Conceive for a moment a "top-heavy" building or an "ill-proportioned" space. No doubt the degree to which these qualities will be found offensive will vary with the spectator's sensibility to architecture but sooner or later, if the top-heaviness or the disproportion is sufficiently pronounced, every spectator will . . . experience a certain discomfort from their presence. . . .

There is instability—or the appearance of it—but it is in the building. There is discomfort, but it is in ourselves. . . . The concrete spectacle . . . has stirred our physical memory. It has awakened in us, not indeed an actual state of instability or of being overloaded, but that condition of spirit which in the past has belonged to our actual experiences of weakness, of thwarted effort or incipient collapse. We have looked at the building and identified ourselves with its apparent state. *We have transcribed ourselves into terms of architecture.*

But the "states" in architecture with which we thus identify ourselves need not be actual. The actual pressures of a spire are downward; yet no one speaks of a "sinking" spire. A spire, when well designed, appears—as common language testifies—to soar. We identify ourselves, not with its actual downward pressure, but its apparent upward impulse. So, too, . . . arches "spring," vistas "stretch," domes "swell," Greek temples are "calm," and baroque facades "restless." The whole of architecture is, in fact, unconsciously invested by us with human movement and human mood. Here, then, is a principle complementary to the one just stated. *We transcribe architecture into terms of ourselves.* (Scott, 1914, pp. 210–213)

However, I reiterate that our reaction to a building may be caused by forms of sensory stimuli other than visual appearance, and that the building offers affordances to us for *our* actions and emotions beyond those emotional responses stirred by the empathy or sympathy of *transcribing ourselves into terms of architecture* or *transcribing architecture into terms of ourselves.* We may view a doorway as "cramped" or "welcoming";

nonetheless, our evaluation will be swayed by whether it works well in providing affordances for the path to our chosen destination. Given our emphasis on the action–perception cycle, the issue remains: no matter how much designers can suggest how the user will "feel into" a building, they must also assess how the feelings so created relate to those aspects of the design that affect how the building will act as an arena for behavior.

To further consider how empathy may or may not relate to our experience of buildings, recall the example (§4.3) of a large impressive courthouse with a grand entrance and then, below it, a mean little door on the steps leading down to the prison beneath, symbolizing the majesty of the law and the crushing weight of justice bearing down on the guilty. How might we express this in terms of Einfühlung? How do we combine separate feelings generated by the observation of forms within the building, and our possible feelings of empathy for (say) the judge who dispenses justice above and the prisoner who is imprisoned below into an inevitably complex, shifting experience of a building? And note how, leaving architecture behind, the nature of one case decided in the law court may leave us with sympathy for the judge and antipathy for the prisoner, while what we know of another case may reverse the polarity of our empathy.

Mallgrave goes back to Schopenhauer[3] to give another sense of how brain processes might inform a reaction to architecture, linking back to our embodied experience of gravity.

> Arthur Schopenhauer . . . argued that perception is no passive process, but one in which the brain actively constructs its world through a complex series of neurological operations. Architecturally, he translated this postulate into the brain reading a building's forms as a conflict between gravity and rigidity. The architect's task was to devise an ingenious system of columns, beams, joists, arches, vaults,

3. See also Smith, M. W. 2017. *The nervous stage: Nineteenth-century neuroscience and the birth of modern theatre*. Oxford: Oxford University Press; and Korab-Karpowicz, W. J. 2012. Schopenhauer's theory of architecture. In B. Vandenabeele (Ed.), The Blackwell companion to Schopenhauer (pp. 178–192). Malden, MA: Wiley-Blackwell. doi:10.1002/9781444347579. ch12.

and domes, through which he deprives these "insatiable forces [of gravity] of the shortest path to their satisfaction." (Mallgrave, 2015, p. 12)

Mallgrave, here, cites Schopenhauer as part of a larger historical perspective, and by no means to endorse the defiance of gravity as *the* key to architecture—any more than we would judge a building solely on whether or not it stays standing. Nonetheless, it is worth spending a moment to consider that some buildings make the "fight" against gravity explicit, whereas others do not.

If we look at the Parthenon (Figure 5.1, left), we can indeed see the upper structure as in some sense imposing weight and the columns opposing this force, but this achievement in itself would not have elicited Le Corbusier's boundless admiration for the building. If we turn around on the Acropolis to view the Erectheion (Right), we see the Caryatids which directly represent women resisting the weight of the pediment.

However, when I look at the columns of the Library of Celsus in Ephesus (Figure 5.2), I have no sense of the columns as bearing weight. Rather,

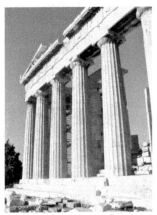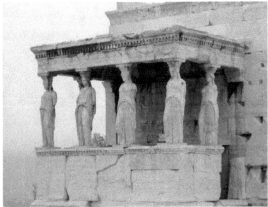

Figure 5.1 A contrast between Greek columns that bear weight but have their own form, and those that represent humans bearing the weight themselves. (*Left*) Parthenon, East Facade, at the Acropolis, Athens (447–432 BCE). (*Right*) Caryatids of the Erectheion, nearby. (*Left*: Photo by Harry Mallgrave, with permission. *Right*: Author's photo.)

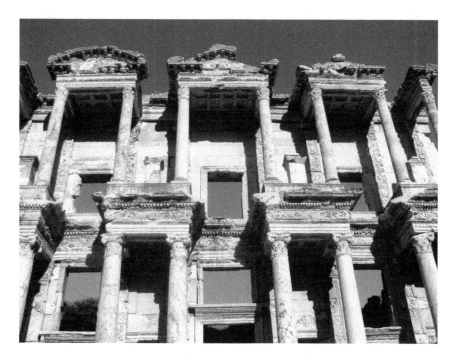

Figure 5.2 Library of Celsus, Ephesus, Turkey, completed 135 CE. (Photo by Harry Mallgrave, with permission.)

I am struck by the grace of the design, the pattern that the columns form. Here, it is the rhythm and the beauty of the facade that has its effect on me, not resistance to gravity. In other words, for some buildings, the architect may indeed choose to display the way certain elements are designed to resist gravity; others will not.

Indeed, neither Mallgrave nor I want to reduce our appreciation of architecture to the battle between gravity and rigidity. Rather, Mallgrave wants to get across the idea that when we see an active process of resisting the force of gravity (and my caryatid example only reinforces this), we have a persuasive example (not an exhaustive one) of where we might imagine something like an embodied person-based empathy for a building. As a complementary example, we may see the spacing of the columns of the Parthenon as providing a spatial rhythm that we could link to toe-tapping or dance. (If architecture is frozen music, then, as diverse authors have asked, is music thawed architecture?)[4] In §5.6, we will see other cases where human actions are implicated in the appreciation of works of art and architecture. The crucial point, though, is that such effects *contribute* to, rather than form the totality of, our appreciation of the building. For example, Le Corbusier's admiration of the Parthenon would have been influenced by the "grace" of its proportions and the subtle visual corrections that achieved them, and the setting atop the Acropolis—though he explicitly decouples this admiration from considerations of use, the very considerations that separate architecture from art more generally.

Whatever one's position on empathy and Einfühlung, a key question remains. As Heinrich Wölfflin asked in 1886 in his *Prolegomena to a Psychology of Architecture* (Mallgrave & Ikonomou 1994), "How is it possible that architectural forms are able to invoke an emotion or a mood?" Consider the following:

> A weeping willow does not look sad because it looks like a sad person. It is more adequate to state that since the shape, direction, and flexibility of willow branches convey the expression of passive hanging, a comparison with the structurally similar psychophysical pattern of sadness in humans may impose itself secondarily. (Arnheim, 1969, p. 64)

But isn't this an abstracted feature of "looking like a sad person"? As in metaphor, only some features carry over from one domain of discourse to another. The notion of empathy in buildings is often seen as carried from people to buildings, but more generally we may carry

---

4. Friedrich von Schelling (1805) asserted that "Architecture is frozen music," to which Susanne Langer (1957) replied ". . . but music is not melted architecture." Her choice of adjective seems crucial, for we might nonetheless agree that music is *fluid* architecture. Here, we contrast the static arrangement (architecture) of most parts of most buildings (without denying the temporal patterns that the building makes possible for its users) with the dynamic arrangement (flowing in time) of the chords of a work of music.

over our impression of grandeur from, say, mountains to buildings. Or consider this:

> Planning atmospheres is an exercise in empathy because it requires us to imagine what a user would feel in this place. (Griffero in Tidwell, 2014, p. 73)

The architect here does not have empathy *for the building*; rather, she is empathizing with how she imagines another person will feel when experiencing the building that is being planned.

For many buildings, the outside sets a context for the interior spaces, and so the architect is not merely thinking of the impact of a room on a person somehow beamed into it without approaching it. What effect would it have for someone who walked up the steps of the building, walked down this corridor, and opened the door before seeing the space? How will they register the atmosphere or the functionality?[5]

To what extent could person--toperson empathy support person-to-building empathy? The latter question seems to me a powerful example of how the conversation between neuroscience and architecture could allow the architect to ask the neuroscientist questions that are intrinsically interesting challenges for neuroscience, not "just" requests for the neuroscientist to help the architect. How can *you* better understand what's going on in the brain, says the challenge to the neuroscientists; then, returning to the conversation, how can *we* get new ways of thinking about the design of a building and the way in which that building will impact people? I don't pretend to have the answers, but at least I can help the architect understand some of the relevant neuroscience. With this, then, the time has come to introduce mirror neurons as a basis for assessing whether they provide the neural mechanisms for "the mind's muscles" that Titchener posited for empathy.

---

5. Tan et al. (2020) highlight the effects of transitional spaces on the mental and psychological health of employees in underground and above-ground offices and suggests specific design interventions to enhance employee well-being.

5.2. MIRROR NEURONS AND THEIR
LARGER SETTING

"The thinking hand and its brain" (§2.6) was based in great part on collaboration with Marc Jeannerod, Giacomo Rizzolatti, and Hideo Sakata, but the major impact of that collaboration came with the discovery of *mirror neurons* by Rizzolatti's group (di Pellegrino et al., 1992). Some of the hand-related neurons in area F5 in monkey premotor cortex (introduced in §2.6) are active not only when the monkey carries out certain manual actions but also when the monkey observes an other (monkey or human) carrying out a similar action. This discovery *in the brains of monkeys* has had an immense impact on the way cognitive neuroscience has come to explore mechanisms for social interaction in the human brain. Let's start, then, with a brief account of the monkey study.

Studying the monkey brain

A standard lab setup for neurophysiology has the electrodes that monitor individual neurons not only feed a computer program which can record each time the cell fires, but also connect to a loudspeaker. One day an experimenter was placing a piece of food on the tray before passing the tray over to the monkey to record its neurons' responses when he noticed that the loudspeaker started clicking away. How could that be when the monkey was not yet doing anything? After trying out various scenarios, the team concluded—as shown in Figure 5.3—that some of the F5 neurons fired not only when the monkey acted in a certain way but also when he observed someone else acting in a similar way. And thus, *mirror neurons* were discovered: neurons that fire vigorously not only during execution of a limited set of actions but also during observation of similar actions.

An important point: Yes, some neurons fire both when the monkey executes a movement and when the monkey observes someone else making a similar movement. But this does *not* mean the set of neurons active when the monkey performs is the same as the set of neurons active when

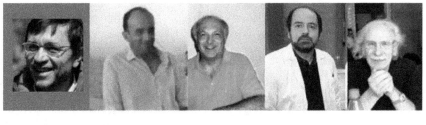

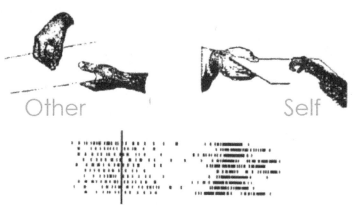

Other   Self

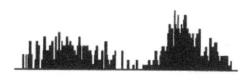

Figure 5.3 (*Top*) The team that put together the first report on mirror neurons: di Pellegrino, Fadiga, Fogassi, Gallese, and Rizzolatti. (*Bottom*) Firing of a mirror neuron that has a preference for the precision pinch. It fires vigorously when the monkey performs a precision pinch to grasp a piece of food ("Self") and (though somewhat less vigorously) when the monkey observes the experimenter perform a similar action ("Other"). The two columns of lines of *dots* show the time course of the cell's firing on 10 different occasions for the two conditions. In both cases, the rasters are aligned on the moment the grasp contacts the food. The histograms sum the rasters to show how "interested" the cell is in the two situations. For this cell, there would be little activity when the monkey is executing or observing a different kind of manual action. (*Bottom*: Adapted from Gallese, V., Fadiga, L., Fogassi, L., & Rizzolatti, G. [1996]. Action recognition in the premotor cortex. *Brain*, 119, 593–609, by permission of Oxford University Press.)

the monkey observes the action. The discovery of mirror neurons shows only that these two populations overlap. F5 also contains so-called *canonical neurons* that fire when the monkey executes an action but not when observing it—and, as the FARS model (§2.6) showed us, many regions besides F5 are involved in planning an action and setting up the parameters specified by the affordances. Similarly, there are distinct sets of neurons active in the recognition process.

Natural actions typically involve both a visual and an audio component. And indeed, some of the neurons in area F5 of the macaque premotor cortex were found to be *audiovisual mirror neurons*. They are responsive not only for visual observation of actions associated with characteristic noises (such as peanut-breaking and paper-ripping) but also for the sounds of these actions. They constituted 15% of the mirror neurons Kohler et al. (2002) studied in the hand area of F5.

Of course, there are many actions that do not have a distinctive sound, but for those that do, the audio information is inherently actor-invariant, and this allows the monkey to recognize that another individual is performing that action when the associated sound is heard. Obviously, the auditory response to paper-tearing cannot start until the peanut actually breaks to emit a characteristic sound, whereas the visual response can commence earlier. A key observation: It is implausible that the monkey brain evolved to have neurons specifically equipped to recognize paper-tearing. For this reason, we postulate that mirror neurons are not genetically specified—rather, the genes specify learning mechanisms that support the emergence of mirror neurons. A computational model for such learning will be provided in §5.4.

Crucially, there are mirror systems for actions other than manual ones, and these will be located in regions of the brain other than the hand-related area discussed so far. One such system involves orofacial neurons in an adjacent area within macaque F5. The majority of these *orofacial mirror neurons* become active during the execution and observation of mouth actions related to *ingestive* functions, such as grasping with the mouth, sucking, or breaking food. Others discharge during the execution of ingestive actions, yet have *communicative* mouth gestures as their most effective visual stimuli. The observed communicative actions (with the effective executed action for different "mirror neurons" in parentheses) include lip-smacking (sucking and lip-smacking); lips protrusion (grasping with lips, lip-smacking, grasping with mouth and chewing); tongue protrusion (reaching with tongue); teeth chatter (grasping with mouth); and lips/tongue protrusion (grasping with lips and reaching with tongue; grasping). Ferrari et al. (2017) show that, unlike the F5 neurons for reaching and hand-grasping within the traditional parietal-premotor circuits, the F5 neurons for orofacial motor control are connected with limbic structures involved in communication/emotions and reward processing. The fact that the hand and mouth mirror networks partially overlap suggests the importance of hand–mouth synergies not only for praxic actions like eating and drinking but also for communicative purposes in order to better convey and control social signals.

Learning about humans from studying the monkey brain

How do we bridge from monkey studies to human insights? While mirror neurons are individual neurons whose activity can be monitored in monkeys, it is impermissible to monitor single neurons within the human brain except when justified in mapping the exposed brain to plan where to cut in neurosurgery (and, more recently, in the design of neural prostheses), and only one such study of mirror neurons exists (Mukamel et al., 2010). Instead, researchers turned to human brain imaging to look for mirror *systems*. A brain region is a *mirror system for a class X of actions* if—against a baseline set by control tasks—the area is more active (e.g., shows a significantly greater blood-oxygen-level-dependent [BOLD] signal in functional magnetic resonance imaging [fMRI] studies) both when the subject performs an action from X and when the subject observes an other performing an action from X. For example, brain imaging has revealed that the *human* brain has a *mirror system for grasping*—regions that are more highly activated both when the subject performs a range of grasps and when the subject observes a range of grasps, compared to simply looking at objects (Grafton et al., 1996, Rizzolatti et al., 1996). Such an area in humans is often posited to contain networks of mirror neurons, each tuned to various actions in the class X—but, given the paucity of human single-neuron data, this is a commonly invoked hypothesis rather than a proven fact. Note that we lose here the precision of the monkey studies where we can discriminate between neurons that are more active for one type of grasp than another. Together, these neurons constitute a mirror system for grasping.[6]

Beyond the mirror

Mirror neurons have elicited great excitement because they offer a key contribution to social neuroscience. The suggestion is that if one can recognize what someone else is doing, then that recognition may be valuable in two ways: you may use that recognition and your understanding of why the person is doing it to better guide your interaction with them; moreover, if you recognize the other person's action but cannot immediately understand why they are doing it, then, when you figure that out, this may enrich your own capability to deploy that action, exploiting its effect in ways that were previously unavailable to you. The latter case may be particularly relevant when you are trying to learn how to behave in a novel environment—you observe how others deploy their actions so that you may learn how to deploy your own.

However, having mirror neurons alone does not guarantee the ability to imitate. *Monkeys do not imitate to any great extent, and so mirror neurons by themselves do not support imitation.* Indeed, mirror neurons are defined only for recognition of actions *in the observer's repertoire.* They may thus play a role within larger circuits when mimicking another's action if one

6. Although activation of a region in some conditions may show mirror system properties, relatively high activation of the region in other conditions is no guarantee that the latter activation is due primarily to the firing of mirror neurons. In other words, it can be misleading to name an area for just one of the functional modes it may exhibit (here, "mirroring"). Dinstein et al. (2008) and Turella et al. (2009) offer related critiques.

has already mastered that action—but mirror neurons alone cannot support adding a new action to one's repertoire as a result of observing another perform it. (I will discuss this latter form of imitation in Chapter 8—the point here is that evolution did not so much expand the power of mirror neurons as such, but rather expanded the brain's capability to work with them.) If a mirror neuron could talk, it might say, "Here's a behavior already in my repertoire. I know what my hands are doing when I carry out this behavior, and I have learned to recognize when somebody else moves their hands that way." But it could not say, "I see somebody doing something that gives them a reward, but I don't know how to perform this skill. I will develop the skill to carry out that behavior myself so I too can get that reward."

John Tenniel's drawing for Lewis Carroll's *Through the Looking Glass and What Alice Found There* John Tenniel's drawing (Figure 5.4) inspires

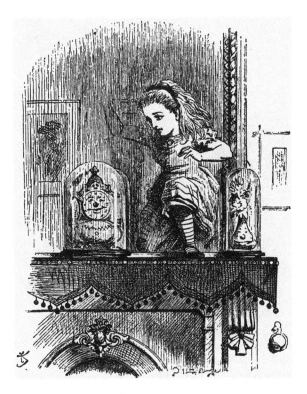

Figure 5.4 Beyond the mirror. Illustration for Lewis Carroll's *Through the Looking-Glass and What Alice Found There* by John Tenniel. (Common domain.)

my slogan that "mirror neurons are important, but if we want to understand their role in behavior we have to understand how they interact with other systems *beyond the mirror.*" Figure 5.5 makes explicit that the brain engages many regions beyond F5 in the monkey and corresponding mirror systems in the human for understanding the world and planning how to act.

An imaging study from Parma (Buccino et al., 2004) helps us go beyond the mirror, while also making the point that there are multiple mirror systems in addition to the basic one for hand movements (Figure 5.6). The mirror system considered here is for orofacial movements involved in both biting food and in communication. fMRI was used to scan the brains of humans in six conditions. In three, the subject saw videos (without sound) of a person taking a bite of food, a monkey taking a bite of food, or a dog taking a bite of food. The finding is that whether looking at human, monkey, or dog, the subject can map the act of biting onto his own actions

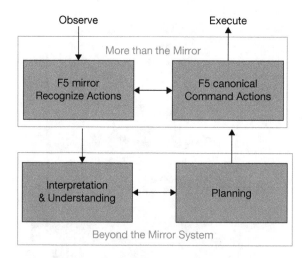

Figure 5.5 The F5 region of macaque premotor cortex contains both mirror neurons (firing both when the monkey performs certain actions and when it observes similar actions performed by others) and canonical neurons (firing when the monkey performs certain actions but not when it observes actions performed by others), and more. However, many brain regions "beyond the mirror" in addition to F5 are required to plan which actions to perform and to understand the behavior of others.

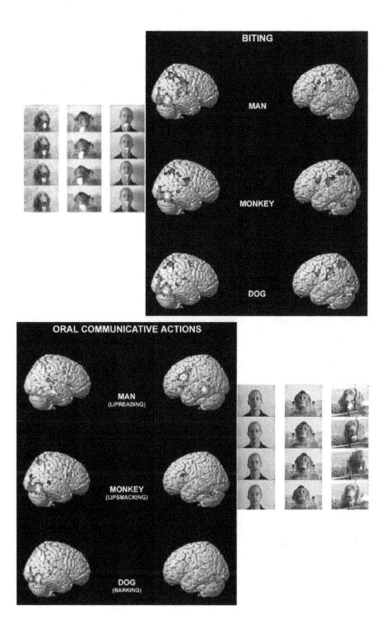

Figure 5.6 Human participants were presented with six videos (no audio) as the basis for fMRI imaging of brain regions involved in the recognition of actions performed by humans and nonconspecifics (monkey and dog). (*Top*) Observing biting, whether by human, monkey, or dog, elicited mirror system activity. (*Bottom*) Observing orofacial movements associated with communication elicited strong mirror system activity when observing the human, minimal mirror system activity when observing the monkey, and no mirror system activity when observing the dog. And yet the participant recognized the action in all six cases! (Adapted from Buccino, G., Lui, F., Canessa, N., Patteri, I., Lagravinese, G., et al. [2004]. Neural circuits involved in the recognition of actions performed by nonconspecifics: An fMRI study. *Journal of Cognitive Neuroscience*, 16[1], 114–126, with permission from MIT Press Journals.)

and that this yields similar activation of the mirror system *for biting*. In the second series, the subject sees a video (again, no sound) of a person talking, a monkey making communicative orofacial movements like teeth-chattering and lip-smacking, and a dog barking. The fMRI shows vigorous mirror system activity when the subject views the human, only modest activity when viewing the monkey, and none when viewing the dog. Now why is that crucial to my argument? This suggests that *we don't need mirror neurons to recognize actions, but that mirror neurons can enrich perception of actions when they fall within our own repertoire.*

I regret that Buccino et al. didn't also study fMRI responses for the tasks "imagine that you are imitating the monkey" and "imagine that you are imitating the dog" for the second set of videos. In this case, the subjects would have been seeking to map the observed behaviors onto their own muscular activity. I suspect that, if they recognized that the dog was barking, the new task might have involved vigorous mirror system activity that is missing in the "just observe" scenario.

In summary, mirror neurons may *inform* one's comprehension, but do not provide the full account:

1. Mirror neurons are active when one executes certain actions and when one observes such action performed by another, *but actions in our own repertoire do not exhaust the actions we may recognize.*

2. Canonical neurons are active when one executes certain actions but *not* when one observes that action performed by another. This suggests that they relate to the recognition of an affordance (executability) as the basis for self-action rather than recognition of another's action.

3. Recalling the distinction (§2.6) between the dorsal "how" system (setting motor parameters on the basis of affordance details) and the ventral "what" system (gathering data on relationships relevant to planning), we note that mirror neurons form just part of the dorsal pathway, whereas the ventral pathway and prefrontal cortex serve as systems beyond the mirror that support a huge range of perceptions, assessment, and planning.

Two more examples from the mirror neuron literature: Aglioti and his colleagues (Abreu et al., 2012; Aglioti et al., 2008) conducted both behavioral and brain imaging studies of people watching videos of basketball throws. They had three populations: fans, sports commentators, and expert basketball players. Mirror neuron activity was well established in all three populations, but if you just showed the first part of the video clip, the athletes could tell you whether or not the ball would go in the basket, whereas the commentators and fans could not. This may seem surprising, but the commentator's job is not to say, "This is the first split second of the throw. I think it's going to succeed," but rather to tell the audience whether or not it succeeded. Recognizing that a throw has succeeded is different from a player's judging in advance whether a throw will be successful and preparing to take appropriate action. Another study (Tomeo et al., 2012), this time with soccer players, found that the goalkeeper had a very different response to videos from that of other players. This suggests that mirror neurons may be implicated in "what one does next" perhaps even more than in emulating the observed action. This would certainly seem to be the case for monkeys.

Mirror systems have also been implicated in empathy—but before considering this, I devote two sections to further discussion on the computational modeling of brain.

5.3. HOW NEURAL NETS ENABLE US TO LEARN AND REMEMBER

We learn from experience. Neuroscience seeks to understand the neural mechanisms that make this possible. Brains function as highly parallel *adaptive* computers, which can adapt to changing task demands, in great part because synapses, the connections between neurons, can change dynamically to support learning on the basis of sensory, motor, and integrative experience. In this section we focus on *three styles of synaptic plasticity for learning*, namely, three different ways synapse may change with experience: *unsupervised learning*, *supervised learning*, and *reinforcement learning.* As we shall see in the next section, two of these are involved in the study of mirror neurons.

Different learning rules may apply to different parts of the brain. For example, Doya (2000) suggested that the cerebellum, the basal ganglia, and the cerebral cortex are specialized for supervised learning, reinforcement learning, and unsupervised learning, respectively. Such ideas have recently been updated by Caligiore et al. (2019). In the EvoDevoSocio framework, we may say that Evo yields the genes that in turn specify the various regions of the brain in terms of their initial synaptic connectivity (both within each region and between regions) and their learning rules; then development (Devo) within a certain social milieu (Socio) will change those synapses to yield brain and behavior and a physically maturing body that reflects the individual experience of each creature.

The treatment of learning rules here is very brief because many readers may not be interested in the details. Indeed, such readers may wish to, at most, skim this section or jump to the double lines near the end and pass rapidly to the next section. Those who do wish to learn more about the relevant mathematical specifications and biological correlates can find chapters on each learning mode (and much more) in the book, *From Neuron to Cognition via Computational Neuroscience* (Arbib & Bonaiuto, 2016).

==

Unsupervised learning

A strengthening of synapses induced by the coactivation of two neurons is called *Hebbian plasticity* in honor of Donald Hebb (1949) who, on the basis of neuropsychological studies of people with intact and damaged brains, hypothesized that, each time a cell B fires, there will be multiple inputs that contributed to that firing, and that on each such occasion any synapse A that contributed to that firing will be strengthened (Figure 5.7).

Hebb's idea was that the repeated coactivation of different neurons in a network—e.g., each time we encounter a banana—will ensure that the

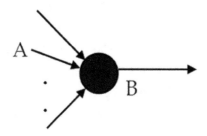

Figure 5.7 An abstract view of a neuron. Hebb's rule for synaptic plasticity (there are others) is that on each occasion when input A and neuron B are active together, the synapse from A to B will be strengthened.

connections between the simultaneously active neurons will be strengthened. In this case, the memory concept "banana" could be formed and represented by the set of strongly connected cells, called a *cell assembly* (Hebb, 1949).

Hebbian learning in this sense is an *unsupervised* learning rule, or "learning without a teacher": There is no notion of good or bad, successful or unsuccessful, rewarding or painful. Hebbian learning is suitable to detect correlations in the input and can therefore be used to explain developmental processes such as the formation of neurons in the early stages of the visual system that capture features that occur statistically often in the visual patterns to which the young child or animal is exposed. Neurophysiology has also implicated Hebbian learning in the learning mechanisms of the hippocampus.

Supervised learning

In *supervised learning*, we have a network in which there are input neurons (receiving signals from outside the circuit) and output neurons (whose axons can send signals outside the circuit). The desired behavior is specified by a *teacher* who provides a training set—this consists of a set of (input, output) pairs. The aim is to get the circuit to respond to each input pattern in the set by having the output neurons produce the cor-responding output pattern specified by the teacher. Each time a training pattern is supplied at the input, the "teacher" has to give the target value for each output neuron. Successful learning here will yield input–output behavior as close as possible to that provided by the teacher. The power of the method is that the learning generalizes to novel inputs as well because all patterns are processed by the setting of the synaptic weights that results from training.

Frank Rosenblatt (1958) introduced an important version of this notion to psychology with a model he called the *Perceptron*. The key idea is this:

- if a neuron fires when the teacher specifies that it should have been silent, reduce the weights of the synapses whose active inputs had contributed to the firing; whereas
- if a neuron is silent when the teacher specifies that it should have been active, increase the weights of the synapses with active inputs that nonetheless failed to yield firing.

A breakthrough for machine learning (but a departure from neuro-biology) came with the invention of *backpropagation*, an algorithm for "structural credit (or blame) assignment" that could be used to guide adjustment of synapses for neurons in "hidden layers" (i.e., neurons, other than output neurons, and thus for which no training signal was available) in a feedforward network (Rumelhart et al., 1986). In the context of these neural networks, "feedforward" simply means that there are no loops in the network, so that signals flow "forward" from inputs to outputs without ever looping back in the opposite direction.

Reinforcement learning

Reinforcement learning does not require a "teacher" that specifies the "cor-rect" strategy (correct firing of individual output neurons in response to the current input pattern). Rather, a *critic* rates the overall behavior controlled by the network, and provides a positive or negative reinforcement signal to *all* neurons. The method then specifies how each synapse in the network will change on the basis of this global evaluation. This is the problem that faces an animal foraging for food, or a human practicing to ride a bicycle.

There is now a mathematically grounded theory of reinforcement learning that makes strong contact with neurophysiology, showing how reinforcement may serve to alter the wiring of the brain—but at a non-conscious level because we cannot consciously monitor our 10^{15} synapses! The theory of reinforcement learning provides insights into one of the ways—not the only way—that the brain can change so that we may learn.

A crucial contribution to the theory was *temporal difference learning* that addressed *temporal* credit assignment in cases where reinforcement was intermittent (Sutton, 1988; Sutton & Barto, 2018). If you do something and immediately get punished, it's "easy" for learning mechanisms to adjust synapses to make it less likely that that you will do it again. Similarly, reinforcement learning can adjust synapses to make you more likely to repeat actions that are immediately rewarded. However, we often work long and hard before we succeed or fail. In playing a game like draughts (aka checkers), it may well be moves made quite early in the game that were responsible for our eventual victory or defeat. But which moves? The *temporal credit-assignment problem* is to determine, when a goal state is finally reached, to what extent decisions made earlier deserve credit (or blame) for the resulting reinforcement—so that reinforcement can be shared out among earlier actions, not just the action that immediately precedes success or failure.

Let me briefly present the essential idea—but not the mathematical details. A novice learning to play checkers may first learn to recognize those states where they are "doomed"—almost nothing can be done to avoid the negative reinforcement of losing the game. Similarly, they may come to recognize states close to the end game where the chances of the positive reinforcement of winning the game are high, as long as they choose their moves with care. As they play more and more games, they become better able to estimate which actions will lead from the current board setting toward success, and which are more likely to move toward failure. The theory formalizes this learning process by showing how an *adaptive critic* can be designed over time to better predict the *expected reinforcement* for situations and actions. The larger and more positive the expected reinforcement, the more likely will future actions lead to success; the more negative the expected reinforcement, the more likely will future actions lead to failure. And as the adaptive critic comes to better estimate the expected future reinforcement, so will the actor come to better select its next action as one that that "moves in the right direction."

One more wrinkle. An action may be desirable if it leads to reward and undesirable if it leads to punishment (in this example, losing the game). However, an action that leads to immediate reward is *more* desirable than one that will only yield that same reward after an extended delay. Thus, the calculations in the temporal difference learning include *discounting* to model this effect—the expected reinforcement discounts future rewards and punishments, and the longer the time before they can be expected, the greater the discount.

At the heart of the operation of the adaptive critic is the notion of the *prediction error*. As further actions are made, the adaptive critic can compare the prediction it made about the expected reinforcement with the actual reinforcement it has since received plus the new prediction for reinforcement it may receive during subsequent actions. The actual computations rest on some subtle equations, but the general idea is this:

- If the prediction error is positive, it indicates that the true reward *may be* greater than the estimate supplied by the adaptive critic (prospects may be better than estimated).
- If the prediction error is negative, it indicates the that the true reward *may be* less than the estimate (prospects may be worse than estimated).
- If the prediction error is equal to zero, it indicates the true reward *may be* equal to the estimate (the adaptive critic should not adjust its estimate at this time).

Why "may be"? Because future actions may still yield positive and negative reinforcement that was not anticipated in the current prediction. Since the error is calculated after each step, the cumulative reward may yet to be experienced.

The adaptive critic uses this prediction error to adjust its estimate of the expected reinforcement of states it encounters—but it does this by adjusting the synapses in its own network, and so the changes affect how reinforcement will be estimated for other states as well.

To get another perspective on these ideas, consider that reward-directed learning depends on the predictability of the reward. If you get what you expect, then there is nothing new to be learned. The reward has to be surprising or unpredicted for a stimulus or action to update what you have learned. The degree to which a reward cannot be predicted is indicated by the discrepancy between the reward obtained for a given behavioral action and the reward that was predicted to occur as a result of that action. We have thus seen, in outline, how such a prediction error enters into the theory of temporal difference learning.

After this excursion into theory (though without the mathematics), there is a surprise. Behavioral roles of dopamine (§4.2) range from purely motor to highly cognitive. The loss of midbrain dopamine neurons results in the symptomatology of Parkinson's disease, and abnormal dopaminergic signaling has been implicated in schizophrenia and addiction. But the surprise is that neuroscience experiments showed that the prediction error of the theory of reinforcement learning (specifically that involving estimation of expected reinforcement when reward and punishment are intermittent and cumulative) seems to correlate with the release of dopamine in the input regions (the striatum or caudate) of the basal ganglia (Hollerman & Schultz, 1998; Schultz, 2016; Schultz et al., 1997). In §4.6, we saw studies that indicated that learning to trust partners may be predicted and reflected in activation of the dorsal striatum, suggesting that this region is also actively involved in evaluating future rewards dependent on interpersonal reciprocity.

From brain to machine: deep learning

Although AI turned its back on learning techniques for several decades, one of the great early papers in AI (Samuel, 1959) anticipated temporal difference learning by developing a technique for machine learning while playing the game of checkers, where reinforcement comes only when one wins or loses the current game. The current resurgence of AI has been made possible by advances in "deep learning," exploiting the simulation of artificial neural networks (ANNs) whose learning is loosely based on the biological lessons concerning synaptic change—but augmented by varying "tricks" that augment the computations that support the learning. Intriguingly, the key techniques were in place by the mid-1990s (there are diverse articles by some of the key researchers collected in Arbib, 1995), but their impact on AI long remained limited. It is only recently that increasingly powerful computers and immense databases have made this technology widely applicable and commercially compelling.

We will return to deep learning when we consider robot emotions in §7.4, assessing its possible impacts on neuromorphic architecture, the design of buildings with "brains."

Having now examined three forms of synaptic plasticity, I should stress that the human brain has evolved mechanisms to extend learning in ways that exploit the large-scale memory systems we met in §3.3. A crucial aspect of human behavior is that it can privilege long-term plans over immediate satisfactions. For example, the design of a building may extend for years, but this long-term goal will involve attention to details at many levels, some of which will be a pleasure to work on, whereas others will be tedious and yet will be motivated by their part in the overall project. Humans learn to apportion credit to different activities. They have evolved not simply to use reinforcement learning based on adjusting active synapses, but to ask, "What went wrong this time? What should I do next time?"—generating plans by analogy as much as by logic. The ability to ask and answer questions rests on our sensory and motor experience but in the end is bound up with the evolution of language—with its ability to negate, generalize, state counterfactuals . . . and ask questions—and the changes in consciousness that accompany it.

We humans work with imperfection, but like other animals we have neurons of a diversity and complexity that are unmatched by the artificial neurons whose learning is exploited in current AI, and we have a highly variegated anatomy of brain regions, with distinctive neurons and connectivity that is related to that of other creatures (Kaas, 2017)—but with innovations that support unique abilities such as language. However, these neural and neurological subtleties have yet to factor into AI.

5.4. MODELING HOW MIRROR NEURONS LEARN AND FUNCTION

In the general spirit of action-oriented perception, it must be stressed that mirror neurons are as much perceptual as motor. For example, recognizing a manual action from visual observation requires, in general, recognition of the affordance of the object upon which the action is to be executed and of the spatiotemporal pattern of the hand's movement relative to the object. My group's models of the mirror system for grasping, to which we now turn, show how neurons may *become* mirror neurons by learning to recognize the trajectory of the hand in an object-centered reference frame for self-execution of an action. This representation then supports recognition of the action when performed by others and, in many cases, will allow confident recognition of the action relatively early in the trajectory of the hand toward the object.

While I hope many will want to read about the workings of the models, I have separated these from the exposition of "what it's all about" in the next section, as I occasionally do elsewhere. Many of my architect friends have tended to skip even these gentle descriptions of the neuroscience when reading earlier drafts of the text. However, I think the exposition of a number of cog/neuroscience studies focused on architecture (as in §4.5 or in §5.7) will demonstrate that serious collaboration between architect and scientist does require some serious engagement with the other's subject matter, at least to the point where focused discussion of the design and results of an experiment become possible, even while each participant leaves certain of the details in the safe hands of their colleagues. Of course, for the reader (whether architect or general reader) not seeking future collaborations, no such considerations apply.

A model of learning in the mirror neuron system

As noted earlier, monkeys have mirror neurons specifically responsive for breaking peanuts *or* for tearing paper, and such neurons could not have been "wired up" on the basis of a genetic blueprint. The MNS Model (Oztop & Arbib, 2002) provided the first computational demonstration of mirror neurons, focusing on the learning capacities that form mirror neurons.[7] We modeled the situation where the monkey (or, equally well, the human child or adult) has first acquired the ability, perhaps by trial and error, to perform a certain kind of action (Oztop et al., 2004, modeled infant grasp learning) and then extends that capability to recognize that others are performing a similar action.[8]

The key point is that the learning must transform neurons that are not mirror neurons for an action into neurons that are. Putting this another way, there is *a pool of neurons that can become mirror neurons, but are not initially mirror neurons.* Let's call them *quasi-mirror neurons* before they become mirror neurons.

Readers uninterested in further details of the MNS model may jump to the next double lines to see the implications of the model for the ongoing discussion.

---

7. Bonaiuto et al. (2007) extended the MNS model to train up *audiovisual mirror neurons* as well as neurons responsive specifically to viewing a manual action.

8. The ability to recognize manual actions and the further ability (absent in monkeys) to exploit such recognition in the imitation of complex skills should not be confused with "neonatal imitation," the ability of the newborn human to respond to some basic facial expressions of a caregiver with a similar facial expression, such as tongue protrusion (Meltzoff & Moore, 1977; Ferrari et al., 2006).

The main points about the model are as follows:

1. After the monkey has mastered a manual action, call it A, there will be "canonical neurons" whose activity controls performance of that action.
2. The activity of these neurons will also activate certain quasi-mirror neurons. However, these are not yet mirror neurons for A. At this initial stage, they require the monkey's own execution of A, as encoded by the activity of the corresponding canonical neurons, to be activated.
3. A crucial hypothesis is that the quasi-mirror neurons also receive inputs encoding how the hand is moving toward the relevant affordance of an object when the monkey itself performs A. Of course, the actual hand trajectory may vary from occasion to occasion.
4. The further hypothesis is that the activation of a quasi-mirror neuron by canonical neurons when A is being activated serves as the training signal for the quasi-mirror neuron to learn to recognize trajectories similar to those that accompany the monkey's own performance of A.
5. After sufficient learning, the neurons can be activated when the monkey observes such a hand-to-affordance trajectory whether or not the hand is that of the monkey. *The quasi-mirror neurons have become mirror neurons for action A.*

The particular version of learning included in the model has the important property that the model may not need to see the whole trajectory to recognize the grasp—as learning progresses, the system recognizes the trajectory from its initial segments "as early as possible," rather than waiting for the grasp to be completed. Moreover:

- When the monkey observes an other performing action A, it is only the trajectory of the hand relative to the object that can activate the mirror neurons for A.

- However, when the monkey itself performs A, the mirror neurons for A can be activated in one of two ways—by the canonical neuron activity for A, or by observation of the hand's trajectory—or by both together.

It is not necessary for the arguments that follow to recall the details of the FARS and MNS models. What is important is to understand that many different neural populations must work together for the successful control of hand movements, for the successful operation of the macaque mirror system for grasping, and for the learning that supports them.

Mirror neurons are not just for social interaction

As discussed earlier, mirror neurons have come to play an important role in *social* cognitive neuroscience: if we can recognize the actions of others as similar to our own, then we may be able to interact with them more fruitfully, especially if we can exploit "tells"—recognizing an action just as it starts rather than having to see it through to completion. Moreover, they may help us recognize that our own actions have uses and implications that we had not discovered hitherto. This has led many researchers to suggest that mirror neurons evolved under adaptive pressure to improve social interaction. However, I argue that mirror neurons *initially* evolved so that we could learn from monitoring *our own* behaviors. The further argument is that when this ability was in place, their capacity could be exploited (with no necessary change in the circuitry) to *give us the skill to track the behaviors of others*—and thus, but secondarily, to become evolutionarily advantageous for social interaction. To bolster this argument, I offer an example of modeling that is important because it looks—as almost none of the other neuroscience literature does—at *the role of mirror neurons in tracking one's own behavior* rather than the behavior of others.

Bror Alstermark is a Swedish neuroanatomist who studied the connections from the spinal cord to different parts of the musculature. In one study (Alstermark et al., 1981), he found specific axons coming out from the spinal cord that controlled the paw of the cat (grasping) as distinct from the arm of the cat (reaching). The top of Figure 5.8 shows a normal cat able to coordinate arm and paw, that has learned to reach into a glass tube to grasp a piece of food and bring it to its mouth. At bottom, we see a cat that had received a transection that blocked the neural control of the paw. Amazingly, within just four or five trials, this cat developed a new behavior with no need for a protracted period of learning by trial and error. He would reach into the tube but couldn't grasp the food. Instead, he just batted the food out and then, after it fell to the ground, he could efficiently grab it with his jaw.

We (Bonaiuto & Arbib, 2010) explained this by developing the Augmented Comp[etitive Queuing (ACQ) model, which addresses the *flexible scheduling* of actions to achieve some overall goal. Unlike most of the mirror neuron literature, *ACQ emphasizes the utility of a mirror system in recognizing one's own actions.*

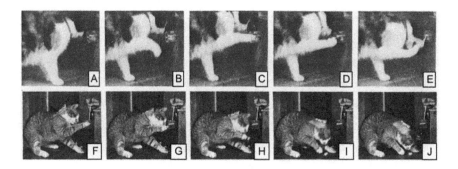

Figure 5.8 Alstermark's cat—flexible action patterns and their rapid reorganization. *A* to *E* show a normal cat that has learned to reach into a glass tube, grasp a piece of food, bring it to its mouth, and eat it. *F* to *J* show a cat that had mastered this task but had then received surgery that disabled its ability to control grasping. In only a few trials, it dramatically restructured its behavior, batting the food out of the tube then using its mouth to grasp it from the floor. (Reprinted by permission from Alstermark, B., Lundberg, A., Norrsell, U., & Sybirska, E. [1981]. Integration in descending motor pathways controlling the forelimb in the cat: 9. Differential behavioural defects after spinal cord lesions interrupting defined pathways from higher centres to motoneurones. *Experimental Brain Research, 42,* 299–318. © 1981, Springer-Verlag.)

At any time, one may have to choose which of many possible actions to execute next. In ACQ, competition to determine the next action is based on priorities that are updated each time an action is executed. Specifically, separate subsystems in ACQ assess

- the *executability* of actions (the availability of suitable affordances and—possibly—the ease of exploiting them); and
- the *desirability* of actions (an estimate of the expectation that executing that action will lead on to attainment of the distal goal).

ACQ chooses the action with the highest value of *priority = executability * desirability*, and that action is then executed to completion.

Executability and *desirability* are then updated, and the action with the resultant highest priority is executed. This process continues until the overall goal is attained.

Before applying this to Alstermark's cats, let's relate it to our own experience. If you are watching TV, and you want a cup of tea, then drinking that tea becomes most desirable. However, if there is no cup of tea by your side, then drinking the tea is not executable. Over time, you have acquired various actions to solve this problem that can only be executed if certain prior actions have set up the appropriate affordances. Here is one such sequence where each requires prior actions to become executable, and where the earlier actions are not necessarily desirable in and of themselves, but become desirable within the context of drinking a nice cup of tea:

> Go to the kitchen → put water in the kettle → set the kettle to boil → put a teabag in a cup → pour water on the teabag (after the water has boiled) → remove and discard the teabag (after it has steeped long enough) → carry cup back to the living room → drink some tea.

If the kettle has just boiled, one can skip the second and third actions— they no longer have higher priority than any of the later actions. To refine the discussion, one may note that another possible sequence might get the teabag in place before attending to the kettle. In each case, early actions are less desirable in themselves than later actions. But for now, let's return to those cats.

When the normal cat sees the food, the most desirable action is to eat it. But the cat can't do that until it has put the food in its mouth. Its behavior is then to perform a chain of actions, each one setting up the affordances for later ones to become executable—and each one being more desirable than the one that preceded it because it brings the animal closer to its goal of eating the food:

Reach into the glass tube → grasp the food → bring the food to the mouth → eat.

The relative desirability of each action would have been learned by *temporal difference learning* (§5.3). In the present example, a "win" is getting to eat food, and we use the term "desirability" for the expected reinforcement of carrying out various actions when affordances are available for their execution. However, temporal difference learning includes a discount factor so that, even if an action will normall lead to that "win," its desirability will be discounted as the delay until eating the food is increased.

The previous sequence for the normal cat involves executing increasingly desirable actions when they are executable. However, the lesioned cat cannot succeed with this sequence. It may try repeatedly, but it swiftly learns that *grasp the food* is no longer executable. Nonetheless, in four or five trials, the animal comes up with a new and successful strategy:

Reach into the glass tube → bat the food out of the tube so it falls to the floor → grab the food with the jaws → eat.

According to ACQ, the key to this is that the mirror system can also monitor *self*-actions to assess whether an *intended action* proceeded as expected or whether the output resembled another action, the *apparent action*.

While the MNS model focuses on manual actions, we here exploit the MNS hypothesis of the previous section in a form that applies to any visually observable action. We saw in the previous subsection that mirror neurons for a self-action can be activated via two pathways: by the canonical code for the movement and by an appropriate trajectory as observed via the visual system.

The key insight is this: In general, these two pathways will activate the same mirror neurons—*but only if the action is successful.* If the action fails, then two sets of mirror neurons may be activated: one set for the *intended* action, activated by the canonical code; and a distinct set for the *apparent* action if the unsuccessful action happens to resemble an action in the mirror system repertoire. For this reason, we titled the ACQ paper, "What Did I Just Do? A New Role for Mirror Neurons."

In the case of the lesioned cat, it would reach into the glass tube and try to grasp the food. Grasping would fail, but the effort to grasp would dislodge the food, which then fell to the floor, where the cat could retrieve it. The ACQ argument is that, each time this happened, not only did grasping become increasingly recognized as nonexecutable, but also the mirror system recognized the failed grasp as a successful action of batting the food out of the tube. Thus, over a few trials, the batting action, hitherto irrelevant, became more and more desirable and soon gained the priority to be executed as soon as the cat had its paw in the tube.

Scheduling with scripts

Let's return to the cup-of-tea sequence where each requires prior actions to become executable, and where the earlier actions are not necessarily desirable outside the context of preparing tea:

> Go to the kitchen → put water in the kettle → set the kettle to boil → put a teabag in a cup → pour water on the teabag (after the water has boiled) → remove and discard the teabag (after it has steeped long enough) → carry cup back to the living room → drink some tea.

However, the alert reader may have noted that, even though it was introduced as an example of "flexible scheduling," the sequence can also be read as an example of a *script*. And, indeed, different people may have variations on this script if they prefer a mug to a cup, or use sugar, or want lemon or milk (not both) in their tea.

However, the ACQ (flexible scheduling) and the script accounts are *not* two descriptions of the same mechanism. Rather, this duality illustrates that the brain may achieve similar ends by different means. In the first account, diverse actions actively compete to be executed; in the latter, there is chaining in which the successful completion of one action triggers the next (though with the ability to recognize when one can start partway along the chain). The further claim would be that that the script could have been learned in one of two ways: either because repeated flexible scheduling of a novel chain (as in the case of Alstermark's lesioned cat) could have supported the strengthening of associative links between one action and the next, or because one had explicitly been trained to perform the actions in the given order. The first mechanism emphasizes learning what actions succeed working back from the last; the latter requires learning a sequence working forward from the first element without there necessarily being any access to the desirability of what can be achieved when performing the whole sequence in some appropriate context. Alstermark's cat received no training of the second kind in order to develop its markedly different script for eating the food it could see in the glass tube.

We will encounter another dichotomy when we consider wayfinding in Chapter 6. For habitual navigation, we simply follow a habitual route, a detailed script for finding affordances and executing prescribed actions (when you see the supermarket, take the next left turn). However, when our habitual route is blocked, or we want to get to a habitual destination from some other place, then we need a cognitive map to provide the underlying knowledge base that allows us to apply flexible scheduling skills to find our way.

Ideas like this will resurface in Chapter 10 when we consider how a room or building may provide the necessary affordances to allow users to perform a varied set of scripts, and how the architect may design the places in spatial relationship that will support users of a building in acting in ways that exemplify those scripts, and yet may also support exploration and discovery.

Learning and disability

Of course, learning can do much more than train up mirror neurons, support decisions on what to do next, or develop new scripts. The example of correcting for a prism in aiming at a target (§2.2) involves supervised learning in the cerebellum, whereas Hebbian learning has been implicated in the formation of "feature detectors" that match the statistics of the environment in sensory processing, as well as Hebb's original notion of recognizing instances of a general category. I do not know whether these particular examples will prove essential to the A↔N conversation, but I do know that the future growth of that conversation will increasingly engage with areas of neuroscience whose relevance is not yet apparent. Thus, I have augmented my various tours of brain mechanisms whose relevance to architecture has already been established with a number that you will, I hope, in any case find interesting and that may stimulate you to consider whether they may prove relevant in ways not charted in this book.

The study of the cat that was unable to grasp food with its paw raises the issue of whether such experiments and the related computational modeling can offer insights into the design of spaces for people with certain physical disabilities. How can we help people through adaptable designs based on the learning mechanism of the brain? Such questions made me realize that I had been engaged in related issues long before I became seriously engaged in linking neuroscience and architecture. In the late 1980s, my work on the neural mechanisms of motor control somehow led to my becoming a "guru" for the two departments of *Physical Therapy* and *Occupational Therapy* at USC. Physical therapy traditionally focused on exercises designed to gain mastery over muscle movements, restoring or substituting "degrees of freedom" following a stroke or an accident or disease. Occupational therapy focused not so much on the muscles as such but on the tasks of everyday living, seeking to provide strategies that would be effective even if the original effectors were impaired. In each case, the focus was on manipulations of the body to improve function. My role was to help my colleagues build on their initial efforts to expand practice and research to more fully link with the findings of cognitive science and neuroscience, a transformation that has by now been long embedded in the fabric of both departments. This effort may be seen as a precursor of my current concern with how a subject like architecture could be enriched by cog/neuroscience, but the key point is that it was only the commitment of my within-discipline colleagues to expand their own work and to hire new people with whom they could collaborate that made possible the expansion of curriculum and research to better integrate neuroscience into their vision of their fields.

For example, note that physical therapy may involve repeated and tedious practice to regain control of muscles when, for example, the cortical circuitry for that control has been grossly affected by stroke. In one study, Cheol Han modeled how forced practice might lead to rewiring of a remnant population of cortical neurons to more fully cover the spectrum needed for effective muscle control. Our modeling (Han et al., 2008) predicted that the "dosage" of therapy constraining the patient to use only the affected hand could reach a threshold such that the patient's use of that hand would be competent enough that they would no longer avoid using it so that the "natural" use would thereafter obviate the imposition of forced use during therapy. Led by collaboration of neuroscientist Nicolas Schweighofer (one of the new hires) and clinician Carolee Winstein, the clinical implications of this finding have been widely discussed (Schweighofer et al., 2009).

Separately, we may see parallels between the way architects have already learned to design buildings and the case of the disabled cat. The cat's task was to get the food into its mouth, and here it learned how to switch from trying to grasp the food with its paw to achieving a state in which it had available the affordances for grasping the food with its mouth. In the same way, a person who is unable to climb stairs may be catered to by providing a ramp with a handrail to support effortful walking to a destination, or to support someone in a wheelchair.

The latter case points to an increasingly powerful symbiosis between robotics and architecture. The wheelchair may be considered as a relatively simple example of an assistive robot. The ramp offers affordances that the "extended human"—the human in a wheelchair—can exploit even if the human cannot ascend the ramp unaided (recall the extendibility of the body schema, §2.4). But, as we shall emphasize in Chapter 7, the combination of human "extension" and responsive buildings will be of increasing concern for architecture in general, not just in catering for people with disabilities. As the base case for this, consider how many of us now feel "disabled" if we do not have the "extension" of a smartphone in hand, and an environment that affords us constant Wi-Fi access to the Internet.

5.5. EMPATHY AND THE BRAIN

In Chapter 3, we assessed two proposals that link neural circuitry to aesthetic judgment of *visual* form, one based on neural circuitry of early visual cortex in humans and the other on visuomomotor mechanisms in the frog's brain. In this, we were building on the distinction between *general-purpose vision* (as exemplified in the study of initial stages of processing in mammalian visual cortex) and *action-oriented vision* (as exemplified in the study of "prey detectors" in the frog retina). But we will now explore evidence that mirror systems (human brain systems that, presumably, function in part through activity of mirror neurons) are implicated not only in action recognition but also in empathy that includes the ability to in some sense "feel" another's emotions. With this, we will be well prepared to loop back to "Empathy and Einfühlung in life, architecture, and art" and consider how scholars have linked this to the brain's motor system in general and mirror systems in particular. A reminder: We must not talk of *the* mirror system but rather seek to understand the roles of, and interactions, between, multiple mirror systems and systems "beyond the mirror."

Gazzola et al. (2006) used fMRI to search for brain areas that respond both during motor execution and when individuals listened to the sound of any action made using the same effector. (Recall the earlier mention of audiovisual mirror neurons in macaques.) They found two such systems: one more involved during listening and execution of hand actions, and another more involved for mouth actions. So far, not so surprising. But Gazzola et al. tested a further notion. Would people with stronger mirror system activity for these two classes of actions tend to show more empathy for others? To test this, they employed a standard questionnaire for assessing how empathic each subject was and, indeed, found (statistically, rather than in every case) greater activation of the mirror systems in those individuals who scored higher on the empathy scale. This suggests a link between the mirror systems and empathy. However, empathy cannot be reduced simply to mirror system activity. Differences in mirror system activity explained 40% of the variance on the empathy test. Thus, this particular correlation suggests that people who are more observant of others' (visible and audible) actions may be somewhat better at inferring their mental states—but other systems beyond the mirror are also involved. For example, their study did not examine other parts of the brain involved in recognizing emotional expression.

With this, we turn to a study of a human mirror system for an emotion, in this case *disgust*. This study brings another region of the cerebral cortex into play, the insula. This is folded deep within the fissure separating the temporal lobe from the parietal and frontal lobes. The insulas (one on each side of the brain) are believed to play a role in diverse functions usually linked to emotion or the regulation of the body's homeostasis. Wicker et al. (2003) found a mirror system for seeing and feeling disgust. For their fMRI study, participants inhaled odorants that smelled disgusting. The same participants also observed video clips showing the emotional facial expression of disgust and other emotions. Wicker et al. say, "Observing such faces and feeling disgust activated the *same* sites in the anterior insula and to a lesser extent in the anterior cingulate cortex. [My italics.]" But examination of Figure 5.9 shows this to be misleading. There are many voxels activated for seeing disgust registered on another's face, and there are many activated while smelling the disgusting smell. The overlap is

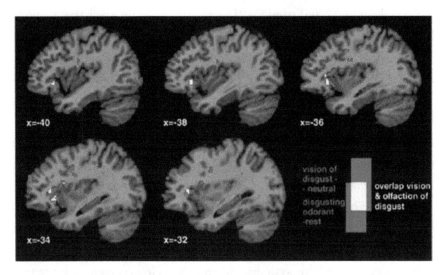

Figure 5.9 Possible fMRI evidence for a mirror system for disgust. *Red and white* voxels relate to activity when the participant smells a disgusting odorant; *blue and white* voxels relate to activity when observing facial expressions of disgust by another. Note that the overlap of these, the *white* voxels—the putative "mirror system for disgust"—forms only a small proportion of the "action" and "recognition" subsets. (Reprinted from Wicker, B., Keysers, C., Plailly, J., Royet, J. P., Gallese, V., & Rizzolatti, G. [2003]. Both of us disgusted in My insula: The common neural basis of seeing and feeling disgust. *Neuron*, 40[3], 655–664, © 2003, with permission from Elsevier.)

relatively small. For this reason, one must qualify one's support for their claim that "observing an emotion activates the neural representation of [experiencing] that emotion [and this] finding provides a unifying mechanism for understanding the behaviors of others." We come to understand these emotions only in part from recognizing how others experience them, and this requires tapping into memory structures that go beyond mirror neurons as narrowly conceived. This idea relates to the distinction (§4.4) between the internal role of emotion (in providing a general emphasis for one's current behavior) and the external role of emotion (providing cues about one's current disposition that may inform others about if and how to interact with you).

Let's do an experiment. Unfortunately, I cannot conduct this experiment with you in a controlled way, but please assess your own reaction and compare it to what I find happens with an audience:

Here are three frames (Figure 5.10). I ask you to read the slides down from top to bottom to simulate watching a video.

Did you feel the emotion of the person as expressed in the first "video"? Most people in my audiences experience at least a momentary twitching of the lips into a smile. In this case, then, the mirror neuron theory of empathy—we recognize an emotion by feeling that emotion—seems to gain some support. However, my concern is that this ignores context. In general, our reactions (recall the action–perception cycle) depend on our current mental state as much as (perhaps more than) our current sensory input. So before we look at a second "video," let me first establish a context. Imagine the following. "You have spent the day cooking a superb dinner.

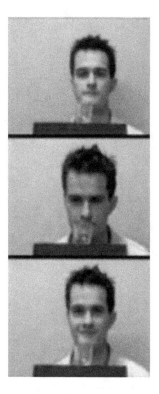

Figure 5.10 The first "video." (Adapted from Wicker, B., Keysers, C., Plailly, J., Royet, J. P., Gallese, V., & Rizzolatti, G. [2003]. Both of us disgusted in My insula: The common neural basis of seeing and feeling disgust. *Neuron*, 40[3], 655–664, © 2003, with permission from Elsevier.)

You've really put your heart into producing this wonderful dish. You really want to please your guests, and you chose a very special and expensive wine to complement the meal. You have just poured a glass of the wine and your guest has picked it up." The second "video" (Figure 5.11) shows how he reacts.

When I try this out on an audience, nobody feels the disgust that the subject is registering. Rather disconcertingly, their usual reaction is to burst into laughter. However, they tend to agree that if this had really happened to them, their reaction would be anger or disappointment or embarrassment, not disgust. In short, any theory of empathy (or

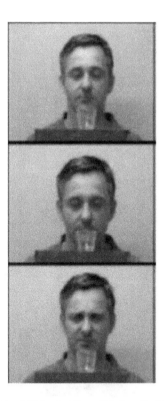

Figure 5.11 The second "video." (Adapted from Wicker, B., Keysers, C., Plailly, J., Royet, J. P., Gallese, V., & Rizzolatti, G. [2003]. Both of us disgusted in My insula: The common neural basis of seeing and feeling disgust. *Neuron*, 40[3], 655–664, © 2003, with permission from Elsevier.)

human behavior in general) must integrate the study of mirror neurons with the study of systems beyond the mirror to better explain how our interactions with the social and physical world around us unfold over time.

More generally, our emotional response "is not just empathy." Feeling disgust when stepping on dog shit while walking down the street is very different from registering someone else's disgust. Their expression may elicit an empathic reaction, or it may simply help turn one's attention to the source of that disgust, which will lead one to avoiding stepping in it oneself, and then may, or may not, elicit one's own disgust through direct observation rather than empathy. Sadly, too, in many cases one's reaction may be laughter rather than sympathy—a reaction exploited in the "comedy" of the *Three Stooges*, among many others. Recall my assessment that the Buccino et al. data show that mirror neurons are just part of a larger brain system for recognition. My further point is that such recognition may be the basis for reactions that bypass empathy.

Here's another example. If you are walking down the street and a passing stranger smiles at you, you may smile back without any explicit reflective mediation—as if the mirror neurons that recognize the smile were to play directly into your motor system to produce that smile of your own. But life in general is more complicated. If someone whom you think of as untrustworthy smiles at you, you might think, "What's that bastard smiling at?" and not smile back. There might be, who knows, a fraction of a second in which the mirror neurons might register that this is a smile, but that does not entail that you must smile back reflexively. Other brain mechanisms are at work, and they can take the lead in determining your reaction. We thus need to distinguish the "gut semantics" of emotion in which mirror neurons link activation in, for example, amygdala, orbitofrontal cortex, and insula to the embodied (somatic/visceral) feeling of emotions from the "disposition semantics" of being able to recognize that a certain facial expression may betoken another person's behavioral disposition without feeling the attendant emotion oneself.

5.6. EINFÜHLUNG AND THE MOTOR COMPONENT
OF CONTEMPLATION

What might all this mean for art and architecture? Enriched by our under-standing of mirror systems, it is now time to explore their role in relating aesthetic experience to activity of the motor system and mirror neurons. To this end, we consider two chapters (Gallese & Gattara, 2015; Mallgrave, 2015)[9] from the book, *Mind in Architecture: Neuroscience, Embodiment, and the Future of Design* (Robinson & Pallasmaa, 2015). Gallese and Gattara state:

> The experience of architecture, from the contemplation of the decorative element of a Greek temple, to the physical experience of living and working within a specific architectonic space, can be deconstructed into its grounding bodily elements. Cognitive neuroscience can investigate of what the sense of presence that some buildings possess is made. This approach can also contribute a fresher empirical take on the evolution of architectonic style and its cultural diversity, by treating it as a particular case of symbolic expression, and through identifying its bodily roots. (Gallese & Gattara, 2015, p. 164)

However, their chapter says very little about "living and working within a specific architectonic space." They focus on the contemplation of archi-tecture but not on *use* (as in distinguishing architecture from sculpture). With Mallgrave, they recast the "feeling into" of Einfühlung as "neurologi-cally simulating" objects of artistic contemplation, with mirror neurons as the key neural correlate. However, mirror neurons respond to actions, not objects, so neurologically simulating the *object* of artistic contemplation is

---

9. A somewhat overlapping treatment is provided in Tidwell (2015), *Architecture and Empathy*, with contributions from Juhani Pallasmaa, Harry Francis Mallgrave, Sarah Robinson, and Vittorio Gallese. I should also note that both Gallese and Mallgrave have published many writ-ings relevant to our concerns since 2015. Here, let me just single out a more recent book by Mallgrave (2018), *From Object to Experience: The New Culture of Architectural Design*.

somewhat different from neurologically simulating some *action* involving that object.

Gallese and Gattara stress that "[t]he neurophysiological and behavioral evidence of [the] early phase of aesthetic experience is strikingly similar to that which underlies the mundane perceptual experience of non-artistic objects," but this is unsurprising since they here employ "aesthetic experience" as covering sensory experience *in general*, as distinct from my use of the term specifically for *the combination of sensory experience with aesthetic judgment*. However, we agree that one cannot reduce perception to only the sensory portals such as vision and audition—one must take the motor system into account.

David Freedberg and Vittorio Gallese (2007) challenged "the primacy of cognition in responses to art":

We propose that a crucial element of esthetic response consists of the activation of embodied mechanisms encompassing the simulation of actions, emotions and corporeal sensation, and that *these mechanisms are universal*. This basic level of reaction to images is essential to understanding the effectiveness both of everyday images and of works of art. Historical, cultural and other contextual factors do not preclude the importance of considering the neural processes that arise in the empathetic understanding of visual artworks. [My italics.]

Yes, precognitive as well as conscious cognitive processes affect our response to art—and, indeed, to our everyday environment. However, the notion of "universal mechanisms" must be treated with some care. They stress that "[h]istorical, cultural and other contextual factors do not preclude the importance of considering the neural processes that arise in the empathetic understanding of visual artworks." I respond by stressing (EvoDevoSocio) that many of those neural processes reflect our individual experiences, and that these are shaped in part by our social and cultural networks. In aesthetic *judgment*, historical, cultural, and other contextual factors may play the crucial role. On the other hand, our treatment of

motivation and emotion in Chapter 4 (and, indeed, the "initial conditions" for learning in MNS) make clear that Evo provides a strong biological framework for these developments. None of these caveats deny that
mirroring mechanisms play a role for empathetic responses to works of
visual art and architecture, but they do question their primacy.

In the *Laocoön* sculpture (Figure 5.12), the emotional impact is very
much in terms of seeing the posture of the bodies and the anguished

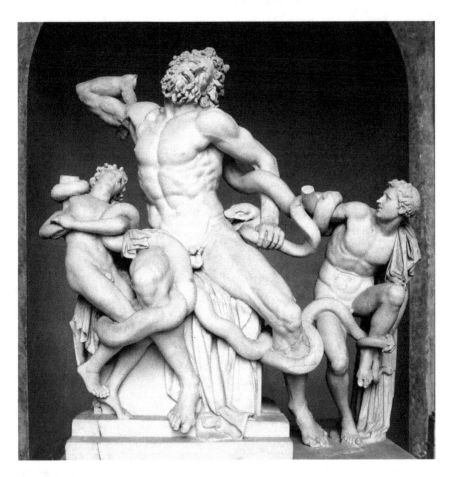

Figure 5.12 Sculpture of *Laocoön and His Sons* suffering the wrath of Athena. This
ancient sculpture was excavated in Rome in 1506 and has since been on public display
in the Vatican Museum. (https://commons.wikimedia.org/wiki/File:Laocoon_and_His_
Sons.jpg, Creative Commons Attribution-Share Alike 4.0 International license.)

expression on the faces of the father and his sons. Further visual exploration lets us recognize (nonmotorically) the serpent as being the source of the struggle, taking us beyond mirror neurons because fear of snakes is probably an innate part of our emotional repertoire. Gallese and Gattara (2015) observe that the Russian movie director Eisenstein (1937/1991), when commenting on the *Laocoön* sculpture, wrote that "the lived expression of human suffering portrayed in this masterpiece of classical art is accomplished by means of the illusion of movement. Movement illusion is accomplished by means of a particular montage, condensing in one single image different aspects of expressive bodily movements that could not possibly be visible at the same time." I agree that this is a crucial point. Whereas in witnessing a movie or a play, we see the actual movements, when we look at a drawing or painting or sculpture, we may (or may not) interpret the static image as a dynamic episode.

Further, let's note the distinction between having an object evoke a sense of movement and the aesthetic judgment of whether, and if so how, that object is emotionally compelling. Imagine a variation on the *Laocoön* where context is provided by a Christmas tree and opened boxes and the snake is replaced with gift ribbons. The motor activity expressed in the bodies and faces of the three figures remains the same, but the aesthetics has changed completely from great art to kitsch.

A bird in flight may be beautiful even though it cannot *directly* activate mirror neurons (these are restricted to actions within our own repertoire), and our appreciation of the beauty of a peacock's tail is evoked by the static display of its iridescent patterns, not by movement. In short, mirror neurons may—as in the *Laocoön*—contribute to aesthetic experience, but—as in seeing the peacock's tail on full display—they are not necessary for it.

However, Gallese and Gattara ask us not only to consider figurative works of art, such as the sculpture of *Laocoön*, with which we may possibly form some powerful emotional or empathic attachment with the subjects portrayed. They argue further that we can read the work in terms of the actions of the artist in creating the work. However, the skill of the sculptor of the *Laocoön* is such that there is no visible trace of his creative gestures. By this, I mean that there is no trace of the work of the chisel.

The surface has been smoothed to remove all such traces. You might thus appreciate that this is incredibly skillful work, but that is totally different from recognizing traces of the actions of the sculptor in creating the work. Nonetheless, this duality between production and result has crucial implications for aesthetics. It also reminds us that our aesthetic experience will in general integrate diverse dimensions, whether or not they are embodied simulations of the efforts of the artist or the artwork's protagonists.

Gallese's group conducted electroencephalographic (EEG) and behavioral studies where they had people look at pictures to show that the perception engaged a possibly subliminal motor component. Heimann et al. (2013) recorded beholders' brain responses when looking at a letter of the Roman alphabet, a Chinese ideogram, or a meaningless scribble, all written by hand. They found that these activated the hand-motor representation in beholders. However, the issue for me is not that perception of some objects can invoke a (possibly subliminal) motor response; the issue is when and whether these responses are crucial to how the stimuli are experienced (even leaving aside aesthetic judgment for the moment). Many readers of this book can recognize letters of the Roman alphabet; relatively few can recognize (m)any Chinese characters yet may be able to recognize that certain scribbles might possibly be Chinese characters while others cannot. This knowledge seems at least as relevant to the perceptual experience as the ghost of the effort that might be involved in retracing the pattern. Similarly, seeing a room or object may activate affordances that can prime motor cortex, but this need have little to do with aesthetic judgment.

With this, let's turn to studies that used EEG to suggest that a similar "motor simulation" of hand gestures was evoked in subjects beholding photographs of "cuts" on canvas (Figure 5.13) by Lucio Fontana (Umiltà et al., 2012), or the dynamic brushstrokes on canvas by Franz Kline in his *Chief* (1950, oil on canvas, held by the Museum of Modern Art, New York; Sbriscia-Fioretti et al., 2013). But is one actually simulating the motor activity of the artist if, for example, the Fontana work elicits a subliminal action of cutting? I had the pleasure of seeing a related Fontana piece at an exhibition on art from Latin America at the San Diego Museum of Art

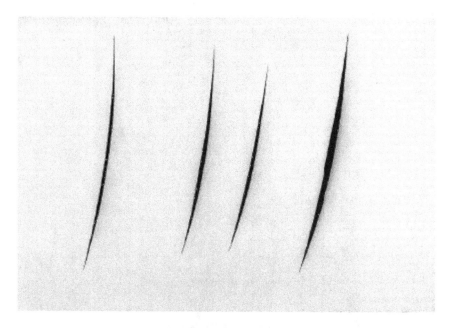

Figure 5.13 Lucio Fontana, *Spatial Concept* #2, (1960, Oil on Canvas, The Philadelphia Museum of Art), an artwork suggested by Gallese and Gattara to elicit strong motor components in aesthetic experience. (© 2020 Artists Rights Society [ARS], New York/ SIAE, Rome.)

(Figure 5.14). Getting up close, I could see that there are no cuts in the canvas. Rather, the canvas is not flat, and the "cuts" are actually depressions carefully molded into the canvas and highlighted with black acrylic. What about the painting by Kline? It seems to be all about placing evocative black brushstrokes on the canvas so that "mirroring" those brushstrokes is crucial to appreciating the work of the artist. And yet, when I saw a similar Kline painting at the Nelson-Atkins Museum of Art in Kansas City, Missouri, I found that Kline had achieved his effect not only by the bold black brush strokes already noted but also by painting in white.

One may still argue that Fontana wanted to make us think of slashes and Kline of bold brushstrokes, but recognizing and even "mirroring" these actions is different from empathy with specific actions of the artist as he produced the piece. In other words, the suggestion here is that—as in the *Laocoön*—to the extent that the experience of action was part of

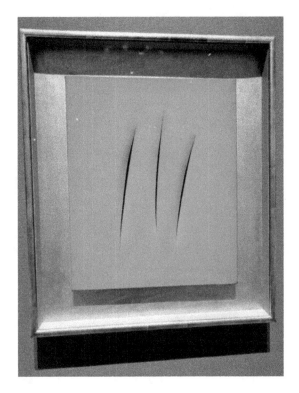

Figure 5.14 Lucio Fontana, Argentinian/Italian, 1899–1968. *Spatial Concept, Expectations.* Acrylic on canvas, 1963–1964. Author's photo of the painting as seen at the exhibit, *Modern Masters From Latin America: The Pérez Simón Collection*, San Diego Museum of Art, October 21, 2017 through March 11, 2018. (© 2020 Artists Rights Society [ARS], New York/SIAE, Rome.)

the viewer's aesthetic experience, it was because of the "high-level" design of the piece, not because of traces of the artist's actions in producing the work. Further aesthetic judgment of Fontana's work rests more on the orientation and placement of the slashes than on the "motor illusions" that may be created by the individual slashes.

Few of us can distinguish the brushstrokes of a Rembrandt or a Vermeer even though we can often classify correctly an artwork of these two masters on the basis of both the subject of the painting and various "higher level" characteristics in the choice, shaping, and disposition of colored forms. These are intended effects of the painter's actions, not the direct traces of the movements of the master's hand. In other words, to the extent that our appreciation of the work depends on insights into the artist's intentions (and it need not do so), the relevant intentions may reside at a level far above that of individual manual actions. When I had my house remodeled, we discovered that there were many horrible odds and ends in the walls as they were being built, and then someone slapped on "mud" to get a smooth surface—hiding rather than revealing the messy details of construction.

None of this is to deny that *some* artworks may enhance their effect by making the artist's actions manifest. As Mallgrave noted on viewing the Assyrian bas-relief (Figure 5.15):

We may read these panels as a narrative history depicting the proud warrior in victory but when we go to the British Museum we "study

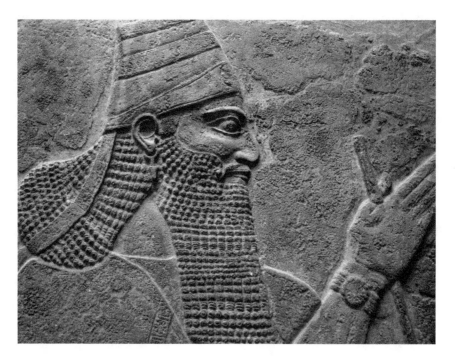

Figure 5.15 Assyrian panel (detail). (Photo by Harry Mallgrave, with permission.)

the delicate chisel marks that create the composition; we admire the intricacy and detail of the author's hand, the skill that is always present in a great work of art. We are simulating our own hand carrying out this work."

Mallgrave (personal communication) adds: "The craftsmanship in delineating the exquisite forms of this composition drew me into it. Skillful chisel marks may not in themselves make a great work of art, but I agree with both Ingold and Sennett that craftsmanship is central to a masterly production of any work of art."[10] However, as noted with the *Laocoön*, our admiration of that craftsmanship may depend in many cases on rendering this effort invisible in the final product. We may wonder why this Assyrian has a wristwatch, but our appreciation is enriched, in this case, not only by close-up examination of the traces of skillful chisel use but also by a feeling of awe at how long ago the panel was made, a sense of deep time. Moreover, note that Mallgrave himself in no way reduces his appreciation to mirror neuron activity. While he eschews using the term "beauty," he does speak of exquisite forms of composition and masterly production of works of art. These, for me, count as aesthetic judgments and reinforce the discussion, already initiated in §3.1, that "beauty" is but one form of aesthetic judgment—and "beauty" takes many forms, with some more subjective than others. Neither the linkage of aesthetic judgment to visual mechanisms in §3.5 nor to motor mechanisms here can tell the whole story.

Another example from Mallgrave goes some way to supporting this analysis, and begins our transition from painting and sculpture to architecture. Commenting on the chapel of the Church of the Monastery of Jesus in Setubal (Figure 5.16), Mallgrave writes:

a twisted column might induce a state of tension within our bodies, as our mirror systems viscerally simulate the twisting of

10. See, for example, *Making: Anthropology, Archaeology, Art and Architecture* (Ingold, 2013), and *The Craftsman* (Sennett, 2008).

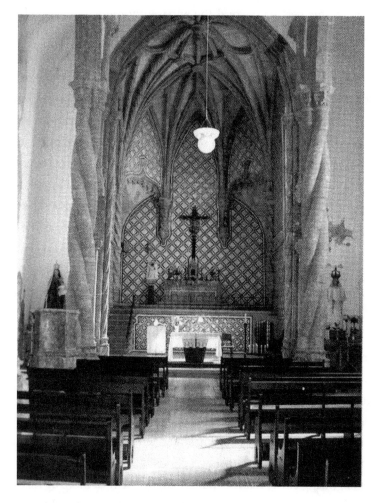

Figure 5.16 Chapel of the Church of the Monastery of Jesus, Setubal, Portugal, c. 1498. (Photograph by Harry Mallgrave, with permission.)

the column. . . . [S]uch simulation can be read *both symbolically and emotionally.* Symbolically, the twisting visually strengthens the supports for assuming the load of the heavy vaults, while emotionally this tense gesture seems entirely appropriate in a chapel that was designed specifically to house the ritual sacrifice of Christ. (Mallgrave, 2015, pp. 25–26)

Crucially, this gets us beyond the apparently reductive view of Gallese and Gattara because Mallgrave not only evokes visceral simulation of the effort of twisting the columns but also symbolically links the twisting of the columns and their support of a heavy load to the ritual sacrifice of Christ. Consider, by contrast, Figure 5.17 where our swift visual appreciation of the skein of wool evokes neither visceral simulation of the effort of twisting nor Christian symbolism. Were we to see a photo cropped to show just part of a column, it might equally evoke schema instances for a forcefully twisted object and for a skein of wool. It is the Christian context that provides the top-down influence that definitively emphasizes the former schema and removes all conscious trace of the skein schema. But where is the mirror system in this? Where does embodied simulation leave off and symbolism take over? Or, perhaps more appropriately, when and how does embodied simulation play an important role in aesthetic experience or judgment?

Based on the data of Buccino et al. (2004) on the recognition of actions performed by nonconspecifics, I postulate that schemas for recognizing actions are part of the ventral pathway, and that mirror neurons for recognizing the fine details of actions *that are within the observer's action repertoire* are part of the dorsal pathway. A major implication of the examples used by Gallese and Gattara and by Mallgrave is that not only can we recognize details of *ongoing* actions, but we also have schemas that can recognize patterns that may be *traces* of actions. My further suggestion is that these may be more ventral (as in recognizing chisel marks, and adjudging them as more or less skillful) or dorsal, activating a parametrized representation that may yield, if not overt

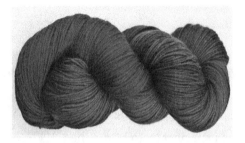

Figure 5.17 A skein of wool.

action, at least a subliminal trace in the motor system that may be detected by EEG. However, I reiterate that when we are actively engaged with our world, rather than contemplating artworks, our recognition of (traces of) the actions of others will in general serve more to help determine our own course of action rather than subliminally mimic the observed action. Consider your reaction to recognizing that the lock on your front door has been broken. In this case, the emotion evoked is an angry or despairing response to the breakage; there is no empathy for the experience of the intruder breaking the lock.

Thus, while we have gained a deeper appreciation of possible roles of the motor system in contemplation of art and architecture—looking at a sculpture, a painting, or a single view of a building—we must continue to explore the relevance of such contemplation to the experience within the action–perception cycle in moving through the building and using it in various ways. Even as contemplation remains part of our experience, we seek affordances for our own actions, rather than responding (usually or primarily) to the actions of the artist in creating the work or the actions represented within the work.

In designing an atmosphere for a building, the architect seeks to evoke the emotion of those who experience the building, not the emotions the architect experiences as they elaborated the details of how best to support such evocation. A building is a setting for each user's behavior, and this involves the setting up of actions within the integrated setting of the user's motivation and current tasks and (consciously and unconsciously) perceived aspects not only of the building but of others with whom the space is shared. The building is a setting for interaction with other people as well as for exploiting the affordances of the building itself. Our attention not only wanders around the visual scene but also seeks to enter the minds of those around us while tapping our own memories and intentions—and hence our subsequent emotions and actions may rest on a focus on but one of these aspects, or a synthesis of many of them. The inference here is that aesthetic judgment—of which the judgment of beauty in some form may or may not be a component—is not a single separable dimension of experience. Many different factors come into play in aesthetic judgment, and—no matter how important or unimportant the motoric component—,the relation between them is of the essence.

To close, let's pose the challenge of understanding the aesthetic reaction to a complicated building, the Public Library in downtown San Diego (Figure 5.18). To my mind it is a pastiche, a collection of pieces rather than a unified building. Different parts have very different feels. There's a children's area where everything is designed to engage the child—the books on display have colorful covers; there are tables where they can play with objects as well as look at the books. There is a genealogy section where all the tools are provided for anybody seriously interested in finding out their (more or less) local family history. Some of the rooms are engaging; others simply do their job. One can debate, then, whether the architect should set an overall tone or simply provide the various functions piecemeal, where each room may be given a distinctive use-focused character unrelated to that of others.

Some, unlike me, may find the building beautiful; others may appreciate the merits of the children's room or the genealogy section and make no assessment of the building as a whole. In either case, they may judge the building by the affordances it offers for their own activity, not by any Einfühlung for the building itself. The building, unlike the sculpture or painting, must

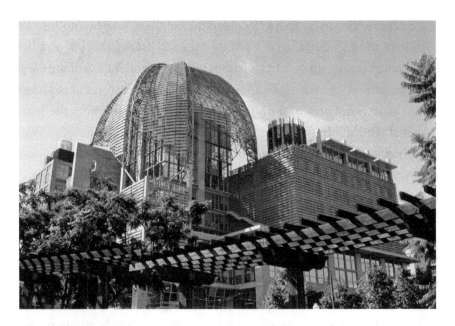

Figure 5.18 San Diego Central Library. Architect: Ross Quigley. (https://en.wikipedia. org/wiki/San_Diego_Central_Library#/media/File:San_Diego_Central_Library.jpg. Creative Commons Attribution-Share Alike 3.0 Unported license.)

perform, and the successful performance must involve a dynamic balance between multiple factors, both utilitarian and aesthetic—a balance that may perhaps be evaluated similarly by many users, but will not satisfy everyone.

5.7. NEUROAESTHETICS REVISITED, AND MORE

The present section delivers on my promise in §3.1 to sample a number of contributions to neuroaesthetics. This will allow me to comment on the gap between such studies and the need for future *focused* studies linking cog/neuroscience and architecture.

The results reviewed next will mention a number of brain regions not discussed elsewhere in this book. For example, anterior cingulate cortex is a region strongly responsive to the reward properties and emotional salience of objects. However, rather than offer an exposition of these regions, I leave their names as placeholders for those readers who wish to explore further.

Kirk et al. (2009) studied fMRI correlates of aesthetic judgments of visually presented architectural stimuli and control stimuli (faces) for a group of architects (architectural students) and a group of nonarchitects. (Their study was noted in §3.1 as the only architecturally oriented study cited in two early books on neuroaesthetics.) When looking at buildings, architects had more neural activity than nonexperts in some parts of the reward system, the medial orbitofrontal cortex as well as the anterior cingulate, suggesting that the students' architectural experience modulated their pleasure. By contrast, there was more neural activity in the nucleus accumbens for attractive faces and buildings irrespective of viewers' level of expertise. However, architects had more neural activity in the hippocampus when they looked at buildings than when they looked at faces. Kirk et al.'s interpretation was that pictures of buildings activated the experts' memories of buildings. However, another interpretation is possible. Since the hippocampus is engaged as much in wayfinding (Chapter 6) as in episodic memory (Chapter 10), it may be that buildings were more likely to encourage "mental wayfinding" than would faces, and that this would increase with expertise. We see again the challenge of data interpretation that we already noted for the contemplative-building study of §4.5.

Oshin Vartanian and colleagues conducted studies on the impact of certain key variables on architectural judgments, based on reaction to photographs. Vartanian et al. (2013) found that participants were more likely to judge spaces as beautiful if they were curvilinear rather than rectilinear, and fMRI showed that curvilinear contours activated the anterior cingulate cortex. *Pleasantness* accounted for nearly 60% of the variance in beauty ratings. However, contour did not affect approach–avoidance decisions, although curvilinear contours activated the visual cortex. Moreover, Vartanian et al. (2015) examined the impact of ceiling height and perceived enclosure (e.g., as defined by doors and windows) in aesthetic judgments and approach–avoidance decisions in architectural design. They found that rooms with higher ceilings were more likely to be judged as beautiful, and (again shown by fMRI) they activated structures involved in visuospatial exploration and attention in the dorsal stream. Open rooms were more likely to be judged as beautiful, and they activated structures underlying perceived visual motion. Additionally, enclosed rooms were more likely to elicit exit decisions, and they activated the anterior midcingulate cortex—the region within the cingulate gyrus with direct projections from the amygdala. They suggest that a reduction in perceived visual and locomotive permeability characteristic of enclosed spaces might elicit an emotional reaction that accompanies exit decisions.

One challenge for the architect is that when one assesses a set of pictures designed around a couple of variables, the general conclusions may have less importance in architectural designs where diverse utilitarian and aesthetic factors are at play. For example, a prison cell is designed to block exit decisions; but the decision of whether to include (shatterproof) windows with an attractive view might involve a tradeoff between punishment (depriving the prisoner of a view beyond the cell) and rehabilitation (biophilia can be restorative). A neuroscience challenge is to assess to what extent fMRI findings may be illuminated by findings on low-level circuitry of vision—such as the aesthetic assessment of contours by Albright, or the linkage of approach–avoidance in frog to judgments of placement of visual forms (§3.5).

Coburn et al. (2020) had participants rate 200 images of architectural interiors on 16 aesthetic response measures. They analyzed the data to identify three components that explained 90% of the variance in ratings.

The first two, *coherence* (ease with which one organizes and comprehends a scene), and *fascination* (a scene's informational richness and generated interest) are well-established dimensions in response to natural scenes and visual art. The third, *hominess* (extent to which a scene reflects a personal space), was a new dimension related to architectural interiors. They also reanalyzed data from the Vartanian et al. (2013) study to demonstrate that, regardless of task, the degree of fascination covaried with neural activity in the right lingual gyrus, coherence covaried with neural activity in the left inferior occipital gyrus only when participants judged beauty, and hominess covaried with neural activity in the left cuneus only when participants made approach–avoidance decisions.

Ed Vessel, Gabrielle Starr, and their colleagues again use photos and fMRI in their studies, but they offer tantalizing ideas about the difference between landscapes and the built environment. But first I need to introduce the default mode network (DMN). This comprises brain regions that are most active when the subject is simply lying in the MRI scanner, rather than performing the tasks of an experiment. Based on my experience of lying in the scanner during a nonbrain MRI, I think of this as the "mind-wandering system," engaged as one tries to distract oneself from the intense sounds made by the machine and possible claustrophobia. However, since the brain evolved long before MRI machines, the question arises as to the role of the DMN. Belfi et al. (2019) enriched prior fMRI studies of aesthetic experience of static visual art by assessing the temporal dynamics of this engagement. They showed that, in the first few seconds following image onset, activity in the DMN (and high-level visual and reward regions) was greater for very pleasing images, while DMN activity counteracted a suppressive effect that grew longer and deeper with increasing image duration. For very pleasing art, return of the DMN response to baseline was time-locked to image offset. Conversely, for nonpleasing art, the timing of this return to baseline was inconsistent. This differential response seems, to me, consistent with the mind-wandering hypothesis—if the art is not compelling, the mind tends to wander.

In a related study, using photos from different domains such as cultural artifacts versus landscapes, Vessel et al. (2019) found fMRI data that they interpret as supporting a model of aesthetic appreciation whereby domain-specific representations of the content of visual experiences in ventral occipitotemporal cortex feed into a "core" domain-general representation of visual aesthetic appeal in the DMN. However, since the DMN is a network, I am unclear why the data supports the notion of a core representation, rather than a distributed network of coupled representations. Indeed, the 2019 study identified additional prefrontal regions containing information relevant for appreciation of cultural artifacts (artwork and architecture) but not landscapes.

An earlier study (Vessel et al., 2018) tested whether there are systematic differences in the degree of shared taste across visual aesthetic domains, using photographic images of real-world content. Preferences for images of faces and landscapes showed a high proportion of shared taste, while preferences for images of exterior architecture, interior architecture, and artworks reflected strong individual differences. A further study compared the two most well matched domains—natural landscapes and exterior architecture. Agreement across individuals was significantly higher for natural landscapes than exterior architecture, with no differences in reliability. Consistently with our EvoDevoSocio framework, this suggests that humans may have evolved circuitry especially suited to perception of naturally occurring domains (e.g., faces and landscape), whereas these must engage with other regions—through learning via enculturation—to variations in response to artifacts of human culture (e.g., architecture and artwork).

The problem with fMRI studies is that the subject must lie immobile in the scanner. Various researchers have thus switched the emphasis from response to pictures to response to three-dimensional interiors simulated in a CAVE system. This, basically, is a cube in which the subject can move, but with each wall a giant computer screen to create the illusion of being in some architectural or other environment (similar studies can employ virtual reality). Since there are no portable fMRI scanners, they switched to EEG recording. (Recall the tradeoff: temporal data at a much finer grain than fMRI, but losing the localization of activity that fMRI provides.) Vecchiato et al. (2015a, 2015b) had participants judge three-dimensional interiors according to dimensions of familiarity, novelty, comfort, pleasantness, arousal, and presence. A correlation analysis on personal judgments showed that scores of novelty, pleasantness, and comfort are

positively correlated, while familiarity and novelty are negatively correlated. EEG revealed correlations of these factors with different cortical
rhythms, including those related to action as well as perception. This led
the authors to suggest, in harmony with the guiding theme of this book,
that people's experience of architectural environments is intrinsically
structured by the possibilities for action. Jelić et al. (2016) offer an *enactive perspective* as their take on the action-oriented approach to the A↔N
conversation. Note, however, that the Vecchiato et al. studies do not assess
the brain activity correlated with the subject's use of a building—they are
responding to visual qualities, but now in a space in which they can move,
rather than responding to a static view projected on a flat screen.

Where Bermudez turned to neuroscience to enrich his understanding of
architected spaces, Colin Ellard turned from the neuroscience of vision in
gerbils—as in "Spatial Cognition in the Gerbil: Computing Optimal Escape
Routes From Visual Threats" (Ellard & Eller 2009)—to the application of his
scientific methodology to a number of cognitive studies of great interest to
architects, such as offering (Ellard, 2017) "out of the laboratory and onto the
street" as a new slogan for urban psychology. He sees his work as within the
tradition of environmental psychology, but takes advantage of new instrumentation. One such study (Negami et al., 2018) looked at the effects of
urban design interventions, such as colorful crosswalks and greenery, on
participants' "mental well-being, sociability, and feelings of environmental
stewardship." Each participant was equipped with a smartphone and led on
walks of Vancouver's West End neighborhood, stopping at six sites to indicate their emotional response to, and perception of, the environment using
an app on their smartphone. This study revealed that spaces with greenery
and spaces with a colorful, community-driven urban intervention were associated with higher levels of happiness, trust, stewardship, and attractiveness
than their more standard comparison sites. They conclude that this demonstrates that a number of simple urban design interventions can increase
subjective well-being and sociability among city residents.

We see here a novel environmental–psychological field methodology
for collecting empirical affective and cognitive data on how individuals respond to urban design. However, this study focuses on perceptual
and affective response to various urban scenes as the subjects are simply

walking and occasionally stopping to answer questions. The subjects are not "living in" or "using" the city. Ellard has other studies that probe some forms of urban engagement (e.g., stress in crossing a busy street), but I want to close this section by asking, "What might be involved in adapting his methodology to taking focused A↔N studies 'out of the laboratory and into the building as it is being actively used and experienced'"?

For example, one might imagine instrumenting people as they execute a certain range of activities in a particular building, such as entering a bank to make a simple transaction with a teller rather than an ATM, or shopping for a particular garment in a clothing store. In each case, one cannot assume a fixed route, and one cannot expect subjects to stop what they are doing and tap into a cell phone when their hands may be engaged in some activity. Here, one might gather three kinds of data. The room might be instrumented with cameras and microphones to track how each subject moves around the space and the actions in which they are engaged ("intelligent" rooms are the subject of Chapter 7). The subject could wear a portable EEG helmet so that evoked response potentials could be time-locked to specific actions and shifts of attention. And (whether time-based, or based on the room's action recognition) voice interaction over a smartphone could elicit participants' subjective analysis of their behavior and their cumulative response to the environment. Such data would offer a trove of insights into the experience and use of architecture—and would also set important challenges for protecting the privacy of subjects.

REFERENCES

Abreu, A. M., Macaluso, E., Azevedo, R. T., Cesari, P., Urgesi, C., & Aglioti, S. M. (2012). Action anticipation beyond the action observation network: A functional magnetic resonance imaging study in expert basketball players. *European Journal of Neuroscience*, 35, 1646–1654.

Aglioti, S. M., Cesari, P., Romani, M., & Urgesi, C. (2008). Action anticipation and motor resonance in elite basketball players. *Nature Neuroscience*, 11, 1109–1116.

Alstermark, B., Lundberg, A., Norrsell, U., & Sybirska, E. (1981). Integration in descending motor pathways controlling the forelimb in the cat: 9. Differential behavioural defects after spinal cord lesions interrupting defined pathways from higher centres to motoneurons. *Experimental Brain Research*, 42, 299–318.

Arbib, M. A. (Ed.). (1995). *The handbook of brain theory and neural networks*. Cambridge, MA: Bradford Book/MIT Press.

Arbib, M. A. (Ed.). (2013). Language, music and the brain, a mysterious relationship. *Strüngmann Forum Reports*, 10. Cambridge, MA: MIT Press.

Arbib, M. A., & Bonaiuto, J. J. (Eds.). (2016). *From neuron to cognition via computational neuroscience*. Cambridge, MA: MIT Press.

Arnheim, R. (1977). *The Dynamics of Architectural Form*. Berkeley, Los Angeles: University of California Press.

Belfi, A. M., Vessel, E. A., Brielmann, A., Isik, A. I., Chatterjee, A., et al. (2019). Dynamics of aesthetic experience are reflected in the default-mode network. *NeuroImage*, 188, 584–597.

Bonaiuto, J. J., & Arbib, M. A. (2010). Extending the mirror neuron system model. II: What did I just do? A new role for mirror neurons. *Biological Cybernetics*, 102, 341–359.

Bonaiuto, J. J., Rosta, E., & Arbib, M. A. (2007). Extending the mirror neuron system model. I : Audible actions and invisible grasps. *Biological Cybernetics*, 96, 9–38.

Buccino, G., Lui, F., Canessa, N., Patteri, I., Lagravinese, G., et al. (2004). Neural circuits involved in the recognition of actions performed by nonconspecifics: An FMRI study. *Journal of Cognitive Neuroscience*, 16, 114–126.

Caligiore, D., Arbib, M. A., Miall, R. C., & Baldassarre, G. (2019). The super-learning hypothesis: Integrating learning processes across cortex, cerebellum and basal ganglia. *Neuroscience and Biobehavioral Reviews*, 100, 19–34. https://doi.org/10.1016/j.neubiorev.2019.02.008

Coburn, A., Vartanian, O., Kenett, Y. N., Nadal, M., Hartung, F., et al. (2020). Psychological and neural responses to architectural interiors. *Cortex*, 126, 217–241.

Dinstein, I., Thomas, C., Behrmann, M., & Heeger, D. J. (2008). A mirror up to nature. *Current Biology*, 18, R13–R18.

di Pellegrino, G., Fadiga, L., Fogassi, L., Gallese, V., & Rizzolatti, G. (1992). Understanding motor events: A neurophysiological study. *Experimental Brain Research*, 91, 176–180.

Doya, K. (2000). Complementary roles of basal ganglia and cerebellum in learning and motor control. *Current Opinion in Neurobiology*, 10, 732–739.

Eisenstein, S. (1937/1991). Laocoön (English translation by Michael Glenny from the Russian of c.1937). In M. Glenny & R. Taylor (Eds.), *S. M. Eisenstein. Selected works, Vol. 2: Towards a theory of montage* (pp. 177–178). London: British Film Institute.

Ellard, C. (2017). A new agenda for urban psychology: Out of the laboratory and onto the street. *Journal of Urban Design and Mental Health*, 2, 3.

Ellard, C., & Eller, M. C. (2009). Spatial cognition in the gerbil: Computing optimal escape routes from visual threats. *Animal Cognition*, 12, 333–345.

Ferrari, P. F., Gerbella, M., Coudé, G., & Rozzi, S. (2017). Two different mirror neuron networks: The sensorimotor (hand) and limbic (face) pathways. *Neuroscience*, 358, 300–315.

Ferrari, P. F., Visalberghi, E., Paukner, A., Fogassi, L., Ruggiero, A., & Suomi, S. J. (2006). Neonatal imitation in rhesus macaques. *PLoS Biology*, 4, e302.

Freedberg, D., & Gallese, V. (2007). Motion, emotion and empathy in esthetic experience. *Trends in Cognitive Sciences*, 11, 197–203.

Gallese, V., & Gattara, A. (2015). Embodied simulation, aesthetics and architecture: An experimental aesthetic approach. In S, Robinson, & J. Pallasmaa (Eds.), *Mind in architecture* (pp. 161–179). Cambridge, MA: MIT Press.

Gazzola, V., Aziz-Zadeh, L., & Keysers, C. (2006). Empathy and the somatotopic auditory mirror system in humans. *Current Biology*, 16: 1824–1829.

Grafton, S. T., Arbib, M. A., Fadiga, L., & Rizzolatti, G. (1996). Localization of grasp representations in humans by positron emission tomography. 2. Observation compared with imagination. *Experimental brain research*, 112, 103–111.

Han, C. E., Arbib, M. A., & Schweighofer, N. (2008). Stroke rehabilitation reaches a threshold. *PLoS Computational Biology*, 4, e1000133.

Hebb, D. O. (1949). *The organization of behavior*. New York: John Wiley & Sons.

Heimann, K., Umiltà, M. A., & Gallese, V. (2013). How the motor-cortex distinguishes among letters, unknown symbols and scribbles: A high density EEG study. *Neuropsychologia*, 51, 2833–2840.

Hollerman, J. R., & Schultz, W. (1998). Dopamine neurons report an error in the temporal prediction of reward during learning. *Nature Neuroscience*, 1, 304–309.

Ingold, T. (2013). *Making: Anthropology, archaeology, art and architecture*. Routledge.

Jelić, A., Tieri, G., De Matteis, F., Babiloni, F., & Vecchiato, G. (2016). The enactive approach to architectural experience: A neurophysiological perspective on embodiment, motivation, and affordances. *Frontiers in Psychology*, 7, Art. 481.

Kaas, J. (Ed.). (2017). Evolution of nervous systems (2nd ed.; in 4 volumes). Elsevier.

Kirk, U., Skov, M., Christensen, M. S., & Nygaard, N. (2009). Brain correlates of aesthetic expertise: A parametric fMRI study. *Brain and Cognition*, 69(2), 306–315.

Kohler, E., Keysers, C., Umilta, M. A., Fogassi, L., Gallese, V., & Rizzolatti, G. (2002). Hearing sounds, understanding actions: Action representation in mirror neurons. *Science*, 297, 846–848.

Langer, S. K. K. (1957). *Problems of art*. New York: Charles Scribner's Sons.

Mallgrave, H. F. (2015). "Know thyself" or what the designers can learn from the contemporary biological sciences In S. Robinson, & J. Pallasmaa (Eds.), *Mind in architecture* (pp. 9–31). Cambridge, MA: MIT Press.

Mallgrave, H. F. (2018). *From object to experience: The new culture of architectural design*. London: Bloomsbury Visual Arts.

Mallgrave, H. F., & Ikonomou, E. (Eds.). (1994). *Empathy, form, and space: Problems in German aesthetics, 1873–1893*. Santa Monica, CA: Getty Center for the History of Art and Humanities.

Meltzoff, A. N., & Moore, M. K. (1977). Imitation of facial and manual gestures by human neonates. *Science*, 198, 75–78.

Mukamel, R., Ekstrom, A. D., Kaplan, J., Iacoboni, M., & Fried, I. (2010). Single-neuron responses in humans during execution and observation of actions. *Current Biology*, 20, 750–756.

Negami, H., Mazumder, R., Reardon, M., & Ellard, C. (2018). Field analysis of psychological effects of urban design: A case study in Vancouver. *Cities & Health*, 2, 106–115.

Oztop, E., & Arbib, M. A. (2002). Schema design and implementation of the grasp-related mirror neuron system. *Biological Cybernetic*, 87, 116–140.

Oztop, E., Bradley, N. S., & Arbib, M. A. (2004). Infant grasp learning: A computational model. *Experimental brain research*, 158, 480–503.

Rizzolatti, G., Fadiga, L., Matelli, M., Bettinardi, V., Paulesu, E., et al. (1996). Localization of grasp representations in humans by PET: 1. Observation versus execution. *Experimental brain research*, 111, 246–252.

Robinson, S., & Pallasmaa, J. (Eds.). (2015). *Mind in architecture: Neuroscience, embodiment, and the future of design*. Cambridge, MA: MIT Press.

Rosenblatt, F. (1958). The perceptron: A probabilistic model for information storage and organization in the brain. *Psychological Review*, 65, 386–408.

Rumelhart, D. E., Hinton, G. E., & Williams, R. J. (1986). Learning internal representations by error propagation. In D. Rumelhart & J. McClelland (Eds.), *Parallel distributed processing: Explorations in the microstructure of cognition* (Vol. 1, pp. 318–3620. Cambridge, MA: MIT Press.

Samuel, A. L. (1959). Some studies in machine learning using the game of checkers. *IBM Journal of Research and Development*, 3, 210–229.

Sbriscia-Fioretti, B., Berchio, C., Freedberg, D., Gallese, V., & Umiltà, M. A. (2013). ERP modulation during observation of abstract paintings by Franz Kline. *PloS One* 8, e75241.

Schultz, W. (2016). Dopamine reward prediction error coding. *Dialogues in Clinical Neuroscience*, 18, 23–32.

Schultz, W., Dayan, P., & Montague, P. R. (1997). A neural substrate of prediction and reward. *Science*, 275, 1593–1599.

Schweighofer, N., Han, C. E., Wolf, S. L., Arbib, M. A., & Winstein, C. J. (2009). A functional threshold for long-term use of hand and arm function can be determined: Predictions from a computational model and supporting data from the Extremity Constraint-Induced Therapy Evaluation (EXCITE) trial. *Physical Therapy*, 89, 1327–1336.

Scott, G. (1914). *The architecture of humanism: A study in the history of taste*. Boston and New York: Houghton Mifflin.

Sennett, R. (2008). *The craftsman*. London: Allen Lane.

Sutton, R. S. (1988). Learning to predict by the methods of temporal differences. *Machine Learning*, 3, 9–44.

Sutton, R. S., & Barto, A. G. (2018). *Reinforcement learning: An introduction* (2nd ed.; 1st ed., 1998). Cambridge, MA: MIT Press.

Tan, Z., Roberts, A. C., Lee, E. H., Kwok, K.-W., Car, J., et al. (2020). Transitional areas affect perception of workspaces and employee well-being: A study of underground and above-ground workspaces. *Building and Environment*, 179, 106840.

Tidwell, P. (Ed.). (2015). Architecture and empathy: A Tapio Wirkkala–Rut Bryk Design Reader (with contributions from Juhani Pallasmaa, Harry Francis Mallgrave, Sarah Robinson, and Vittorio Gallese). Espoo, Finland: Tapio Wirkkala–Rut Bryk Foundation.

Tomeo, E., Cesari, P., Aglioti, S. M., & Urgesi, C. (2012). Fooling the kickers but not the goalkeepers: Behavioral and neurophysiological correlates of fake action detection in soccer. *Cerebral Cortex*, 23(11), 2765–2778.

Turella, L., Pierno, A. C., Tubaldi, F., & Castiello, U. (2009). Mirror neurons in humans: Consisting or confounding evidence? *Brain and Language*, 108, 10–21.

Umiltà, M. A., Berchio, C., Sestito, M., Freedberg, D., & Gallese, V. (2012). Abstract art and cortical motor activation: An EEG study. *Frontiers in Human Neuroscience*, 6, 311.

Vartanian, O., Navarrete, G., Chatterjee, A., Fich, L. B., Gonzalez-Mora, J. L., et al. (2015). Architectural design and the brain: Effects of ceiling height and perceived enclosure on beauty judgments and approach-avoidance decisions. *Journal of Environmental Psychology*, 41, 10–18.

Vartanian, O., Navarrete, G., Chatterjee, A., Fich, L. B., Leder, H., et al. (2013). Impact of contour on aesthetic judgments and approach-avoidance decisions in architecture. *Proceedings of the National Academy of Sciences*, 110(Suppl. 2), 10446–10453.

Vecchiato, G., Jelic, A., Tieri, G., Maglione, A. G., De Matteis, F., & Babiloni, F. (2015a). Neurophysiological correlates of embodiment and motivational factors during the perception of virtual architectural environments. *Cognitive Processing*, 16, 425–429.

Vecchiato, G., Tieri, G., Jelic, A., De Matteis, F., Maglione, A. G., & Babiloni, F. (2015b). Electroencephalographic correlates of sensorimotor integration and embodiment during the appreciation of virtual architectural environments. *Frontiers in Psychology*, 6, 1944.

Vessel, E. A., Isik, A. I., Belfi, A. M., Stahl, J. L., & Starr, G. G. (2019). The default-mode network represents aesthetic appeal that generalizes across visual domains. *Proceedings of the National Academy of Sciences*, 116, 19155–19164.

Vessel, E. A., Maurer, N., Denker, A. H., & Starr, G. G. (2018). Stronger shared taste for natural aesthetic domains than for artifacts of human culture. *Cognition*, 179, 121–131.

Vischer, R. (1873). *Ueber das optische Formgefühl: ein Beitrag zur Aesthetik*. Leipzig: H. Credner.

von Schelling, F. W. J. (1805). *Vorlesungen über Philosophie der Kunst*. Leipzig: Felix Meiner Verlag.

Wicker, B., Keysers, C., Plailly, J., Royet, J. P., Gallese, V., & Rizzolatti, G. (2003). Both of us disgusted in My insula: The common neural basis of seeing and feeling disgust. *Neuron*, 40, 655–664.

From libraries to wayfinding, waylosing, and symbolism

D ifferent building typologies offer different challenges for extending the A↔N conversation. Schools challenge us to understand how buildings affect the emotional and intellectual development of children and adults, thus tapping deeper insights into how brain mechanisms for learning and memory interact with those for emotion and motivation at different ages. Other studies look at the impact of hospital design on the healing process, or at how an understanding of the progression of Alzheimer's disease may enter into the design of homes that complement lost memory to support the routines of everyday life. It would take a chapter or more on each typology to do justice to the relevance of neuroscience to better understanding the experience of buildings of that type and the lessons such findings may offer architects. Instead, then, the book explores relatively few typologies in developing and exploring its general themes. This chapter starts with a focus on libraries but ends with a cathedral.

The focus on encourages us to think about three topics of general importance in architecture:

> *Function and the action–perception cycle*: Comparing library functions and forms of sensory experience offers a matrix of diverse challenges for library design that is exemplary for other typologies.
> *Symbolism*: Several libraries illustrate architectural strategies for creating symbolism that gives a sense of their overall social significance.
> *Wayfinding*: We also consider the challenge of finding one's way through a library. We contrast wayfinding (getting to a known destination) with "waylosing" and exploration (the joy of discovering the unexpected, not to be confused with "getting lost").

A modern library has many functions beyond the classic role of storing books and making them available to readers. Consideration of the diverse ways in which they engage action and perception demonstrates the view of a building as a *system of systems* devoted to various functions. Note that a brain, too, is a system of systems (embedded in a body embedded in an environment). We complement this functional view by examining classic libraries in terms of their *symbolic function*, noting examples in which flights of stairs leading us from the street to the entrance to the reading room may symbolize the notion of ascending to a realm of knowledge. Such stairs also provide examples of architectural strategies for *wayfinding*—or, at least, getting from the street to the reading room. However, when we enter the stacks, it is the Dewey decimal system that guides us: we have moved from symbolism to symbols. Moreover, when we enter the stacks, we may abandon the search for a specific book in favor of exploration and discovery.

The distinction between the grand symbolic entrance and the use of symbols brings us back to the general notion of scripts that can help us exploit architectural cues as well as specific signage to find our way in a new building. We then use the Seattle Public Library to explore the notion of getting lost in buildings in the negative sense before introducing the general idea of a *cognitive map*, the representation in the brain of places and their relationships, and the knowledge of how to find one's way from one place to another. A classic map, that of the London Underground, helps in two ways. It shows us that, in mastering the use of that map, we master a script that lets us navigate subway systems in cities around the world. Further, it helps us approach a particular model of cognitive maps where different regions may serve as different "worlds," each with their own *world graph* (WG). In each such graph, *distinctive* places are represented by *nodes*, corresponding to the stations in the London map, while a path between adjacent nodes is represented by an *edge*. The key distinction is that in the London map, the nodes and edges are external to us, whereas in a cognitive map, these nodes and edges and the knowledge of how to use them are all encoded in the brain. The architect may find this reminiscent of ideas put forth by Kevin Lynch in his classic *The Image of the City*.

A WG can be contrasted with a *locometric map* whose dimensions explicitly represent the locomotor effort in getting from one place to another. Two stations that appear close together on the Underground map may be quite far apart on the streets of London, and vice versa. An interesting question as we return to architecture is to what extent the cognitive map of one floor of a building can provide a shortcut to forming a cognitive map of another floor—and to what extent an architect wishes to design to increase or play off such similarity. A challenge for architects and urban planners, then, is how to provide not only affordances but also distinctive "place-making" to guide navigation, with signage sometimes a necessary option, and to support diverse scripts for the use of the building as well as the aesthetic opportunities it provides.

The chapter then explores further ideas on "how the brain works" in the hope that this can help in moving the A↔N conversation beyond mere generalities about the brain. Specifically, we explore more fully the role of the *hippocampus as part of the brain system for navigation*, thus bringing locomotion more fully into the action–perception cycle. (Chapter 10 explores how the hippocampus works with other systems to support episodic memory and imagination.) Single-cell recording from the brains of rats revealed that the hippocampus contains *place cells* whose activity correlates with the place in which the animal finds itself. However, it is important to note that the use of the word "place" in the rat studies corresponds more to the notion of location on a locometric map, with peaks of excitation shifting continually as the rat moves around, rather than corresponding to the significant places represented by nodes of a WG.

The taxon affordance model (TAM), corresponds to the situation in which one navigates without a cognitive map, but instead moves from one affordance to the next, as in the case of looking for the next turn indicated by a navigation app. Several brain regions are implicated here, but the hippocampus is not one of them. By contrast, the world graph model (WGM) makes essential use of the hippocampus in determining the location of the animal in a locometric map, which can then be exploited in other brain regions processing the relevant WG to estimate the edge or node that characterizes the current location, transforming the details into the high-level cognitive view that makes route planning possible.

We saw that scripts can help us exploit architectural cues as well as specific signage to find our way in a new building. A visit to Oscar Niemeyer's Brasilia Cathedral will exemplify how architects may achieve novel symbolic forms without necessarily invoking those that have traditionally been employed for a particular typology within a particular culture. The mention of symbols and signage reminds us that human cognition has been transformed by the invention of language and the subsequent invention of writing, and these innovations are, as we shall see in Chapter 8, strongly linked to the capability of the human brain to support the explicit design processes that make possible the forms of creativity exhibited in art and architecture.

6.1. LIBRARIES

What are libraries for?

In 2014, I spoke at the Annual Meeting of the American Libraries Association (ALA) with architect Ken Kornberg and then Princeton architecture librarian Hannah Bennett in a session on "Science + Form = Function (The Impact of Neuroscience on Architecture & Design)" organized by Eric Tidwell of Huntingdon College. At the ALA meeting, Ken Kornberg gave a fine exposition of how spaces affect users through diverse senses, giving particular examples of projects for both libraries and research buildings from his firm—and ended up expressing concern over the future of libraries as they become less book-centered buildings.

Figure 6.1, due to Kornberg, offers two lists—one of library functions and one of various systems (primarily perceptual) engaged in experiencing libraries. For each function, one may ask what perceptual processes and actions it engages, and then consider how to design the library to provide affordances for the activities needed to support its diverse functions. Specifically, note that a given space, structure, or object may serve multiple functions. Of course, such a challenge is relevant to all typologies, though the key functions may vary greatly from one typology to another. However, this function list excludes the more general aspects of "experiencing architecture," which, in the words of Robert Lamb Hart (personal communication) are centered on

the sensing of space—whether immediate, remembered, imagined, or just brought to mind by words. In practice, our perception and mapping of space and mass seem to be able to organize other

Library functions	Experiencing architecture
Contemplation	Vision: shape, color, order ...
Data collection	Smell: flowers, books, wood ...
Meeting, conference	Taste: coffee plus
Presentation: art, books	Sound: quiet, loud, distracting ...
Reading	Touch: texture
Refuge	Pressure; heights, humidity, HVAC
Storage: stocks, archives	Temperature; comfort, attraction
Studying	Motion: time, space
Teaching	Pain: emotional, physical

Figure 6.1 Library functions and sensory experience—implicitly defining diverse challenges as we ask which types of experience are relevant to each type of function. (Adapted from a slide of Ken Kornberg, with permission.)

concurrent inputs into coherent wholes or stories—the order we try to impose on our environments. Like a sculptor's armature, space and the masses that shape it become a kind of unifying core or framework for the on-going experience of a built environment.

Back to library functions. Some are in terms of its "memory function" of maintaining and expanding a storehouse of knowledge—and this reminds us that for modern humans, memory is a system distributed between our own brains and diverse external memory systems. Others are in terms of meeting the needs of patrons for resources, with digital media in increasing demand compared to paper. Yet others involve uses of the library as a public space. Figure 6.1 lists nine functions, which we might group as follows:

Memory function: data collection; storage:—stacks, archives
Meeting resource needs: presentation: —art, books; reading; contemplation; studying
Public space: meeting, conference; teaching; refuge

The list can be continued but already makes clear that the architect must see the library as a network of interconnected spaces, with overlapping functions (while addressing the wayfinding involved for the user in finding where to exercise desired functions).

This view of a building as a *system of systems* devoted to various functions is a crucial one—and is shared with our approach to schema theory, where a given schema may be implemented by patterns of competition and cooperation of different brain regions, while many brain regions may be involved in diverse functions. Thus, a brain, too, is a system of systems, both functionally and structurally (embedded in a body embedded in an environment). In the case of a building, the design requires careful analysis of the affordances needed for each function specified in the program for the building to satisfactorily meet the needs of its users. Consider, for example, the design of the auditorium of a theater. One may start with the creation of a space in which seating can be arranged along with walkways that provide access to the seating, and with each seat having good sight-lines to the stage. But this requires coordination with the design of the stage in terms of not only sightlines but also, more subtly, the acoustics—both for the audience and for the performers. However, the sightlines must not only provide a good view of the performance on the stage, they must also exclude a view of the activity in the wings and the stage machin-ery. Meanwhile, the walkways within the auditorium must be linked to the lobby and hallways to ensure smooth passage of the audience before and after the performance and during the intermission. Thus, the different functions—access and egress for the audience, the audience experience, the needs of the performers and their support by stagehands, and so forth, each impact several spaces within (and, possibly, around) the building, and many functions require the coordinated design of multiple spaces and the affordances they provide.

By invoking all the senses, including vision of shape and color, touch, pressure, temperature, and perhaps even the smell and taste of coffee, Kornberg reminds us that the architect must go beyond the pure func-tionality of the building to take account of the multimodal experience of the embodied user. Figure 6.1 encourages us to think through each use of a building in relation to the many different brain systems involved, includ-ing sensory systems, motor systems, associative systems, and systems for memory and recall.

A complementary issue for librarians concerns strategies for mak-ing libraries relevant in the age of the computer, and this has drastically changed the typology of the library. Yes, books still have a role, but they have become much less important. Before I went to the Las Vegas meeting, I met with a group of librarians at the University of Southern California (where I was on the faculty from 1986 to 2016). One major issue was the setting up of places for people to really concentrate on their own work versus places where people could use the library's resources while work-ing together on a project. And how do the library's functions change in the 2020s and beyond in an age of smartphones and the World Wide Web, when far more people are viewing their computers than are within reach-ing distance of a physical book? In one response, the library must support reference librarians in helping clients find resources on the Web more often than providing access to the library's physical holdings. Meanwhile, downtown libraries are not only expanding their role as cultural centers but also must increasingly meet the challenge of providing a refuge from the streets for the homeless—doing this in a way that does not disturb other patrons, and that also encourages the homeless to go beyond shelter to make good use of the information resources of the library. Of course, security is another concern that affects the design of buildings like libraries focused on relatively unfettered public access in a different manner from banks, say, or government buildings.

Symbolic impact

As we turn to the notion of *symbolism* in architecture, an immediate question is the relation between symbolism and atmosphere. I can offer no definitive analysis of how they may be distinguished and where they may overlap. Instead, I offer the following as a placeholder: Symbolism is more cognitive—this is what the building "means"—whereas atmosphere is more emotive—this is how it "feels." One's first response may be spontaneous sensing of atmosphere that leads almost immediately to a growing "awareness" of symbols, followed by a re-evaluation of each that continues as one spends time in the space, and the relative influence of each merges into a total experience (as was the case for Turner's *The Slave Ship*, §4.4).

Another distinction is that between symbolism and symbols. Consider the way in which the shape of a "traditional" European Christian church,[1] including the relation to its spire and its high roof, provides a distinctive generic form for this typology that is in some sense symbolic of Christian

---

1. The notion of "a traditional European Christian Church" is of course a simplification—a Norman church is very different from a Gothic cathedral or from Orthodox churches. Here, I appeal to the general scheme shared by many modest-sized churches as well as Cathedrals with bell towers, a high nave, stained-glass windows, and more, each with its own Christian symbolism. A similar discussion could be applied to places of worship for diverse religious traditions.

faith—just as an arrangement of domes and minarets may characterize traditional mosques to provide a symbol of Islamic faith. Note, however, that height of the bell tower and the height of the minaret share the function of calling to the faithful—in one case broadcasting the sound of the bells, in the other the voice of the muezzin. Thus, the repeated use of an architectural feature to serve a dedicated function may cause that feature to become crystallized as part of a particular symbolic form that may then evoke a certain meaning for the informed observer even when that function is not in play.

This last observation may offer one more twist to the earlier attempt to distinguish symbolism and atmosphere. The former is based more on the conventions of a particular culture or community; the latter is based on more "primal" responses, such as the evocation of awe. This, of course, has lessons for international architects, or for those developing buildings for a diverse populace—that one must study relevant communities to understand what symbolism will engage people positively, and what (possibly unintended) symbolism to avoid.

But now, following Hannah Bennett's themes at the Las Vegas meeting (and see Bennett 2013), let's focus on the *symbolic value* of libraries in, for example, providing architectural expression of the library as a repository of knowledge. This symbolism may be conveyed not only by mere visual impression but also through the building's engagement of the action–perception cycle of its visitors. For example, the ascent from the street to the entrance of the Stockholm Library designed by the Swedish architect Erik Gunnar Asplund (Figure 6.2) is followed by the even more dramatic staircase that encloses you and obscures your view from all but a glimpse of the books that await you, finally revealed in the great cylinder of the reading room, where knowledge is laid out before you. Together these stairways declare that you are ascending to a palace of knowledge.

In Chapter 4, we noted Le Corbusier's description of the Green Mosque in Asia Minor, and I suggested that this exemplified the drama of transitions (whether from inside to outside or from room to room) rather than showing the primacy of interior to exterior in planning. Asplund's second transition creatively combines the unexpected with the sense that

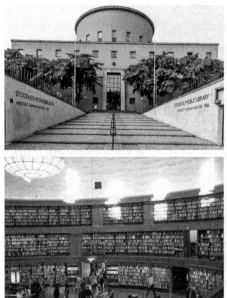
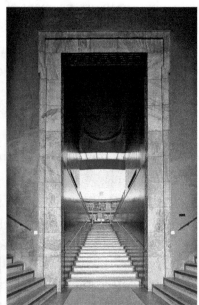

Figure 6.2 The symbolic value of architecture: The Stockholm Library of Erik Gunnar Asplund, and its two ascents to the realm of knowledge. (*Top left*: https://www.picfair. com/pics/010817246-exterior-view-of-stockholm-public-library-designed-by-asplund. Picfair license. *Right*: © Sebastien Poncelet, with permission. *Bottom left*: Photo by Holger Elgard. https://upload.wikimedia.org/wikipedia/commons/c/c2/Stadsbiblioteket_ 2008e.jpg. Attribution-ShareAlike 3.0 Unported license, CC BY-SA 3.0.)

the change is part of a dramatic plan, rather than part of a haphazard assemblage.

Contrast this with Lina Bo Bardi's art gallery, where the entrance was nondescript (head up the stairs or catch the elevator), but the placement of a plaza under the building declared that the space was for the use of the broad public, not just the privileged few—a different symbolism.

When I was an undergraduate, I would visit the Mitchell Library in Sydney. Its great reading room (Figure 6.3) is rectangular rather than circular, with tiers of books accessible via balconies. Walking along, inspecting the books, taking out one here, one there to browse, finally selecting a few to take down to a table on the floor below, gave me a strong feeling that there is so much to know in a very different way from the feeling

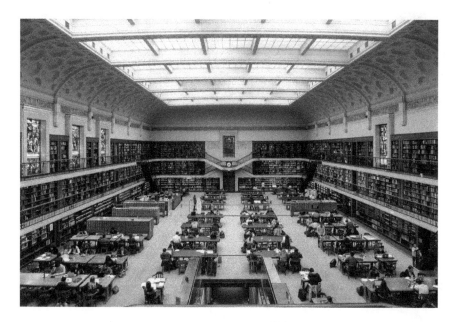

Figure 6.3 The reading room of the Mitchell Library in Sydney. (https://commons. wikimedia.org/wiki/File:State_Library_of_New_South_Wales_Reading_Room_2017.jpg, licensed under the Creative Commons Attribution-Share Alike 4.0 International license.)

one now gets when surfing the Web—the difference between a panoramic view and the view through a pinhole, albeit a pinhole that can be rapidly shifted from place to place. The latter gives you no sense of the whole and may offer too many distractions from any sustained quest to understand a specific subject. And yet, I confess, the Web is invaluable to me in my own pursuit of knowledge; the frequent visits of my youth to libraries are long behind me.

Bennett (2013) also discusses the Philology Library of the Free University of Berlin (Figure 6.4). The library was designed by Norman Foster to look like a brain. The floors are shaped to somewhat resemble horizontal sections through human cerebral cortex and are thus symbolic of the building as a repository of knowledge. Note, here, that the symbolism is not the established symbolism of some class of buildings within a particular typology, but rests on invocation of an unusual association— that between the shape of the building and familiar caricatures of sections

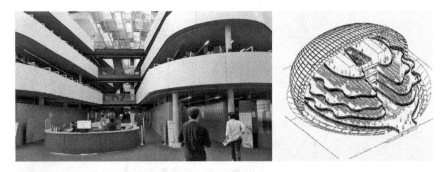

Figure 6.4 "The Brain"—the Philological Library of Free University of Berlin. (*Left*) The interior view as seen from the entrance, showing the "cerebral slices" of the "left and right hemispheres." (*Right*) Schematic view of the "slices" with cutaway of the enveloping shell of the "brain." (*Left*: Author's photo. *Right*: From Werner, K. U., & Diecks, M. [2004]. "The Brain"—The Philological Library, Free University of Berlin. *LIBER Quarterly*, 14[2]. Open access CC by 4.0. © Klaus U. Werner and Monika Diecks.)

through the human brain. Unfortunately, though, this symbolic choice in itself—as distinct from its exemplification of associative processes supported by the brain—contributes nothing to our quest to understand how neuroscience may help us better understand the experience and design of architecture.

My visit to the library in 2017 further illustrated the changing function of libraries. I was lent a device to carry around to get narration describing the different parts of the building. What was especially poignant was Foster's account of how he went about designing it. The shaping image was as follows: "Imagine oneself sitting under a tree reading a book. How might the library recapture some of that experience of immersion in reading in a tranquil environment?" The irony, of course, was that, as I walked around, maybe only one person in ten had a book with them. Everybody else had only a computer. Indeed, the screen image that appears on my iPad when I open the Kindle app to read an electronic book depicts a boy reading a book while seated under a tree. Perhaps the distinction between book and screen is not so important for the reading experience, but the relevance of this distinction to the function of libraries as localized buildings rather than distributed Web resources certainly is.

From symbolism to wayfinding and waylosing

We now enter the Doheny Memorial Library of the University of Southern California (USC), aided by photos by Ruth Wallach and her discussion at the USC library meeting. Figure 6.5 (*top*) exemplifies, on a more modest scale, Asplund's ascent to the temple of knowledge via two flights of stairs. After ascending the second flight of stairs, you find yourself in what Wallach describes as "the Great Hall, symbolic of the realm of wisdom and truth" (*bottom left*).

But Wallach moves us beyond this symbolic space. Entering the doorway at right, you find yourself in "an unprepossessing entryway, a narrow door into a compressed space, the stacks. One feels like an animal

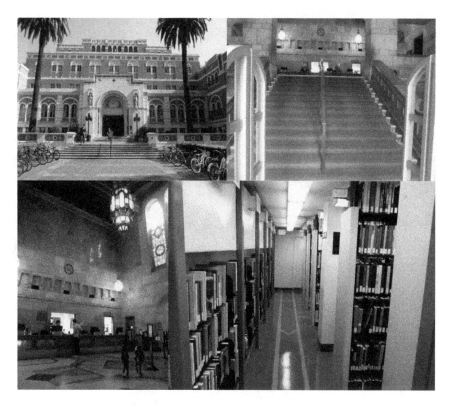

Figure 6.5 Four views of the Doheny Memorial Library of the University of Southern California. (Photos by Ruth Wallach, with permission.)

burrowing underground. No natural light, compressed space, low ceilings" (*bottom right*). She doesn't like it! In defense of the library's architect, one should note that the building was commissioned at a time when the stacks were closed—a place to store the books so that they could be retrieved by a librarian when a reader wanted them, not a place for the general public. It provides, if you will, pure functionality without aesthetics.

My son Benjamin Arbib (he who visited the Therme in Vals) was an undergraduate at USC and is now an architect in Austin, Texas. He had a very different view of the Doheny stacks. He enjoyed the low ceiling, isolated desks in nooks and crannies, the drum of the air conditioning, because he could experience "being lost and then finding yourself, finding unexpected books as you scan the stacks." We are not saying the ugliness and bad lighting noted by Wallach are required for this positive experience, but rather emphasizing that exploration, leaving familiar territory and then finding something new, can be as desirable as swiftly reaching a known destination. Architects can make "good" stacks that also support exploration. Whatever the architect's choices, the rooms and the shelves are augmented by the tactility of the books, the smell of the books, the embodied experience of turning pages to browse. Moral: Whatever the shift to e-resources, don't give up on the book or on large assemblages of books. The book and the assemblage each support a vital kind of immersion and exploration.

This positive sense of exploration is what we might call *waylosing* and is defined in contrast to the well-established notion of wayfinding. The term is employed on page 49 of *Wayshowing > Wayfinding: Basic & Interactive* (Mollerup, 2013); and Mollerup repeats his argument in a later interview:

> I am not advocating waylosing on the way to the maternity ward, but in less stressed situations it can be great fun. Waylosing is . . . one of the great attractions of Venice. . . . Also, we should not forget serendipity, the luck of finding something unexpected and useful when looking for something else. After all, America was found by some guys who lost their way to India. (Per Mollerup, April 21, 2014. https://segd.org/wayshowing-and-waylosing-mollerup)

I thought I had coined the word *waylosing* before I found this citation, and had indeed applied it to the experience of walking in Venice (Figures 6.6 and 6.7). Walking down a street (no cars) you may want to get to the other side of a canal. You get to the canal to find there is no bridge, but you see one to the right. Since there is no footpath along that stretch of canal, you go back and wander around the alleys and finally get back to the canal—and the bridge is to your left. You're in no hurry to get anywhere, and it is an absolute delight to explore this city in this somewhat random way, far from the madding crowd in Piazza San Marco.

To clarify, "waylosing" involves a deliberate intention to leave familiar territory (whether in a building, a town, or elsewhere) with the aim of enjoying new experiences. "Getting lost," by contrast, is the failure of navigation when one has the intention of reaching a more or less specific destination. In the latter case, losing track of how to get to familiar territory becomes stressful rather than enjoyable.

The "joys" of exploration presumably evolved as a survival strategy, to support hunting and foraging, and the search for shelter—and this in turn evolved to support a "drive" to learn more generally, as in building a cognitive map. While "waylosing" has positive affect, we still have a primal fear of being lost or separated from "our group," even panicking, and monkeys have been observed to use special calls to maintain "contact" when they

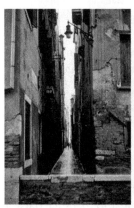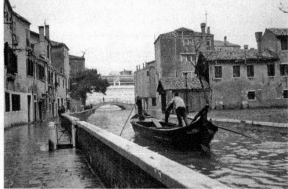

Figure 6.6 Waylosing in Venice, 1957 (Author's photos).

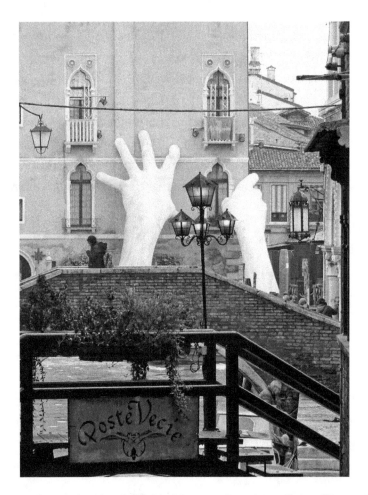

Figure 6.7 What are these hands thinking? Lorenzo Quinn's installation, "Support," for the 2017 Venice Architecture Biennale was designed to highlight the devastation of climate change. But are the hands preventing the Ca' Sagredo Hotel from sinking into the water, or are they trying to dismantle and drag it down? (https://www.abc.net.au/news/2017-05-19/giant-hands-emerge-from-venice-canal-highlight-climate-change/8542652. Photo courtesy of Craig Panner, with permission.)

lose sight of each other (Rendall, Cheney, & Seyfarth, 2000). More broadly, maintaining a sense of the location of "home" is a very ancient evolved trait—even ants have neural mechanisms for *path integration*, keeping track over a long period of exploration of the heading and distance back to the nest (Müller & Wehner, 1994). This provides an evolutionary basis for the importance of wayfinding in designing physical environments where an underlying biological sense may prove less reliable for many modern-day humans needing to keep track of diverse locations as well as finding their way to designated places they have not visited before.

Neither in the library stacks nor in Venice was waylosing part of the design program. In the stacks, the bookshelves were clearly labeled with the range in Dewey decimal notation for the books they contained, and so one could easily navigate to find a book for which one had retrieved the call number from the catalog. In Venice, the waylosing resulted from the need to make full use of the space between the canals and to promote access by boat, so that only in some cases was space there given over to pathways. Thus, if one asks the architect to consider waylosing, this would add a specific concept prescribed by the client to free the user to explore, and to pleasingly discover the unexpected.

To return to the Mollerup quote, if one gets lost on the way to the maternity ward, that is the result of bad design that cannot be excused by an appeal to the joys of exploration. If you are designing a hospital, you need to ensure people can promptly get to emergency or pediatrics or the X-ray or other department, and so will invest much effort into what Mollerup calls *wayshowing*, using signs or colored lines or other techniques to ensure that wayfinding is as simple as possible—helping people get very quickly where they want to go.[2] But in designing a shopping mall, it may be better not to make it too orderly, and to encourage exploration. Indeed, designing retail space to encourage exploration has become its own art and science with well-thought-out experiments—for example, Spence, Puccinelli, Grewal, and Roggeveen (2014) review scientific evidence related to visual, auditory, tactile, olfactory, and gustatory aspects of the store environment and their influence on the consumer's shopping behavior.

---

2. A brief aside on hospital design. I visited a very attractive new hospital a few years ago. The lobby was spacious and airy and had a Starbucks café from which the aroma of coffee drifted tantalizingly. But my guide commented that this last was a bad feature. "All the patients come in through the lobby and many have been fasting in preparation for their procedure. The smell of coffee just makes the fasting worse."

If one has a specific need to get to the European collection or the Far East Asian collection in a museum, directions or a map should be available. But if one has a broader interest in art, the art gallery should be more a place you wander through and make unexpected discoveries rather than a place. Using the Louvre as our example, if you go just to see the Mona Lisa and take a selfie with her if the crowds permit, then wayfinding is crucial – but you are hardly making the best use of this great museum. In other words, wayfinding is an important challenge for architecture, but the balance between wayshowing and waylosing may be more important than usually noted. This example reminds us that we can talk of affordances for contemplation and aesthetic appreciation (whether admiring a painting or standing in awe of a landscape or a sunset), and not only of affordances for action and other forms of navigation. The latter may say "this is the way to travel"; the former announces, "this is a special place. This is not just any affordance. You're very lucky to be here."

6.2. A COGNITIVE ACCOUNT OF WAYFINDING

This section introduces two notions—that of the cognitive map considered as a world graph (WG), and that of a locometric map—that can be linked back to wayfinding in cities as well as buildings. These notions will also play a crucial role in our excursion in §6.3 into developing a cognitive model to chart the role of the hippocampus and other regions in diverse forms of spatial navigation.

Getting lost in buildings

Carlson, Hölscher, Shipley, and Dalton (2010) conclude their account of "Getting Lost in Buildings" with a critique of wayfinding problems in the Seattle Central Library.[3] The library, designed by Rem Koolhaas/OMA of

3. Dalton and Hölscher (2017) have teamed up recently to edit a book of diverse essays, *Take one Building: Interdisciplinary Research Perspectives of the Seattle Central Library.*

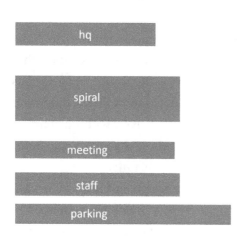

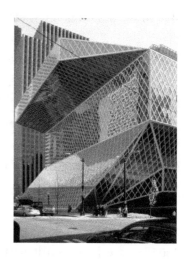

Figure 6.8 The Seattle Public Library. (*Left*) A schematic view of the functions of various floors. We see the relative size and altitude assigned to each function. (*Right*) A view of the facade. (*Left*: Author's diagram. *Right*: https://upload.wikimedia.org/wikipedia/commons/8/8a/Seattle_Central_Library%2C_Seattle%2C_Washington_-_20060418.jpg. Attribution-ShareAlike 3.0 Unported, CC BY-SA 3.0.)

the Netherlands in collaboration with the Seattle firm LMN Architects, has a steel and glass exterior arranged in angular folded planes. Koolhaas claimed that the building's required functions dictate what it should look like.[4] I find that claim unconvincing. At left of Figure 6.8, we see a schematic view of the separation of the various functions—parking, staff functions, meeting rooms, the book spiral, and the headquarters—indicating their relative size and altitude. The functions do not dictate this schematic, and nothing in the schematic demands that it be wrapped in steel and glass in the particular fashion shown at right. Our earlier discussion of performative architecture suggested that "the building's required functions *constrain* what it should look like," and one can see how the curtain envelope is developed in relation to (rather than dictated by) the schematic shown at left. Further constraints are provided by the choice of the

4. See, for example, https://artsandculture.google.com/theme/discover-the-innovative-buildings-of-rem-koolhaas/awJSsVRdLkcbIA?hl=en.

skin of the building, the tradeoff between daylight and artificial light, and many more.

Moreover, the "spiral" offers a strong commitment beyond the basic function of library stacks, the storage and retrieval of books and other materials. Instead of the usual library design having materials on various subjects segregated on different floors, the collection in Seattle spirals up through four stories on a continuous series of shelves, with no stairs or transits to a different part of the building within it. As with the exterior form, this radical innovation is not dictated by this function.

The library was widely praised for its bold design, but Robin Pogrebin (2004) assessed it (along with other prominent buildings completed in 2004) to see how well it performed. Seattle's city librarian was ecstatic that the aesthetic appeal of the building made staff members excited to work there. However, she noted that wayfinding was among several unexpected kinks:

> By the second or third day, we had to put up signs to help people. The bathrooms needed signs coming out, instead of being flat on the wall. The library's organization makes complete sense to us. But for the public, it's not obvious. One portion of the seventh floor is six feet higher because it spirals around. So if it says something is on seven, what does that mean?

Indeed, the spiral proved to be a mixed blessing. For some, the idea of traversing the spiral and seeing what books they might find along the way could be fun. But for people wanting to get a particular book, separate floors with a clear floor plan based on the Dewey Decimal System classification would be more helpful: "go to the third level, turn left, and go to the third row, and you will find the book halfway down on the top shelf on your left." Of course, one still needs a catalog to translate one's interest into specific ranges of the Dewey Decimal System.

In an earlier study, Hölscher, Büchner, Meilinger, and Strube (2009) studied the effects of spatial structure, task requirements, and metric information on wayfinding. They found that, in a multibuilding ensemble, wayfinding difficulties (e.g., disorientation, frequent stops, and substantial detours) were systematically associated with such building features as insufficient visual access in the lobby, awkward staircase placement, and dead-end corridors. However (and this is not in their paper), apparently awkward placement may sometimes be an intentional "nudge." For example, if a lobby offers high visibility for the stairs but lesser visibility and more effortful access for the elevators, this may encourage those going to the next floor to exercise by taking the stairs rather than an elevator.

Weisman (1981) offered three criteria for evaluating architectural legibility:

1. visual access between key locations;
2. architectural differentiation between different parts of an environment; and
3. layout complexity, or the number of rooms and corridors and their configuration.

Contra criterion 1, more general forms of adjacency—for example, "go to the next intersection"—do not require that it be visible, but you should know it when you get there. Certainly, taking the elevator defies criterion 1. Again, whether or not one can see many things from a given vantage point, one needs to be able to focus on the few that may be salient for wayfinding. Ken Kornberg (personal communication) speaks of the benefit of making corridors curved because having the inside versus the outside on your left gives you an unequivocal cue to which direction you are going on a long corridor, while knowing whether a room is on the inner or outer curve can halve the number of rooms that have to be inspected. Of course, some signage may be required for newcomers if the corridor is an important throughway to a crucial node.

For criterion 2, architectural differentiation is certainly important in terms of the "place-making" that lets one distinguish key decision points (related to what I call *nodes* in a cognitive map; see later). Nonetheless, in large buildings, the set of distinctive places may be limited—in a hotel, for example, getting into the right corridor from the elevator, and getting back to the elevator, both need to be supported (the latter often is not), but within a long corridor, signage, such as visible room numbering, takes precedence over architectural distinctiveness.

For criterion 3, it seems a mistake to identify layout complexity with the number of rooms because "go to the end of the corridor" remains a simple instruction. Complexity corresponds to the difficulty of the wayfinding problem and thus involves the efficacy of long-term memory because different people can master cognitive maps of very different complexity. However, it also involves the capacity of working memory—keeping track of where one is in relation to where one is going. This may also include hierarchical memory—keeping track of local details, but with the ability to pop up to a large-scale cognitive map to plan one's way to the next region for which a local map is available. The architect may vary the design to meet the needs of the users. In a library, the public spaces need to have low wayfinding complexity; in staff quarters, one can expect more training and familiarity to support greater complexity of the staff's cognitive maps.

With this background, we turn to a general definition of cognitive maps, discussing how they take us beyond mere route-following. We then return to architecture to complete this section. In §6.3, we establish the link back to neuroscience, exploring a model of the brain that suggests a crucial function for the hippocampus *in concert with other brain regions* in exploiting cognitive maps, even though the hippocampus is not needed for route following.

Defining cognitive maps

The issue is this: to navigate an area, what is the tradeoff between the knowledge in the head of the user of an environment (their cognitive map of its layout) and the explicit indications, like signposts, that can guide the way of someone unfamiliar with the territory? The most common human use of the word *map* is that typified in a world atlas or a road map. Here the map is a two-dimensional pattern (classically, on paper; increasingly, on computer screen), where points in the pattern correspond to points (and related features) on the Earth's surface or in some neighborhood. Akin to the standard use, a *cognitive map* is an encoding in the brain of spatial relations of places in the external world, supporting the behavior of an animal or human in getting from one place to another as it satisfies its various needs, even when the place it needs to get to is far outside the region of the environment available for current perception. (Contrast the sense of "maps in the brain" in §2.2) We exploit a cognitive map when we find our way around our home (or a familiar art gallery or other building), or drive confidently to work, even figuring out alternative routes when a road on our usual route is blocked.

Kevin Lynch's (1960) *The Image of the City* offers a classic contribution of what may be seen as cognitive science to city planning, with insights concerning the relation of buildings and urban spaces—but these have implications at the level of relating spaces within a building as well. However, rather than review Lynch's ideas explicitly, I will explore a later but eerily similar approach to understanding the cognitive science and neuroscience of rats exploring mazes, the World Graph Model.

But first, let's define the general notion of a cognitive map, by reflecting on the classic map of the London Underground (Figure 6.9).

To use this map you first have to be in London! Then you have to find the station name X for where you are, and the station name Y for where you want to be. You then try to find a path from X to Y on the map, which you then decode to tell you which lines to take and where to change trains to get to your desired destination. This is an excellent map, but it is not quite a cognitive map. Why not? Because, by contrast, a cognitive map is the whole system in the brain that allows you, without looking at a paper map or consulting your smart phone, to find your way to a destination in a known territory.

Before going further, let's note that after you have learned to use the London map (or that of your favorite city with a Metro), you have acquired a *general script* that will let you navigate the Metro in cities you have never encountered before. This is because these cities (well, at least the ones I have visited) all offer maps based on the conventions established by Harry Beck. Thus, with the aid of Figure 6.10, you could easily navigate your way around Moscow (after you have learned how to recognize place

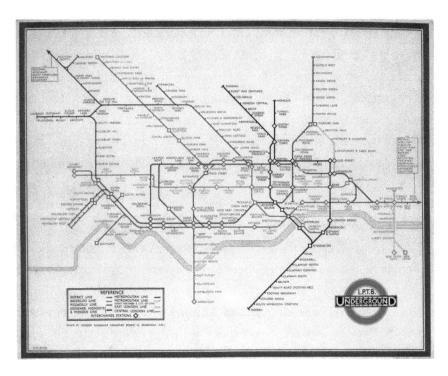

Figure 6.9 The original map of the London Underground (Harry Beck, 1933). (https://www.inyourarea.co.uk/news/harry-beck-the-tube-map-man-was-born-on-this-day-in-1902/. LTM_Image Requests images@ltmuseum.co.uk, with permission.)

names written in Cyrillic). Nonhuman animals have cognitive maps, too, but none can master this script.

Back to the map of Figure 6.9: it is restricted to the Tube stations of London and the connections between them, and covers only an aspect of London "territory" limited both as to region and as to the features that are included. Further, it requires a certain skill to use it, mastering the "script" I have just described. With this, we can define this sort of map—but note the phrase "for a user U":

Definition: *An "ordinary" map M for a user U* is a representation of a limited "sample" of space S such that:

1. U can find in M a representation M(A) of U's current location A
2. U can find in M a representation M(B) of U's desired location B

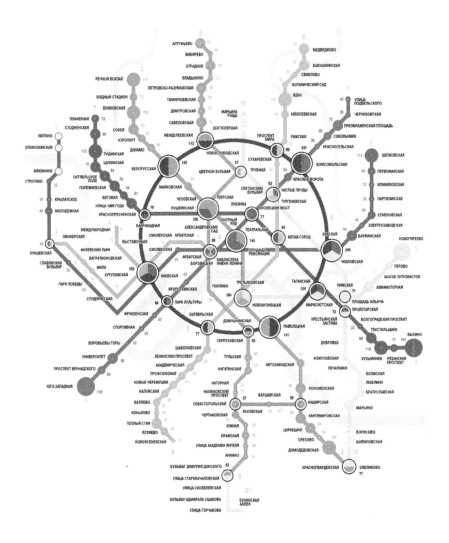

Figure 6.10 The Metro map of Moscow. (Source Aleksei Goncharov, licensed under the Creative Commons Attribution-Share Alike 3.0 Unported license.)

3. U can find a path in M, $P_M(A,B)$, from $M(A)$ to $M(B)$

4. U can transform $P_M(A,B)$ into a path in S, $P_S(A,B)$, from A to B

This makes explicit the limited coverage of such a map (space S), and the fact that it requires some ability (user U) to use it to navigate. Let me then try to distinguish a "paper map" of a region of space from a "cognitive map" as a navigational ability in the brain of an animal or human.

Definition: A *cognitive map* is a *system* that combines a neural encoding of an "ordinary" map with cognitive mechanisms that support the capabilities 1 to 4.

Note that when we use an "ordinary" map, each of the steps 1 to 4 are conscious steps. By contrast, when we "use" a cognitive map to get from A to B, we have no conscious awareness of how $M(A)$, $M(B)$, or $P_M(A,B)$ are encoded in the brain, though we will in general have conscious access to the resulting "path recommendation" $P_S(A,B)$ in terms of being primed to recognize key landmarks (significant places) in S and how to get from one to the next.

In this modern age, we not only have access to maps printed on paper that can be spread out to give a large-scale view in which we can locate places of interest or a route in relation to a range of other well-defined locations; we also have access on computers and smartphones to what I will call *app-maps*. An app-map divorces us from any overall sense of the territory or building in which we seek a path—it just tells us what to do next, and we trust that if we follow each instruction in order, we will finally reach a desired destination. This is comparable to following signage in a building with no sense of the overall layout.

Consider that you are in a strange city (outside China) and want to eat at a Chinese restaurant. You ask the concierge of your hotel, and after she recommends a specific restaurant, you ask for directions. These may come in the form of how to follow a route such as "go down the main street till you get to the second roundabout, then take the second exit and keep going until you see the large red and gold sign with flashing Chinese characters." Or, she may give you a city map with a circle for the hotel and an X for the restaurant, leaving you to relate the map to the city to plan a route for yourself as you walk or drive to dinner. However, in a familiar city, you might just need to be told, "It's a block north of the old Haberdashery Department Store," and in that case you plan a route based on a cognitive map that encodes your prior experience of moving around town. Similar considerations, of course, apply to finding your way around the country-side, or within a building.

Our phenomenological experience may be quite different from the neural representation. Compare the classic *Molyneux's problem*: light reflected from our surroundings projects via each eye's lens to an upside-down image on the retina. How then can we see things "right-side up"? The answer is that our subjective impression is based on our ability to, for example, find that our visual percept and our motor action are in accord—we reach an object when we move our arm to where it appears to be. Our work on adapting to prisms (§2.2) showed that this relationship is shaped by synaptic plasticity in "maps in the brain" (as distinct from cognitive maps) of sensorimotor relations. The adaptation to inverting prisms for Kohler's subjects (Kohler, 1963) was different for the town appearing right-side up while cycling through it, and for the letters on signage in the town "returning to normal." Similar surprises await in our study of the neuroscience of navigation and wayfinding.

Let's add one more wrinkle. Perhaps as a more adventurous traveler in a new town, you decide to set out from the hotel to find that restaurant for yourself. Here, you might use general cues to help you navigate somewhere between a strongly commercial area and endless apartment buildings until you chance upon an area where signs tell you that you have found restaurants but not yet a Chinese restaurant. You use this discovery to look for signs for restaurants to limit your search—until you see a sign for a Chinese restaurant, which you then approach and check the menu. You might stop there or seek another Chinese restaurant—and you might eventually find one that meets your standards, or find that hunger becomes too pressing and settle for a Thai restaurant instead. In this process of exploration, you may notice certain landmarks that enable you to find your way back to the hotel after your meal. The crucial point is that in many ways your adventurous exploration is initially like use of an app-map in that (at first) you may navigate with no overall sense of the territory but simply attend to affordances to determine where to go next. However, your adventurous exploration has two distinctive features:

1. You are having to choose affordances and other visual cues to decide how to act upon each one rather than simply accept the app-map's instruction, "Do x when you reach affordance y." Here, the exploratory drive plays an important role—it is similar to way-losing, but with the emphasis on finding a destination with par-ticular characteristics, rather than finding a path with "interesting" places for contemplation.

2. However, when you are exploring, you are constructing (in more or less detail, with more or less accuracy and more or less memorability) a special-purpose cognitive map, which may suffice for you to find your way directly back to the hotel after dinner, following in reverse a more direct path than the one you took before. That is a key property of cognitive maps—providing knowledge that allows one to plan new routes, not just follow old ones, including the ability to detour around unexpected obstacles that block an established route.

In developing and using a cognitive map, the notion of *distinctive place* (or *node*) becomes at least as important as affordances in guiding naviga-tion. The implication for architects and planners, then, is how to provide not only affordances but also distinctive "place-making." In an urban grid, though, place-making may involve the less architectural solution of pro-viding street signs (you are at the intersection of 49th street and Madison Avenue) to guide navigation between distinctive landmarks. But note where these fall short. If you emerge from the subway, it is not enough to know where you are—you need indicators of orientation. Interestingly, soon after the discovery of place cells in the rat hippocampus (§2.5), head direction cells were found in the nearby postsubiculum (Taube, Muller, & Ranck, 1990).

Affordances signal what you can do in *your immediate environment*. . A map, whether an explicit map on paper or a cognitive map encoded in your head, gives you access to a realm of knowledge *beyond the immediate environment* that can nonetheless let you find your way to some goal. This establishes the difference between "wayfinding by following affordances," which, we shall see, does not involve the hippocampus, and "building and using a cognitive map" so that one can navigate to a desired location even in the absence of destination-encoding cues, which does. This distinction was established by John O'Keefe and Lynn Nadel in their book *The Hippocampus as a Cognitive Map* (O'Keefe & Nadel, 1978), using rather different terminology to define *two systems for navigation*:

- the *locale* (map-based) system for navigation, proposed to reside in the hippocampus (but which we will locate in a set of interacting brain regions, of which the hippocampus is just one); and
- the *taxon* (behavioral orientation) system for route navigation, based on egocentric spatial information (which we view as based on *affordances*, and which need not involve the hippocampus).

The word *taxon* may be unfamiliar, but it is cognate with the word *taxis*—not in the sense of cars and drivers for hire but pronounced tax-iss (*iss* as in *hiss*)—as used in *phototaxis*, going toward the light, or *phono-taxis*, going toward the sound. In the previous example, we might (but would probably rather not) speak of *restaurantotaxis*.

Recall from §2.5 the crucial discovery (O'Keefe & Dostrovsky, 1971) of what are called *place cells* in the hippocampus of the navigating rat—cells that seemed to respond best when the rat was in a particular part of its environment, its *place field*. Because its place field is relatively broad, one cell does not specify the rat's location with much precision. However, we saw that the joint activity of a *population* of neurons can specify that the rat is in the small region (the "location") in which the place fields of active place cells overlap.

We must now resolve an important terminological confusion.

In architecture and in the study of cognitive maps, a *place* is a *distinctive* location. In the studies by O'Keefe and the many who have built on his work, any "point" in space can be a place. Contrast our map of the London Underground. Here, each station is a "place," but neither different locations along the tunnels nor different locations within the station are places in our cognitive sense. If we become familiar with a particular station, then we may develop a *local* cognitive map—and here knowledge of which escalator to take and which turns to take at branch points in the pedestrian tunnels would define a few key "places" for navigation. Meanwhile, hippocampal cells might change their activity as we walk from station entrance to a platform, but the locations—the places in the O'Keefe-sense—that they characterize would not be places at the level of the cognitive map.

The world graph model (WGM)

The notion of "cognitive map" was introduced to cognitive psychology by Tolman (1948), who studied how rats behaved in mazes, but classic studies of maze-running were receiving little attention in the mid-1970s when Israel Lieblich, a psychologist from Jerusalem, spent his sabbatical with me in Amherst, Massachusetts. He posed the challenge of developing a new theoretical framework for considering such behavior. Our key innovation (Arbib & Lieblich, 1977; Lieblich & Arbib, 1982) was the notion of the world graph (WG) as a way of formalizing the notion of a cognitive map, including an account of how a rat might behave differently in a maze based on its motivational state (e.g., hunger versus thirst versus fear), reaching a desired place or avoiding an unpleasant one even when obstacles made detouring necessary.

Many of us are familiar with the use of x-y graphs to represent data relating x and y values representing data on interest. Here, we appeal to another way mathematicians use the term, in which a *graph* comprises a finite set of "nodes," some pairs of which are connected by lines called "edges." (So "edge" here means something different from colloquial use in "the edge of the table.")

A mathematical aside: A classic problem was this: Was there a walk around the Prussian city of Königsberg that crossed each of the seven bridges (shown in blue at left of Figure 6.11) once and only once? The

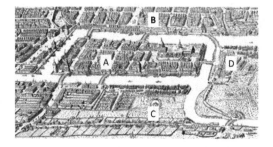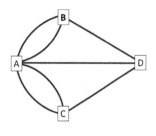

Figure 6.11 The Bridges of Königsberg problem. Is there a walk through the city that would cross each of its seven bridges once and only once? (*Right*) The graph generated by Leonhard Euler as the basis for a general mathematical theorem that implies that no such walk exists. Each land area becomes a node, while each bridge becomes an edge.

genius of Leonhard Euler (1707–1783)[5] was to replace the particularities of Königsberg by the graph shown at right, where each land area becomes a node, while each bridge becomes an edge. The question then becomes: Is there a path through the graph that traverses each edge once and only once? Euler, being a brilliant mathematician, was not content with only answering the original question. Instead he proved (half of) the general theorem:

> For any graph, the degree of a node is the number of edges touching it. A walk of the desired form exists only if the graph is connected and has exactly zero or two nodes of odd degree.

Since all four of the Königsberg map's nodes have odd degree, no path exists that traverses each edge once and only once.

With this theorem, Euler founded the mathematical area called *graph theory*, and also paved the way for *topology*, an area in which the precise measurements of Euclidean geometry are replaced by relationships that

---

5. The Mathematics Genealogy Project (www.genealogy.math.ndsu.nodak.edu) gives the genealogy of each mathematician, with "thesis advisor" in place of "parent." According to the Project, I am an 11th-generation descendant of Euler. However, pleasing though this is, it is hardly a unique distinction: Euler had only six students listed in the Project, but 119,941 descendants. The magic of exponential growth.

would be preserved if the original pattern were drawn on a rubber sheet that was stretched in any way that did not involve tearing it. (Mathematics being mathematics, topology is far more general, not being restricted to two-dimensional patterns.)[6]

Back to cognitive maps: What makes a graph a *WG* is that:

- each *node* corresponds to a *distinctive* place in the animal's world; and
- each *edge* corresponds to a direct path from one distinctive place to another. Sensorimotor features appended to each edge correspond to the associated path.

There is an edge from node x to node x' in the graph for each direct path the animal has traversed from the situation it recognizes as x to the situation it recognizes as x' without passing through another recognizable situation.

In the map of the London Underground, edges are color-coded so that one can factor the cost of changing from one subway line to another into one's navigation plan. Each node corresponds to a station. Unlike Euler's problem, where each bridge can be crossed (edge can be traversed) in either direction, each line between two adjacent stations actually corresponds to *two edges* of the graph, one for travel between the stations in each direction. (Of course, if both stations lie on two different train lines, then there would be distinct edges for each line. Similarly, there could in general be multiple edges between a pair of nodes in a WG.) Moreover, a single place in the world may be represented by more than one node in the graph if, for example, the animal comes upon a place in the maze for the second time but does not recognize that it has been there before.

In our world graph model (WGM), each node not only encodes recognition features but also stores information about the utility of the place (this was related to drives like hunger, thirst, and fear in the rat model).

---

6. For more on this topic, see the Wikipedia article "Seven Bridges of Königsberg," and the chapter "Rubber Sheet Geometry" in *Mathematics and the Imagination* (Kasner & Newman, 1940).

As suggested earlier, many architects will note the relation to ideas in Kevin Lynch's *The Image of the City* (Lynch, 1960). A recognizable "place" is one with *distinctive features* that may make it memorable.

Each of us has many different WGs. There are certain distinctive places in our worlds, and for each of those we have a way of getting to some "neighboring" places. Figure 6.12 represents a fragment of my W for air travel, showing how I get from Los Angeles to Sydney. Thus, when I say, "neighboring places" in a WG, I emphasize that "neighboring" does not mean "nearby." I get on a plane in Los Angeles. I get off that plane in Sydney—that's just one edge of the graph. I need to traverse three edges of this airline WG, corresponding to three flights, to get from San Diego in California to Perth in Western Australia:

San Diego → Los Angeles → Sydney → Perth

Other WGs are on a smaller scale. One helps me get to the airport from my home and serves a range of other needs for road travel in Southern California. When I'm on the plane, I just sit there and eat and drink and sleep and tap away on the computer and watch the flight map or get bored (maybe I develop a small cognitive map for the interior of the plane, to be forgotten after my flight). At the other end, I invoke another WG to get to my friend's house in Perth. The WGs we each have for our home and places of work are on a smaller scale still, and each shrinks to a node in the WG that includes the path for our daily commute, going to the grocery store or the theater, and much more. These last examples remind us that different people may have very different cognitive maps/WGs. A store you

Figure 6.12 Two nodes represent places in the world; each edge represents a direct link from one place to another (in this case, a nonstop flight from Los Angeles to Sydney).

often shop at may be a node in your WG but a barely noticed feature of an edge in mine.

Back to architecture

As in this example of real-life navigation across different scales and in different locales, buildings too are nested environments, and may involve multiple cognitive maps for each user. As we move from one part of a building to another, we may have a representation of relative position in each region, but our overall representation might not be coherent globally, such as when one faces the door of a room but does not know one's orientation with respect to the entrance to the building. With each successive turn, it becomes increasingly difficult to maintain one's sense of direction unless one is in a building or neighborhood structured on a grid like Manhattan's, where one can simply flip between the four directions.

This suggests that in designing a public building, at least, the architect must take into account the way in which newcomers must map the building to make comfortable use of it. Affordances that support learning can play an important role, and their lack can be troublesome. An example. I stayed (pre-Covid-19) at the Intercontinental Hotel in downtown Los Angeles. When I entered, there was no sign of a registration desk, but there was a sign pointing to "Lobby Elevator." Getting on the elevator, I could find no buttons to choose the lobby floor and was discomfited to find that the elevator appeared to be headed to the 70th floor. Fortunately, there was another passenger who explained to me that (a) one had to select one's destination on a touchpad outside the elevator, and (b) the lobby was indeed on the 70th floor. I quickly learned from this how to use the elevators in the building and how to get to the lobby—a mixture of procedural learning and growing a cognitive map. By the time I reached the lobby, this new WG had two nodes (representing the ground floor of the hotel and the lobby) and the edge between them (accessed by the action: press 7-0 before entering the elevator on the ground floor), and I had a new script for elevator use.

The lobby, with its high ceilings, glass walls, and dramatic view across Los Angeles was indeed an attractive, unusual, and memorable feature of the hotel—but the lack of visible affordances for getting to the lobby on first use, while memorable, would have been stressful had no one been using the elevator when I needed it and explained to me how to use it.

This simple example—designing an attractive place, the lobby, but with a poorly thought out approach for helping the first-time guests find their way there—suggests the important complementarity between wayfinding and place-making, a relationship like that between nodes and edges in a WG, that could be developed to provide detailed challenges for evidence-based design.

Locometric maps

When staying in a hotel, we may develop an intuition of how far down the corridor we have to walk from the elevator to our room. By contrast, a subway map helps us navigate a city, but has little if any metric structure. When we exit a station, we return to measuring the world in terms of the actions (walking, driving) whereby we traverse it. I use the term *locometric* for this way of measuring space. The notion of locometric space is particularly relevant to the notion of *path integration* mentioned earlier, the ability of a wandering animal to keep track of the location of its home base relative to its current position, without necessary reference to landmarks.

It is here that the cognitive map may make contact with the O'Keefian version of "place"—a location in a local locometric space, rather than a *distinctive* place as for a WG.

The next section will argue that the distinction between WG-style cognitive maps and locometric maps is neurologically grounded—but in general the diverse maps work seamlessly together in underwriting our experience and behavior. Only occasionally will one map burst into consciousness to question the other, as in "I must have missed that turnoff, I'm sure it couldn't have been this far."

This dichotomy can be illustrated by recalling our discussion of the book spiral in the Seattle Public Library. The problem that many visitors had with the spiral was that it lacked distinctive places, and visitors had no easy way to link what they were looking for to the only map they had available, a locometric map of the effort expended in walking up and down the spiral. Our more general discussion of getting lost in buildings and of the challenge of long corridors may be related to the challenge of "place-making" and the need to have "not too many" distinctive places, but also not too few. I earlier mentioned the design of a mall, and the need to accommodate two modes of customer behavior—being able to browse the distinctive shops when in the mood, and yet having visible landmarks to enable finding one's way to a particular shop when so inclined.

Floors in the argument

Some years ago, some colleagues wrote a proposal with me for new research on place cells in the hippocampus. The starting point was the observation that if a rat is placed in different environments, then place cells change their place fields to link to places in one environment that bear no obvious relation to their place fields in the other. Specifically, Wilson and McNaughton (1993) used ensemble recordings of rat hippocampal neurons to predict accurately the animals' movement through their environment. In a novel space, the ensemble code was initially less robust but improved rapidly with exploration. During this period, the activity of many inhibitory cells was suppressed, which suggests that new spatial information creates conditions in the hippocampal circuitry that are conducive to the synaptic modification presumed to be involved in learning. Crucially, though, development of a new population code for a novel environment did not substantially alter the code for a familiar one when the rat returned to the other environment. This suggests that the interference between the two spatial representations was very small. Two charts, one hippocampus.

This suggests a *chart table* view of the hippocampus—as one changes charts, the place associated with a specific location on the "chart table" will change completely. In our previous terms, a fragment of the current nonmetric WG must become linked to the locometric map currently at play in hippocampus.

This motivated the question: If the rat moves from one environment to a *similar* environment, will the new hippocampal chart exhibit savings by exploiting the "old" place fields to map similar places in the new environment. For the proposal, I suggested testing this by recording from the brains of rats that, instead of running in a planar maze, could instead run in a "doll house" in which the second floor was similar to the first. What would happen when a rat, familiar with the first floor, began to map the second? In honor of Henrik Ibsen's play, "A Doll's House," I proposed that our system be called IBSEN, an *Integrated Brain System for Environmental Navigation*. Alas, despite (or because of) the acronym, the proposal was not funded. Instead, to serve the A↔N conversation, I have recycled the acronym in Chapter 10 to stand for *Imagination in Brain Systems for Episodes and Navigation*.

However, the relation of multiple floors in the design of a building—and the impact this design has on the cognitive map of the user—remains of interest. For example, in a tall building with multiple elevator banks, how might an understanding of their relative placement on the ground floor aid one's navigation on the higher floors? Hölscher, Meilinger, Vrachliotis, Brösamle, and Knauff (2006) observed that participants typically assume that the organization of a given floor extends to all floors and show considerable difficulty with wayfinding when this assumption is violated. However, it goes beyond this. In a public building, the ground floor will probably have a distinctive entrance, a lobby, and stated access via stairways and lifts. Other floors may have the same general layout as each other, different from the ground floor, yet may nonetheless have some distinctive features (recall Sullivan's tripartite division of the *exterior* of tall buildings, §1.1). Still, the issue of cognitive savings in navigating new floors (i.e., the ability to build a local cognitive map quickly be reusing parts of an earlier one) is interesting—unless the floors are truly identical, in which case they become boring even if easily navigable!

In buildings for public use and with multiple floors, a defining vertical axis is the elevator shaft. If you are looking for a restroom in a strange building, you will often go first to the vicinity of the elevator. A standard arrangement would have the room for Men on one side and that for Women on the other. If you find one of the restrooms, but it is not for your gender, you look on the other side of the elevators. In other buildings, restrooms change gender on alternate floors. It is as if you have a few generic "cognitive map-scripts" you can plug in to quickly build a cognitive map of a new environment. Yes, a building need not follow the usual scripts (recall Bo Bardi's art gallery). Nonetheless, this sort of general strategy or script can often speed forming a cognitive map. You now have a little fragment of a map that tells you, no matter what floor you're on, how to satisfy one of your basic needs. Such considerations may in turn guide the architect in trading off between familiarity and novelty in designing a building.

6.3. IT TAKES MORE THAN A HIPPOCAMPUS TO BUILD A COGNITIVE MAP

Earlier, I distinguished between O'Keefe and Nadel's *taxon* (behavioral orientation) system for route navigation, based on egocentric spatial information (location relative to currently perceptible *affordances*), which does not involve the hippocampus, and "developing and using a cognitive map" so that one can even navigate to a desired but out-of-sight location, which does. As always, a reminder that we do not rely only on vision to ground our behavior. Seeking a football stadium, for example, one might get directional cues from the roar of the crowd long before the stadium itself becomes visible.

In this section, I develop an account of how the brain might

1. support navigation based solely on affordances, without recourse to the circuitry of the hippocampus, and then

2. see how these mechanisms may be integrated with hippocampus, basal ganglia, and prefrontal cortex to implement cognitive maps.

While I hope that most readers will read the whole section, I will announce when some may wish to fast-forward, skipping some description of how brain regions work together. Although clarifying the affordance/cognitive map distinction, my model invokes neither the grid cells of the entorhinal cortex (whose discovery led to the Mosers sharing a Nobel Prize with O'Keefe) nor regions like the parahippocampus and retrosplenial cortex that will make an appearance when I discuss episodic memory (Chapter 10). Epstein, Patai, Julian, and Spiers (2017) offer an excellent account of how the hippocampus works with such brain regions to support cognitive maps in humans. There may be treasures hidden there that greatly enrich the relevance of the hippocampus and cognitive maps to architecture, but that is a conversation for another day. A further contribution to that conversation is offered by Kate Jeffery (2019), who integrates ideas from studies of human navigation and rat hippocampus to offer the hope "that architects will reach out to their cognitive neuroscientist colleagues so that the resulting knowledge exchange can productively enhance city design, and make spaces more easily navigable, and less stressful and more pleasing, for an urban population that grows ever-denser."

The hippocampus in context, and the A↔N conversation

A classic cartoon shows a man lost in the desert. He discovers a billboard, but finds it contains only an X with the legend, "You are here." Poor fellow. For a map to be of any use to him, it must help him get where he wants to go. My perhaps unkind parody of the role of hippocampus in navigation is that *in itself* it is *not* a map because the place cells just say, "You are here." Our challenge in this subsection is to suggest how a cognitive map can work with affordances—combining the locale and taxon systems—as an animal or human navigates around its world, and to do so in a way that offers the architect at least a conceptual taste of how one may build computational models of brain systems (and recall the framing discussion in §2.7 of "Design in architecture and in brain modeling").

Our model of navigation (Guazzelli, Corbacho, Bota, & Arbib, 1998) will be presented below in two subsections:

1. "Navigation based solely on affordances" presents the taxon affordance model, TAM.
2. "How the brain could implement cognitive maps" shows how this is integrated with a brain-based version of the world graph model, WGM.

The suggestion here is that to understand how people interact with the world—or, for architects, the built environment—the phenomenology from introspection can be enriched (dissected) by understanding what different parts of the brain are doing, and then, perhaps, we can develop new design approaches that can differentially tap into different aspects of brain function.

Are both WG and the locometric map represented in hippocampus? The classic figure of hippocampus we have from Ramón y Cajal shows the neural circuitry in a *cross section* of rat hippocampus. However, an important finding is that the hippocampus varies greatly along its length in ways that are relevant to our discussion. To understand this more fully, let's learn more about the hippocampus by comparing related data from rat and human brains.

Kjelstrup et al. (2008) reported specialization of the *rat* hippocampus along its longitudinal axis, based on recording neuronal activity in CA3, a region that contains place cells:

[They] recorded neural activity at multiple longitudinal levels of [hippocampus] while rats ran back and forth on an 18-meter-long linear track. CA3 cells had well-defined place fields at all levels. The scale of representation increased almost linearly from <1 meter at the dorsal pole to ~10 meters at the ventral pole. The results suggest that the place-cell map includes the entire hippocampus and that environments are represented in the hippocampus at a topographically graded but finite continuum of scales.

This suggests greater precision and detail in the grain of hippocampal representations and reduced receptive field size of place cells as one moves from ventral to dorsal posterior regions. But does this provide an immediate "plug in" for assessing how architects might approach a design at different levels of detail? Not so fast! These data on locometric maps at different scales for a lab rat whose "world" is restricted to a single runway offer no evidence that WGs are encoded in hippocampus. While some might argue that the locometric map is encoded at the posterior end of hippocampus, whereas the current WG is coded more toward the anterior end, they cannot then (in humans, at least) presume that the same kind of representation holds throughout its length (Figure 6.13).

Another concern is that the place fields in a lab rat may vary greatly as the rat is moved from one arena to another. As noted earlier, a different

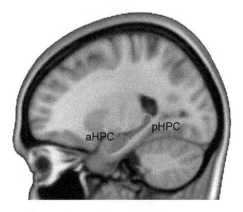

Figure 6.13 A cross section of the human brain, showing the lengthwise division of the hippocampus into the dorsal hippocampus (this is posterior hippocampus [pHPC], both upper and to the rear in primates) and the ventral hippocampus (this is anterior hippocampus [aHPC], lower and toward the front in primates). (From Li, X., Li, Q., Wang, X., Li, D., & Li, S. [2018]. Differential age-related changes in structural covariance networks of human anterior and posterior hippocampus. *Frontiers in Physiology*, 9[518]. Public access.)

"chart" is installed on the "hippocampal chart table" in widely separated locales. Where are the charts stored and how are the relevant ones instantiated? A WG may expand its scope indefinitely, so if all our cognitive maps were encoded in distinct parts along the hippocampal axis, then at some stage along the axis we would have to transition to an abstract level that escapes scale—contrast a map of South Kensington station, a map of the London Underground, or an airline map of the world.

Now consider *human* data on specialization of the hippocampus along its longitudinal axis. Maguire, Woollett, and Spiers (2006) compared London taxi drivers with London bus drivers. They were matched for driving experience and levels of stress, but differed in that taxi drivers had mastered "the Knowledge" of all details of London streets, whereas bus drivers follow a constrained set of routes. Taxi drivers had greater gray matter volume in mid-posterior hippocampus and less volume in anterior hippocampus than bus drivers. Furthermore, years of navigation experience correlated with hippocampal gray matter volume only in taxi drivers, with right posterior gray matter volume increasing and anterior volume decreasing with more navigation experience.

Maguire et al. conclude that spatial knowledge, and not stress or driving, is associated with the pattern of hippocampal gray matter volume in taxi drivers, but speculate that the complex spatial representation that facilitates expert navigation might have come at a cost to new spatial memories and gray matter volume in the anterior hippocampus (a very different longitudinal shift from the change of scales offered by Kjelstrup et al.). Perhaps, however, the issue is not reduced ability to form new spatial memories but rather a reduced ability to form complex spatial representations incompatible with the representational system developed in the taxi driver's brain to encode their expert knowledge.

As a point of comparison, Tichomirov and Poznyanskaya (1966) found that master chess players looked at boards for less time than novices and remembered positions more accurately, with the experts turning their gaze from one significant feature of the board to another, while the novices searched randomly. However, if the pieces were randomly arranged on the board, so that the experts had no meaningful search strategy, their performance in memorizing the board is much like that of the novices. Here, the actions that scan the environment are themselves constrained by the subject's plan of action, the plan to play a winning game of chess. Perhaps analogous considerations apply to the taxi driver's analysis of spatial layouts. We see here the action–perception cycle in full swing—we perceive the environment to the extent that we are *prepared to interact* with it in some reasonably structured fashion (Arbib, 1972).

A more specific concern is whether the "hippocampal chart table" notion is compatible with the observation of enlarged gray matter volume in mid-posterior hippocampus in London taxi drivers. Here are alternative hypotheses:

1. All of "locometric London" is simultaneously present as encoded by place cells of posterior hippocampus.
2. A high-level view of London (and elsewhere) is carried outside hippocampus in the WG (wherever that may be). At any time, the place cells have place fields that correspond to a limited region of London. For different regions, it is a state of the neural network that needs to be "installed" by contextual signals from the WG.

On the latter view (the one I adopt here), posterior hippocampus becomes more complex both to "accommodate more detailed charts" and to "reset accurately for a larger range of contextual cues." Alas, I have not found any serious attempts to assess this idea in the neuroscience literature.

Finally, note that the hippocampus has many roles including the support of episodic memory (see Chapter 10) that still remain active even if we make less use of cognitive maps. Moreover, even if we do use navigation apps, we will still build cognitive maps, though with reduced "coverage"—for example, in our own home and in familiar buildings and neighborhoods.

Recall my earlier comment that neuroscientists and architects who wish to engage in the A↔N conversation need only know enough of each other's field to be able to work together. For the architect interested in the relevance of the hippocampus to wayfinding, it might be enough to understand the basic dichotomy addressed by the TAM-WGM distinction, without an understanding of some basic interactions involved. Here, then, is the place where the reader makes a choice: to read carefully to master the rest of the section, to read more quickly while humming when things seem to be getting complicated, or to move on to the next double lines. Future conversations might then involve updating the details of neurophysiology and neuroanatomy that guided the modeling summarized here to explore their relevance to architectural exploration of wayfinding. A variant of the following exposition appears in the little book, *Meaning in Architecture: Affordances, Atmosphere and Mood* edited by Bob Condia (2020).

Of course, for the architect wanting to build on the neuroscience, this model is only the beginning. In relation to TAM, and working back from the behaviors of users, one can design specific studies of what visual, haptic, and auditory cues can most effectively signal affordances that provide rapid guidance for the appropriate behaviors. For example, a road sign indicating the path to an airport can be confusing if the airplane icon on the sign can be misread as an arrow pointing in the wrong direction.

AIRPORT NEXT LEFT✈

TAM-WGM was based on a wide range of neurophysiological and behavioral data, and its computer implementation offered new insight into some of these observations; a later paper expanded the treatment (Arbib & Bonaiuto, 2012) and adapted ideas on temporal difference learning applied in the augmented competitive queuing (ACQ) model (§5.5) to a form of spatial difference learning that could develop successful paths through the WG.

Navigation based solely on affordances (TAM)

TAM shows how we can navigate based on affordances. Although the model was based primarily on data on the brains and behaviors of rats, I shall use accounts of human behavior to motivate the exposition—and to better suggest its possible relevance to architects assessing the behavior of people in the built environment.

Figure 6.14 shows the stripped-down part of TAM for just choosing an affordance and responding accordingly. There are "boxes" connected by

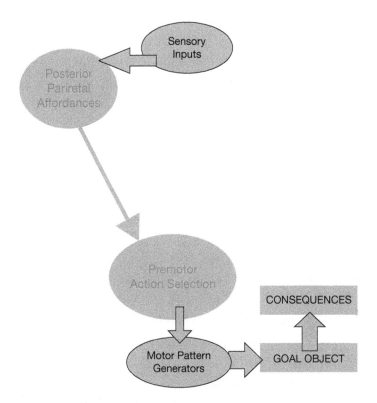

Figure 6.14 The taxon affordance model (TAM), shown without the learning component. The posterior parietal cortex processes sensory input to determine available affordances; these are then sent to premotor cortex where one action is selected for which an affordance is currently available. This encoded selection is then sent to motor pattern generators (MPGs), which carry out the action on the goal object (e.g., locomotion toward an observable landmark). The consequences of this action can then be evaluated.

arrows. Each box is labeled with a function; some are also labeled with the names of brain regions. Some boxes do not have anatomical labels. This could mean either that the relevant brain regions that support the function are not known, or that the modeler can rely on (or hypothesize) the availability of the relevant processes without needing to invoke any data about the neural activity that underlies it. Because of this, the figures that follow omit explicit mention of visual and other sensory areas of cerebral cortex as well as motor cortex and a range of subcortical brain regions and the spinal cord. The association of a function with a brain region, or the claim that an arrow represents connections between the two indicated brain regions, will in general be based on available data, but in some cases will represent hypotheses that suggest new neuroscience experiments.

As sensory inputs are processed, various affordances are detected (posterior parietal cortex). For the case of a walking human, affordances might be offered by a gap in the crowd, an interesting doorway, or a sign that they would like to read. In this example, three affordances are competing. Which one do you locomote toward? The premotor cortex is the one in which it is established which one of those affordances you are going to act upon. Other brain regions outside premotor cortex assist the decision, assessing the priorities of the affordances in terms of one's current task or motivation. (Compare the FARS model, §2.6, for selecting affordances for grasping an object.) This decision is relayed (via motor cortex and other regions outside the scope of the model) to motor pattern generators that convert that decision into the actual footsteps that get you to your next goal. This part of the model concludes with registration of the consequences of the selected action.

The consequences of the action provide the brain with the data it needs to learn from experience. They may be positive (that action would be worth repeating in similar circumstances) or negative (let's not make that mistake again). The original work with Israel Lieblich emphasized that a rat's behavior (like ours) very much depends on its motivational state. If it is hungry, it will look for a place where it can find food. If it is thirsty, it will seek water. If it finds itself near a place where it gets an electric shock, it will avoid it. Figure 6.15 thus focuses on the "motivational schema." The

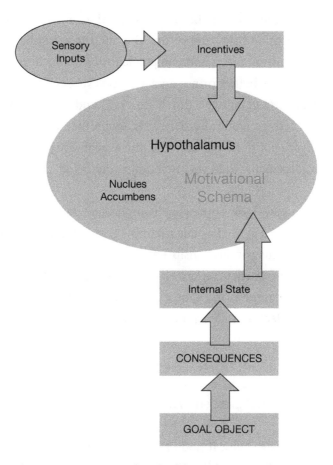

Figure 6.15 The motivation system. The job of the nucleus accumbens is to monitor the latest action and assess to what extent the new location yields positive or negative reinforcement. This reinforcement depends on the current motivational state of the animal—availability of food will be far more reinforcing when the animal is hungry than when it is sated or when it is only thirsty.

linkage of consequences to the internal state encodes such changes as "if you eat you are less hungry," "if you drink you are less thirsty." The incentives box reflects that, for example, the smell of food might increase one's drive to eat even if, in its absence, one might be only moderately hungry. (Compare wafting the aroma of freshly baked bread into a bakery to increase sales; conversely, consider the downside of allowing too "fishy" an aroma in a fishmonger's.)

The hypothalamus has the basic motor routines for handling hunger and thirst and fear and sex, and so on. The nucleus accumbens provides the basic mechanism for reinforcement learning here. It can take the information about whether or not an action was successful in addressing the current drive (e.g., hunger, thirst, fear, sex) and accordingly bias the desirability of acting on one affordance versus another *depending upon the current motivational state.* For example, the availability of food may offer positive reinforcement when you are hungry, but be off-putting if you are feeling full.

Figure 6.16 may look somewhat complicated, but it just combines Figures 6.14 and 6.15. My hope is that now that you have approached it gradually, it remains comprehensible and you can get some sense of how the two subsystems work together. I have added one extra arrow—the one from nucleus accumbens to make explicit that the learning system can modify action selection in the rat or human whose ongoing behavior we wish to study.

How the brain could implement cognitive maps (WGM)

The full WGM shows how, if node x represents the current location and node x′ represents a desired location, the brain can find a path from x to x′ in the current WG, which can then be translated into overt behavior as each edge on the path is read out as the corresponding action. The details are outside the scope of this book. Here, I just want to note how the WG may change over time, as mine did at the Intercontinental Hotel, before outlining some brain regions that interact in underwriting our ability to navigate using cognitive maps.

WGM captures our (or the rat's) exploratory drive as follows: Edges with unknown termini (i.e., unexplored affordances, such as a street or corridor you have not ventured down before) can compete with other edges from a node x. Figure 6.17 (top) shows that if movement occurs along an unexplored edge and leads to a new place *that is memorable*, a new node x′ and a new edge from x to x′ will be added to the graph, and

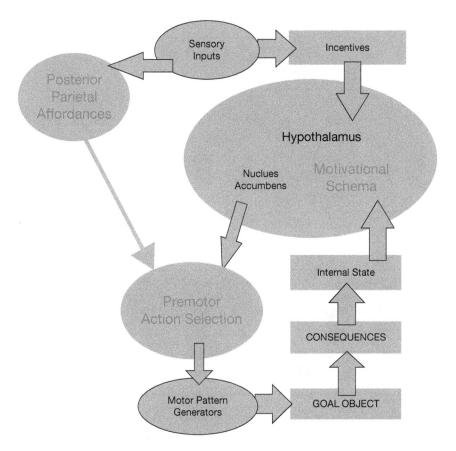

Figure 6.16 The complete taxon-affordances model (TAM). This combines Figures 6.14 and 6.15, but with one extra *arrow* to indicate how the assessment of negative or positive reinforcement by the nucleus accumbens can bias the selection of the future actions.

each will be tagged with the appropriate defining features. The bottom half of Figure 6.17 illustrates the merging of previously distinct nodes in the WGM. If the animal thinks it is at $P(x')$, the place represented by node x', but then recognizes that the place is also represented by a different node x'', then x' will be merged with x''. Just consider exploring an art gallery and finding oneself *unexpectedly* back in a room one had been in earlier. At first it looks different because one has entered it from a new direction, or noticed paintings one had not noticed before, but after a short time there one recognizes it as the same room one visited earlier. One initially

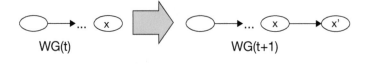

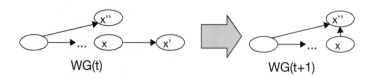

Figure 6.17 Exploration may add new nodes to a world graph (WG) (*top*) or collapse two nodes into one (*bottom*).

added x′ for a "new" room, then it "collapses" into the x″ for the "old" room (whether consciously or not).

An interesting example of a rat "thinking" it is in one place yet being in another goes back to the original O'Keefe style of experimentation. The experimenters put a rat in a radial maze, and measured a variety of place cells to find the place field of each cell (Figure 6.18). In particular, they could use the firing of the cells to identify which arm of the maze the rat "thought" it was on. Olton, Becker, and Handelmann (1980) added a little

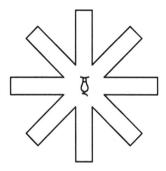

Figure 6.18 Rat in a radial maze. In general, various cues are placed around the maze so that the rat can visually distinguish one arm from another by what it sees as it moves out from the center.

wrinkle. They put food at the end of each arm at the beginning of each trial. The rat develops the optimal strategy—scurry up one arm and eat, return to the center of the maze, then scurry up a different arm. It won't go to the same place twice during a trial because it has learned that the food is not replaced during the trial.

The cognitive map built up for this maze probably has nodes for the center and for the ends of the arms. The place fields in the hippocampus encode the locometric maps of the arms. (Interestingly, there are different place fields for going out and coming back—just like position on a freeway is different depending on the direction you are going in. By contrast, place fields for regions in an open field are activated irrespective of the direction of approach.) But note that the maps are complemented in this experiment by a working memory that updates the knowledge of which nodes still have food.

In another version of the experiment, the rat runs in the dark. Then, instead of visual cues, it uses its own motion to update the firing of place cells that represent where it is in the maze. Every now and again, the rat will make an error and go up an arm it has visited before, and when this happens the experimenter finds that the place cells are coding an arm where food remains, not where the rat really is. This exemplifies a general issue of sensorimotor integration: How do your visual and tactile experiences register with your motor experience in locating yourself in an environment? Under what circumstances do the various cues get out of registration?

With this, we can comprehend the high-level view offered by Figure 6.19. The hippocampus registers where the animal is and updates the relevant node or edge in the WG currently activated in prefrontal cortex. On the basis of some criteria about the goal, prefrontal cortex determines possible paths to a goal and then biases action selection to choose an action that lies on one of the paths and currently has available affordances. As each new significant place is reached, the operation is repeated until the final goal is reached.

Figure 6.20 assembles all the various brain modules. In this integrated model, affordances matter even if we are navigating on the basis of a

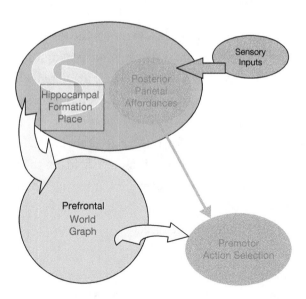

Figure 6.19 Introducing the hippocampus and the world graph for the model. The hippocampus encodes where the animal is in locometric detail. The relevant portion of prefrontal cortex activates the appropriate world graph and recognizes that the animal is at a significant place (encoded by a node) or en route from one place to another (encoded by an edge). Prefrontal cortex then processes the world graph to compute an overall path to get to some desired position; it can thus bias action selection after each new node-encoded place is reached.

(cognitive) map, but the model can also support taxon-based exploration until affordances for achieving the current goal are found. Indeed, recalling Figure 6.17 and the lobby of the Intercontinental Hotel, a cognitive map may be being built even in the latter (affordances only) mode. Whether or not that cognitive map becomes established in long-term memory will depend on contingent factors.

Although it is not part of TAM-WGM, I see ways to extend the model to allow part of the memory in WGM to be externalized to the use of a paper map. By contrast, route following under instruction by an app-map short-circuits the WGM computations, and we are basically reduced to relying on TAM, looking for the next affordance specified by the phone and acting as it directs.

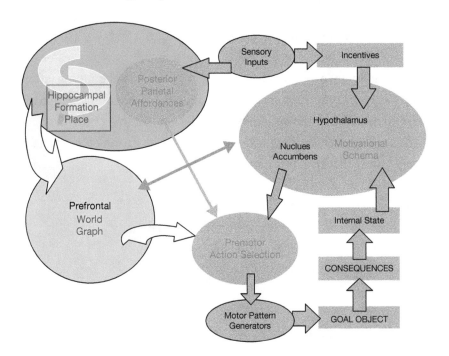

Figure 6.20 The complete taxon affordance model + world graph model (TAM-WGM).

Learning from the integrated model

The ideas embedded in this brain model make clear that it takes more than a hippocampus to build a cognitive map. The intuition provided in the account of visiting Bo Bardi's Sao Paulo art museum (§2.1) adds that, in architectural design, there is an interesting combination between exploiting the underlying "script" for how buildings of a given typology support behavior—what it is that you can expect people to know when they approach the building for the first time—and providing an element of surprise. The visitor to her museum finds famous paintings in elaborate frames. Expectations about being able to admire great art are met, but the visitor's "default" cognitive map proves useless. A joint challenge for architects and neuroscientists, then, is to go beyond the add-a-node-and-an-edge style of building a cognitive map (Figure 6.17) to get a better handle on the "scripts" that allow people to generate cognitive maps when they experience a building *of a given typology* for the first time (such as the restroom-finding strategy discussed earlier). Such a "map" goes beyond wayfinding to incorporate the variety of actions the building affords (which may include interaction with other people, adding a dynamic component to the environment that even a static building provides).

The challenge for the architect is to provide an environment that enables people to map that environment to meet their needs, while offering a measure of aesthetic satisfaction and adding that frisson when expectations are departed from without causing undue frustration in doing so. It takes more than a hippocampus not only to build a cognitive map but also to defy the visitor's initial expectations for a building's cognitive map in an architecturally pleasing way.

6.4. SYMBOLISM AND SYMBOLS

It is now time to find our way back to the discussion of symbolism. We have seen the stairs of Asplund's Stockholm library symbolizing the ascent to the level of wisdom and learning. The arrangement of the grand entrance of a courthouse contrasting with a small door below leading down to the prison beneath symbolized the majesty of the law and the crushing weight of justice bearing down on the guilty. A building may employ forms that traditionally symbolize progress, advancement, or financial power. In contemporary architecture, however, much of the traditional symbolism has become unused, or abstracted to a point where it may not "speak" to most users of the building. The lack of traditional symbolism may also be a response to having a limited budget. For example, a storefront church lacks the spires and bell tower and stained-glass windows that carry the symbolic charge of a "traditional" Christian church simply because there is no budget available for them. Instead, the storefront might bear a simple sign such as "St. Mark Pentecostal Church. All Welcome." Here *the symbolic is replaced by symbols*, in this case words of the local language. Indeed, for such a church, it is the words of the Bible and the uplift of singing hymns, countering rather than being aided by the architecture, that provide the path to inspiration.

Stained-glass windows in a church may combine the bringing of light with the "telling" of biblical stories. However, when I visited the Netherlands in the 1960s, a friend (Mirjam Verbeek) introduced me to the work of her father—creating new stained-glass windows to replace those that had been destroyed during World War II. Moving away from direct depiction, he created wonderful but abstract patterns of stained glass. Here, the symbolism was indirect: the patterns of light were evocative of the light through traditional stained-glass windows and thus (for those old enough to know them) evocative of the biblical associations that the previous windows had evoked more directly, but offered illumination (in both senses) that the faithful could imbue with spiritual meaning.

Such illumination harks back to the "Experiences of ultimacy" of §4.6—evoking religious feeling not through symbols associated with a specific religion, but rather through the evocation of exceptional emotion by an exceptional sunset or other "ultimate" experience. Having first drafted this section at a time when bushfires were ravaging Eastern Australia, let me just add that even such "primal" beauty is conditional—sitting around a safely contained campfire is far different from watching a fire leaping from tree to tree to threaten, and possibly destroy, your home, your livestock, and the wildlife that contribute so much to your sense of place—whether the sight of a kangaroo bounding across a paddock, or the morning chorus of the magpies and kookaburras. This reminds us that when neocortex evokes voluntary actions, it may well inhibit the automatic responses that would otherwise occur, and that such inhibition may itself depend on one's current emotional state.

But here I want to consider one example of modern architecture that does indeed place symbolism at the core of its design, but creating a new symbolism rather than replicating traditional symbolism—Oscar Niemeyer's Brasilia Cathedral (Catedral Metropolitana Nossa Senhora Aparecida).

In an NPR interview with Juan Forero (2010), the then 103-year-old Niemeyer stated that the vital component for his work is concrete. With it, he broke what he calls the tyranny of the right angle—hence the curves in many of his structures. His love of curves may be suggested by the pinup on the wall behind him in Figure 6.21. In the Forero interview, Niemeyer also said, "When I start to design, I have only a vague idea about what I'd like to do"—claiming that he doesn't think about any other building he's built before; he

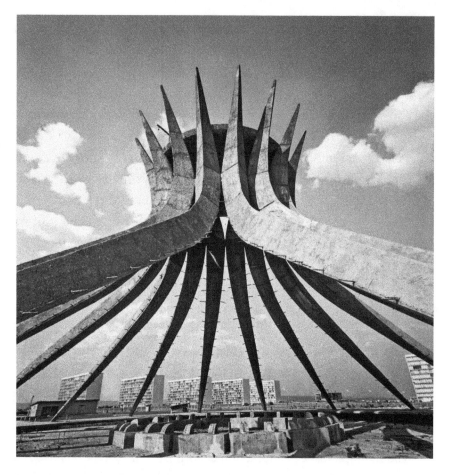

Figure 6.21 Oscar Niemeyer in his office with a model of his Brasilia Cathedral (Catedral Metropolitana Nossa Senhora Aparecida), and another model on the wall. (Photo by Frank Scherschel. The LIFE Picture Collection. Licensed from Getty Images.)

simply starts from scratch. I invite the reader to ponder this apparent contradiction to Zumthor's "images come to mind," but here I want to focus on a *possible* symbolic interpretation of part of Niemeyer's design.

Figure 6.22 shows the view of the incomplete cathedral that was adapted for the cover of the book, *Brazil's Modern Architecture* (Andreoli & Forty, 2004). The structure's 16 columns reach to the sky. Their shape has been compared to a giant orchid, but I want to suggest a different, more relevantly symbolic, interpretation. For me, the structure evoked the image of a pair of hands holding a disk aloft. Figure 6.23 shows the working out of my idea (but is hardly a proof of Niemeyer's intention). At left, we see Pope

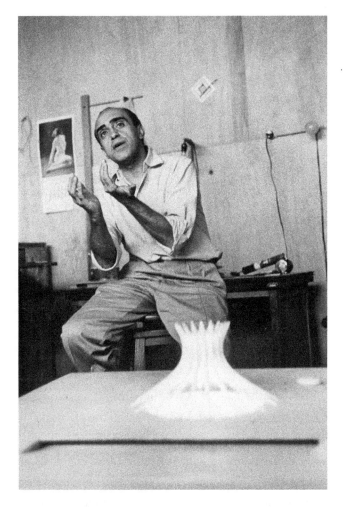

Figure 6.22 An external view of Oscar Niemeyer's Brasilia Cathedral at an early stage of construction, before erecting the stained-glass windows. (© Marcel Gautherot/Instituto Moreira Salles Collection, with permission.)

Benedict holding aloft the host.[7] At right we see a photo of my wife Prue's hands holding a saucer aloft. This is my suggestion for a bridge between the Pope's (and each Catholic priest's) symbolic gesture, and Niemeyer's columnar array.

7. The host is a disk-shaped bread whose substance, Roman Catholics believe, is transformed by the eucharistic prayer that invokes the action of the Holy Spirit into the substance of the Body of Christ, a prayer that at the same time transforms the substance of wine into the substance

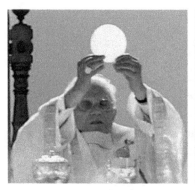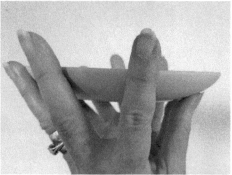

Figure 6.23 From raising the host to two hands holding a disk aloft. (*Left*: Pope Benedict XVI Holds the Host Aloft. Fabio Pozzebom/ABr, CC BY 3.0 BR, via Wikimedia Commons. *Right*: Author's photo.)

Unfortunately, in his autobiography, *The Curves of Time*, Niemeyer is silent about the exterior of the Cathedral. Instead, he says this:

> The search for an unusual solution fascinated me. In the Metropolitan Cathedral at Brasilia, for example, I avoided conventional solutions, which had produced the old dark cathedrals reminding us of sin. On the contrary, I designed a dark entrance hall leading to the nave, which is brightly lit, colorful, its beautiful, transparent stained-glass windows facing infinite space. I always received understanding and support from the clergy, even from the Papal nuncio, who could not contain his enthusiasm upon visiting the cathedral: "This architect must be a saint; only a saint could devise such splendid connection between the nave, heaven, and God." (Niemeyer, 2000, p. 173) (See Figures 6.24 and 6.25).

Pope Benedict's action of holding the host aloft only gains its symbolic meaning for those have been steeped in the Christian Gospels and the traditions built upon them. Although the action is simple, its symbolism

of His Blood. Members of the communion then partake of the Body and Blood of Christ by eating a small piece of the host and taking a small sip of the wine after their transubstantiation. The symbolism of the Pope's gesture may seem incredible to outsiders, but is highly evocative to many Christians.

rests on a web of words and actions. In §2.5, I recalled that Mary Hesse and I, in our book, *The Construction of Reality*, contrasted the perceptual, motor, and other schemas "in the head of the individual" with the "social schemas" that provide a complex social environment that helps shape the individual (by shaping, in part, the individual experience that shapes those internal schemas)—with examples of those schemas including languages, religions, and ideologies, but also many more focused domains of human knowledge and interaction. Our Chapter 9, "The Great Schema," addressed the way narratives are interwoven with belief, citing Northrop

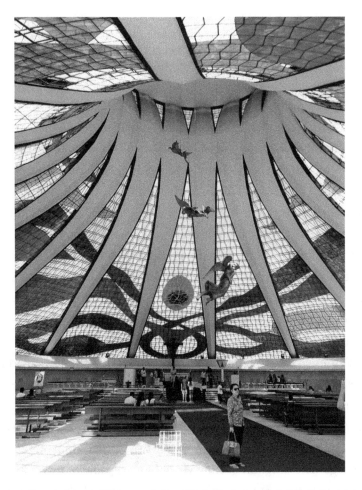

Figure 6.24 Interior view of Niemeyer's Brasilia Cathedral, with bright light shining through the stained glass and the explicit symbolism of the angels. (Author's photo.)

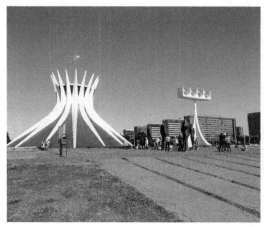
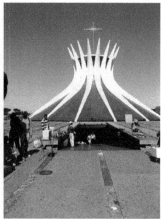

Figure 6.25 Exterior views of Niemeyer's Brasilia Cathedral. (*Left*) The separation of the bell tower from the church, with no resemblance to a conventional campanile. (*Right*) The subterranean entrance to the interior. (Author's photos.)

Frye's (1982) *The Great Code: The Bible and Literature.* Frye noted that so much of European literature contains allusions (whether explicit or implicit) to Biblical stories—and discussed the challenges of teaching literature in an age in which many students had little or no knowledge of what he called the Great Code, namely the Bible.

The point I am trying to make here, however, goes far beyond the design of religious buildings and the way their symbolism rests on complex oral or written traditions and interlinked patterns of behavior—or, perhaps more often, rests on the unconscious residue of such traditions that originally informed those patterns. It is that we, as modern humans, are far more than embrained bodies moving in a physical environment—we move, too, within a symbolic environment that encompasses our own past and the history that framed it. The symbolic enrichment of our physical environment extends into a range of imagined futures that may cause us to behave in ways that seem to fly in the face of our immediate needs and affordances.

Whether we discuss libraries or churches or law courts or schools, architectural symbolism is intertwined with the way modern humans are shaped by language. The question of how we became capable of living in such an expanded environment is a large, even overwhelmingly large, one, but one I shall briefly address in Chapter 8 when I offer my own theory of how biocultural evolution yielded early humans with the brains, bodies, and social structures that made possible the cultural evolution, over tens of millennia, of societies that not only had language but also had a rich array of cultural systems, including (relatively recently) art, architecture, and so much more.

REFERENCES

Andreoli, E., & Forty, A. (Eds.). (2004). *Brazil's modern architecture.* London: Phaidon Press.

Arbib, M. A. (1972). *The metaphorical brain: An introduction to cybernetics as artificial intelligence and brain theory.* New York: Wiley-Interscience.

Arbib, M. A., & Bonaiuto, J. J. (2012). Multiple levels of spatial organization: World graphs and spatial difference learning. *Adaptive Behavior,* 20(4), 287–303.

Arbib, M. A., & Lieblich, I. (1977). Motivational learning of spatial behavior. In J. Metzler (Ed.), *Systems neuroscience* (pp. 221–239). New York: Academic Press.

Bennett, H. (2013). The psyche of the library: Physical space and the research paradigm. *Art Documentation: Journal of the Art Libraries Society of North America,* 32(2), 174–185.

Carlson, L. A., Hölscher, C., Shipley, T. F., & Dalton, R. C. (2010). Getting lost in buildings. *Current Directions in Psychological Science,* 19(5), 284–289.

Condia, B. (Editor) (2020). *Meaning in architecture: Affordances, atmosphere and mood (NPP eBooks. 33).* (with contributions by M.A. Arbib, C.L. Ellard, B. Chamberlain, & K. Rooney) Manhattan, KS: New Prairies Press.

Dalton, R. C., & Hölscher, C. (2017). *Take one building: Interdisciplinary research perspectives of the Seattle Central Library.* London and New York: Taylor & Francis.

Epstein, R. A., Patai, E. Z., Julian, J. B., & Spiers, H. J. (2017). The cognitive map in humans: Spatial navigation and beyond. *Nature Neuroscience,* 20(11), 1504–1513.

Forero, J. (2010, November 12). Celebrating Niemeyer, Brazil's modernist master. *All Things Considered,* National Public Radio. https://www.npr.org/2010/2011/2012/131271636/celebrating-niemeyer-brazil-s-modernist-master

Frye, N. (1982). *The great code: The Bible and literature.* New York: Harcourt Brace Jovanovich.

Guazzelli, A., Corbacho, F. J., Bota, M., & Arbib, M. A. (1998). Affordances, motivation, and the world graph theory. *Adaptive Behavior,* 6, 435–471.

Hölscher, C., Büchner, S. J., Meilinger, T., & Strube, G. (2009). Adaptivity of wayfinding strategies in a multi-building ensemble: The effects of spatial structure, task requirements, and metric information. *Journal of Environmental Psychology,* 29(2), 208–219.

Hölscher, C., Meilinger, T., Vrachliotis, G., Brösamle, M., & Knauff, M. (2006). Up the down staircase: Wayfinding strategies in multi-level buildings. *Journal of Environmental Psychology,* 26(4), 284–299.

Jeffery, K. (2019). Urban architecture: A cognitive neuroscience perspective. *Design Journal,* 22(6), 853–872. doi:10.1080/14606925.2019.1662666

Kasner, E., & Newman, J. (1940). *Mathematics and the imagination.* New York: Simon and Schuster (republished in 2001 by Dover Publications).

Kjelstrup, K. B., Solstad, T., Brun, V. H., Hafting, T., Leutgeb, S., Witter, M. P., . . . Moser, M.-B. (2008). Finite scale of spatial representation in the hippocampus. *Science*, 321(5885), 140–143. doi:10.1126/science.1157086

Kohler, I. (1963). The formation and transformation of the perceptual world. *Psychological Issues*, 3.1–174.

Lieblich, I., & Arbib, M. A. (1982). Multiple representations of space underlying behavior. *Behavioral and Brain Sciences*, 5, 627–659.

Lynch, K. (1960). *The image of the city*. Cambridge, MA: MIT Press.

Maguire, E. A., Woollett, K., & Spiers, H. J. (2006). London taxi drivers and bus drivers: A structural MRI and neuropsychological analysis. *Hippocampus*, 16(12), 1091–1101. doi:10.1002/hipo.20233

Mollerup, P. (2013). *Wayshowing > wayfinding: Basic and interactive*. Amsterdam: BIS Publishers.

Müller, M., & Wehner, R. (1994). The hidden spiral: Systematic search and path integration in desert ants, Cataglyphis fortis. *Journal of Comparative Physiology A*, 175(5), 525–530. doi:10.1007/BF00199474

Niemeyer, O. (2000). *The curves of time. The memoirs of Oscar Niemeyer* (I. M. Burbridge, Trans.). London: Phaidon.

O'Keefe, J., & Dostrovsky, J. O. (1971). The hippocampus as a spatial map: Preliminary evidence from unit activity in the freely moving rat. *Brain Research*, 34, 171–175.

O'Keefe, J., & Nadel, L. (1978). *The hippocampus as a cognitive map*. Oxford: Oxford University Press.

Olton, D. S., Becker, J. T., & Handelmann, G. E. (1980). Hippocampal function: Working memory or cognitive mapping? *Physiological Psychology*, 8, 239–246.

Pogrebin, R. (2004, December 26). Inside the year's best-reviewed buildings. *New York Times*. https://www.nytimes.com/2004/2012/2026/arts/design/inside-the-years-bestreviewed-buildings.html

Rendall, D., Cheney, D. L., & Seyfarth, R. M. (2000). Proximate factors mediating "contact" calls in adult female baboons (*Papio cynocephalus ursinus*) and their infants. *Journal of Comparative Psychology*, 114(1), 36–46.

Spence, C., Puccinelli, N. M., Grewal, D., & Roggeveen, A. L. (2014). Store atmospherics: A multisensory perspective. *Psychology and Marketing*, 31(7), 472–488. doi:10.1002/mar.20709

Taube, J. S., Muller, R. U., & Ranck, J. B., Jr. (1990). Head-direction cells recorded from the postsubiculum in freely moving rats. I. Description and quantitative analysis. *Journal of Neuroscience*, 10(2), 420–435. doi:10.1523/jneurosci.10-02-00420.1990

Tichomirov, O. K., & Poznyanskaya, E. D. (1966). An investigation of visual search as a means of analyzing heuristics. *Soviet Psychology*, 5, 2–15.

Tolman, E. C. (1948). Cognitive maps in rats and men. *Psychological Review*, 55, 189–208.

Weisman, J. (1981). Evaluating architectural legibility: Way-finding in the built environment. *Environment and Behavior*, 13, 189–204.

Wilson, M. A., & McNaughton, B. L. (1993). Dynamics of the hippocampal ensemble code for space. *Science*, 261(5124), 1055–1058.

When buildings have "brains"

Neuroscientists use expressions like "neural architecture" or "the architecture of the brain" to describe the patterns whereby neurons and their connections are arranged in layers, columns, and regions in the three-dimensional structure of a brain. A computer scientist may use the term "neuromorphic architecture" for the circuitry of a computer that, unlike a conventional serial computer, has its components laid out in a fashion inspired in part (often a very small part) by the architecture of the brain. In this book, however, the word architecture is almost always used in the sense of "the architecture of the built environment," with the latter term centered on, but not limited to, rooms, buildings, and the urban environment.

Thus, when I talk of *neuromorphic architecture*, my aim is to explore what sort of buildings it would take for interaction between human and building to proceed in both directions. Neuromorphic architecture charts the future of buildings that in some sense (to be carefully delimited) have "brains." Just as an animal has a body equipped with sensors, effectors, and a brain that controls its response to changes in the environment, so would a building have a "brain" (or a network of "sub-brains") that responds not only to the external environment but also, more challengingly, to the needs of it users in and around the building.

We start by revisiting Le Corbusier' famous dictum that "a house is a machine for living in," but we recall that the machines that inspired him were the airplanes, ocean liners, and automobiles of his day. However, we now live in an age of cybernetic machines, of feedback and feedforward control systems, of computer networks, and of increasingly powerful artificial intelligence (AI) inspired in part by insights from the neuroscience of how neural networks can learn. We thus seek to understand each house— or building more generally—as an *interconnected system of systems* whose spatial layout must be developed in a way that is both functional and harmonious, while serving the needs of multiple users.

Neuromorphic architecture may thus be considered a variant of "smart" architecture in which design of buildings as "machines for X-ing in" is informed by lessons from the study of the brain and of cybernetic machines. This observation requires a short discussion of terminology; some architects reject the term *smart architecture* because a building cannot be smart in the way that a human is smart, while others reject the term *artificial intelligence* because computers are different from people. However, depending on the context, we can say that someone is "smart" because they dress well or because of their intelligence. In a similar fashion, the term "smart architecture" will refer to buildings that can indeed respond in increasingly complex ways to their environment, while "artificial intelligence" is exhibited by certain computers and robots that are able to act in ways that, were we to observe them in humans, we might consider indicative of at least some limited aspect of intelligence. As stressed in earlier chapters, we will learn from *neuroethology*, the study of the way in which different brains and bodies support the behavior of different animals. Just as animals vary widely in their size, appearance, and ecological niche, so do buildings vary widely in their size, appearance, and typology.

The interactive space Ada provides an early example of neuromorphic architecture. It was designed for the Swiss Expo of 2002. Ada was "a machine for experiencing in." Crucially, Ada had sensors for vision, audition, and even a sense of touch mediated by floor panels. Ada could use this information to guide visitors to come together in groups with which Ada could interact before leading them toward the exit. Moreover, there was a sense in which Ada had "emotions" and would interact with visitors in a way that was designed to increase Ada's "happiness." Of course, these terms capture very limited aspects of the richness of human emotions, but they do provide a signpost toward the incorporation of more lessons from neuroscience into architectural design. This leads us to a brief analysis of the back and forth between the study of "emotion" in buildings and robots in relation to the neuroscience of emotions as studied in animals, including humans.

With this, we turn to a general account of neuromorphic architecture, where we distinguish the *physical space*, the body of the animal or the physical structure of a building, from the *neural space* that connects sensors and effectors in providing adaptability to the environment. Whereas we typically emphasize the behavior of the animal in relation to the world around it, much of our emphasis in neuromorphic architecture is on the behavior of the building in relation to the people within it. However, it may engage in *homeostasis*, keeping critical elements in physiological balance, with dynamic elements that go far beyond a conventional heating, ventilation, and air-conditioning system. As in Ada, though, a major capability is for *social interaction* between the building and its users. This may build in part upon insights from the study of mirror neurons as our design exploits action recognition by the building to better set the mood or support the actions of its inhabitants. To complement this, the example of a neuromorphic kitchen grounds discussion of how rooms or buildings may learn through adaptive machinery inspired by the neuroscience of learning, or the deep learning of AI. Such buildings can in some sense be considered as *inside-out robots* or *embrained bodies*.

We temporarily abandon neuromorphic architecture to consider two important ideas. One is the notion of *biophilia*, the idea that human well-being can be improved by buildings that are open to nature. The other, perhaps even more important, factor (and exceptionally poignant when this is being written during the height of the Covid-19 epidemic) is the way in which humans flourish when they have a *sense of community*. To illustrate this, we discuss the Kampung Admiralty project in Singapore, which was designed to provide the benefits of biophilia while also offering a sense of community not only to its residents but also to people in the surrounding neighborhood. Although it does not count as an example of neuromorphic architecture, it nonetheless fits into the overall themes of the book by exemplifying the key idea of comprising a *system of systems*— both in the interaction of subsystems within the Kampung itself, and in its interaction with the city around it and larger systems like the housing system of Singapore. In this way, we make contact with the general relevance of the system of systems idea to studies of interacting systems within the brain, of the competition and cooperation between schemas that underlies our action and cognition, and of the dynamic interactions that constitute our social realities, and the cities and broader regional, national, and international systems that support them in integrating the social, the physical, the natural, and the built environment. Moreover, when we consider a building as a system of systems, we may assess which of those subsystems may be ripe for being cybernetically enabled and possibly coupled into a broader information infrastructure.

The chapter closes by asking where neuromorphic architecture[1] might lead us, while forcing us to confront some of the real issues about privacy associated with the rise of the Internet of Things as it comes to increasingly penetrate the design of buildings, whether the inspiration comes from current developments in AI or engages more directly with the findings of neuroscience as we develop further insights into the ways in which the built environment can support human well-being, or fail to do so.

---

1. My dictation software transcribed this as "near a more fake architecture." I hope that it was mistaken.

7.1. MACHINES FOR LIVING IN, REVISITED

Let's offer a fresh perspective on Le Corbusier's dictum that "a house is a machine for living in" (Le Corbusier, 1927):

> A house is a machine for living in. Baths, sun, hot-water, cold-water, warmth at will, conservation of food, hygiene, beauty in the sense of good proportion. An armchair is a machine for sitting in and so on. Architecture as practiced provides no solution to the present-day [the 1920s] problem of the dwelling-house. . . . It does not fulfil the very first conditions [functionality?] and so it is not possible that the higher factors of harmony and beauty should enter in.

Le Corbusier also refers to a house as a tool. We may celebrate how much the house has changed for many of us since the 1920s, but I suggest that the house is better seen not as a tool but as an *interconnected system of systems* whose spatial layout must be developed in a way that is both functional and harmonious—while also considering the need to accommodate multiple users. Indeed, this multiplicity seems explicit in Le Corbusier's statement of the Problem of the House:

> A house: a shelter against heat, cold, rain, thieves and the inquisitive. A receptacle for light and sun. A certain number of cells appropriated to cooking, work, and personal life.
> A room: a surface over which one can walk at ease, a bed on which to stretch yourself, a chair in which to rest or work, a work-table, receptacles in which each thing can be put at once in its right place.
> The number of rooms: one for cooking and one for eating. One for work, one to wash yourself in and one for sleep.

We might ask whether the functions must have separate rooms, as they do not in some non-Western cultures such as the Japanese style, where "bedrooms" emerge only as one brings out the futons ("resets the furniture") at night – a good example of "room dynamics," even if effected by the users rather than by the room "itself."

Le Corbusier offers "The Manual for the Dwelling," which is very much addressed to bourgeois men and women, including as it does "Demand ... a dressing-room in which you can dress and undress. Never undress in your bedroom" and "Demand that the maid's room should not be an attic." Interestingly, it does bring in olfaction: "Put the kitchen at the top of the house to avoid smells." However, the notion of a "house" or "apartment" that many of the readers of this book will take for granted contains much that remains unattainable for a sizable fraction of the world's population. The issue of providing adequate housing for all humans is absolutely important—but lies beyond this book's ambit. Nonetheless, many of the ideas raised here remain relevant, but with a number of the issues to be addressed by urban planners or the collective actions of villagers. Note especially the system of systems approach; §7.5 will introduce an example from the architectural firm WOHA in Singapore that offers positive ideas for addressing related issues, at least for a community that has risen above the poverty line.

In spelling out ways in which a house is a machine for living in, Le Corbusier lists baths, sun, hot-water, cold-water, warmth at will, conservation of food, hygiene, and "beauty in the sense of good proportion." Our contribution expands this in two ways: (a) by building on our emerging neuroscience-informed framework for reconceptualizing the experience and design of architecture, and (ii) by expanding Le Corbusier's concern with ocean liners, airplanes, and automobiles (recall the discussion in §3.1) as his exemplary machines to include the new machines of the cybernetic age and the computation and communication networks that link them.

The provision of hot and cold water reminds us of how greatly access to utilities has changed the design of the house in diverse cultures. The ready availability of running water transforms kitchen, laundry, and bathroom, a transformation complemented by the presence of sewers to rid the house of excrement and urine. Gas and electricity contribute to cooking and heating, but also—for better and worse—transform the boundary between night and day. The very form of the house reflects these changes—and now we envisage further changes as the Internet becomes a pervasive utility. At present, its impact has been more on bringing new objects into the home, but we can expect further impacts as we allow the house to conform to the needs of its inhabitants, exploiting the Internet of Things, and furniture acting as robotic effectors.

This talk of furniture blurs the line between architecture and interior design, while increasing dynamic interaction blurs the distinction enshrined in French between *meuble* for furniture and *immeubles*, which means both building and immovable. As our example of the Japanese use of futons shows (and one may compare the Murphy bed), while design may to some extent be constrained by the way in which different rooms support different functionality (e.g., bathrooms vs. kitchens), the furnishings can change relatively often, and renovations can occur on a longer time-scale.

We saw (§3.1) that at times Le Corbusier seems to be suggesting that if only houses were built according to engineering principles, they would satisfy our aesthetic needs. However, he still sees it as the task of the architect—but an architect liberated from old styles—to create the necessary aesthetics, ensuring that "the higher factors of harmony and beauty . . . enter in." Architecture must creatively balance the constraints of form and function, offering satisfactions that span all the way from basic needs to the aesthetic emotions.

7.2. CAN ARCHITECTURE BE SMART, CAN INTELLIGENCE BE ARTIFICIAL?

Some of my architect friends dislike the terminology of "smart architecture" or even "artificial intelligence"—and certainly reject the notion that a building could have a "brain," even in quotes. Let me attempt to justify these uses. The key point is that use of these technical terms in no way implies that buildings or machines are smart or intelligent in the same way that humans are.

The term "smart architecture" has come to be used for buildings wherein many elements have an operative nature controlled by computations to yield environments that are "intelligent" in the specific (and very limited) sense that they are able to adapt to—and even anticipate—certain human activities and changing environments in real time. Buildings currently have many "smart" devices like HVAC systems, security systems, and automated lighting, but our neo-Corbusian exploration of buildings as cybernetic machines will take us much further.

Architects have always been able to find smart solutions in their design of buildings, and in most cases these designs have nothing to do with "smart architecture" in the technical sense. Indeed, a solution that does not invoke "smart architecture" may often be smarter than one that does. For example, in certain climates it may be smarter to provide a building with shade trees, breezeways, and operable windows than to install air conditioning and automatic controls.

When we explore the neuroscience of the experience and design of architecture, we are looking to neuroscience to enrich our understanding of how humans experience and how humans design. We seek to understand how the human brain contributes to that totality of brain-in-body-in-society that constitutes a person, and have stressed that the aim is not to reduce the person to a bunch of neural networks but rather to engage in a conversation between person-reality and neuron-reality. However, *we cannot understand the human brain by studying human brains alone.* To probe the mechanisms underlying the evidence we glean from brain lesions, neurological disorders, and even brain imaging in humans, we must exploit comparative studies. Our understanding of the circuitry supporting human vision comes in great part from the study of what we take to be similar (not identical) circuitry in cats and monkeys, as well as pondering the different visual circuitry of the frog. Our ideas about mirror systems in the human brain were initiated by studies of mirror neurons in the macaque brain. A major insight into wayfinding came from the discovery of place cells in the rat hippocampus. Neuroscience gains its power by placing the study of the human brain within a broad framework of comparative analysis that may engage the study of diverse animals at all levels from the molecular biology of synaptic plasticity to the action–perception cycle and social interaction.

Nonetheless, in studying the experience and design of architecture our focus is on the human. However, when we turn to neuromorphic architecture, there is no claim that the *building* must be human-like. In particular, to assert that a building has a "brain" is not to assert that the building has a human-like brain, or human intelligence or feelings, nor that it should be treated like another human being. But it would *behave*. To take a current example: Self-opening doors are actuated by sensors that register a person's trajectory and open in anticipation of the person's going through the door. This is usually helpful, but sometimes incorrect, possibly even annoyingly so.

As stressed many times in this book, our study of animals reveals that their brains and bodies can be greatly varied in form and complexity. In neuromorphic architecture, the "brain" (or "brains") of a building may incorporate design features gleaned from the brain and behavior of a specific kind of animal or general principles abstracted from brains of different species.

In the study of animals, it is often debated whether words that apply to humans also apply to other creatures—but these general terms mask crucial differences. Humans have language—in the sense of a rich lexicon and the grammatical means to combine them to create endless new meanings that others can understand—whereas monkeys and apes (and, presumably, our last common ancestors) do not. But there is a paradox here. In creating electronic computers, we have created machines that can be instructed to behave in more complex ways by following instructions encoded in what we call *programming languages*. The ability to accept and behave according to programs in such "languages" is completely outside the capability of nonhuman animals. On the other hand, endowing robots with the flexibility of movement or the complexity of visual and other forms of perception that animals can muster is at the forefront of current robotics research, and far from satisfactory achievement. Nonetheless, when we use the term "language" for our computers but not for animals, we remain aware that human languages and programming languages are dissimilar in crucial ways.

In a related vein, while some readers may feel uneasy about the word "smart" in conjunction with mobile phones and architecture, it is now in common parlance. We simply need to distinguish this use from what we might consider to be "smart" in a human's behavior—just as we feel free to also apply the word "smart" to some people's choice in clothing. Similarly, it is too late to avoid using the term "artificial intelligence." One may consider it as shorthand for "computers equipped with programs that can achieve something that we used to think was the purview of human intelligence." For example, around 1900 the ability to carry out lengthy arithmetic computations was seen as specific to human intelligence, but by now electronic computers have gone far beyond this; they can even be programmed to "learn" to improve their capability to the point where specific computers have competed successfully with human world champions in chess and Go. Increasingly, household computers (empowered by Internet connectivity) can respond to commands and queries expressed in natural language. Whether this is a blessing or a curse is currently a matter for intense debate, but what is not debatable is that AI will continue to play an increasing role in future buildings (as in many other parts of our environment, including autonomous vehicles). In what follows, we will assess ways in which insights from neuroscience might be factored into that future.

7.3. THE INTERACTIVE SPACE ADA

The interactive space Ada (Figure 7.1) was open to the public at the Swiss Expo in Lausanne for part of 2002 and attracted 550,000 visitors. The design team was led by two computational neuroscientists then in Zurich, Rodney Douglas and Paul Verschure. Ada was not just a space with a few displays, a static functionality to which users must adapt, but was constructed as a perceiving, acting, and adapting entity, interacting with the people inside the space. The space was named for Ada, Countess Lovelace

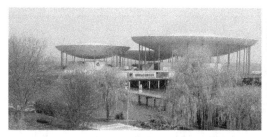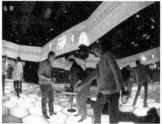

Figure 7.1 (*Left*) A view of the pavilion housing Ada. (*Right*) An internal view of Ada. (Photos courtesy of Rodney Douglas and Paul Verschure.)

(1815–1852), daughter of Byron and the world's first computer programmer, working with Charles Babbage (1791–1871) on his Analytical Engine. "She" (Ada, the space—not the Countess!) had a "brain" based in part on artificial neural networks and, as we will see later, even had "emotions" (in a sense to be explored as the section progresses) and wanted to "play" with her visitors. This was the basis for her patterns of interaction.

The key paper for understanding the workings of Ada (Eng et al., 2003) is, tellingly, titled "Design for a Brain Revisited: The Neuromorphic Design and Functionality of the Interactive Space 'Ada.'" The main title pays tribute to a classic (though to my taste, rather elementary) book on cybernetics, *Design for a Brain*, by Ross Ashby (1952); the subtitle introduces the adjective "neuromorphic" into architecture. In the next section, I will build on Ada to introduce a general perspective on neuromorphic architecture. An organism has sensors whereby impressions of the environment are received, effectors with which to act upon the environment, and, of course, a brain that links action and perception. In the same vein, Ada too had sensors and effectors—one might think of her as an inside-outside robot.

Her sensors include cameras for vision, microphones for audition, and pressure-sensitive floor tiles for touch. (Although Ada existed only in 2002, in what follows I will describe her capabilities using the present tense.) Of course, it requires a "brain" to turn the activity of these sensors into control patterns for the effectors. Ada deployed her sensors and effectors to form visitors into groups and interact with them. The key point

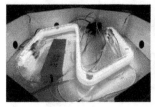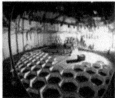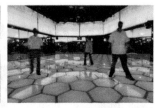

Figure 7.2 The floor is a group of tiles arranged in a honeycomb pattern (*center*). Each tile not only can change color (*left*) but also is touch-sensitive. (Photos courtesy of Rodney Douglas and Paul Verschure.)

here is the bidirectionality of that interaction. Ada does not simply provide static affordances that may invite the visitor to act within the space; Ada *interacts* with her visitors. While some visitors may simply enjoy the light show and varying music within Ada, or observe how other visitors are behaving, the key interaction is that Ada can recognize visitors who are "interesting" in terms of their responsiveness to her signals, "invite" them to form small groups, and then play games with them before it is time for them to leave. This fits into our general theme of multisensory perception—touch, vision, and hearing are combined to keep track of the visitors and assess their behavior.

Crucially, Ada's "skin" (the floor) also serves as her main effector (Figure 7.2). Because Ada can control the colors displayed by the tiles, they allow Ada to "communicate." Ada can assign several nearby people the same colored patterns, and then start moving these patterns together to encourage the people to form a group.

Other visual effectors are ambient lights to set the overall visual emotional tone (atmosphere), while light fingers point at individual visitors or indicate different locations. On the auditory side, Ada uses sound and music composed in real time on the basis of her internal states and sensory input. The composition is generated using a system called Roboser (Manzolli & Verschure, 2005). However, for safety reasons (and unlike humanoid robots), Ada does not have forceful effectors such as robot arms.

Table 7.1 lists a natural progression of the behaviors and interactions of which Ada is capable. Remember that this is a large space with a lot of

TABLE 7.1   A natural progression in visitor interaction.

Sleep	One tile color for all visitors
Wake	Visitors given different-colored floor tiles
Explore	Probe for "interesting" visiotr; deploy light fingers and gazers
Group	Try to direct visitors to a certain location in space
Play	Play game selected on basis for number of visitors in space
Leave	Tile effects show path to exit of space for each visitor

visitors at any one time. Ada can carry on different "conversations," as it were, with different people around the room; but the states in Table 7.1 are global. Visitors are admitted to Ada's space every 5 minutes, and during this period, Ada will progress through the five states in the given order. However, timing of the transition between states depends on Ada's "emotions," and within each state (after Ada "wakes up"), her interactions vary from visitor to visitor.

The base state, "sleep," is passive; one color covers the whole floor. On "waking," Ada begins to assign various colors to the floor tiles on which visitors are standing. "Exploring" seeks to find visitors who are "interesting" in that they respond to stimuli provided by Ada, such as shifting the coloring of tiles in a particular way, or moving where the light fingers are pointing. When nearby visitors are found to be interesting, they can then be formed into a group, and Ada can play a variety of games with each such group. Finally, the colored pattern or the light fingers can be used to gently direct people toward the exit, because if you are going to welcome 550,000 visitors in the space of a few months, getting visitors to leave before too long is as important as bringing them in and making them feel engaged and entertained. I am reminded of an anecdote about P. T. Barnum and his museum of curiosities. There was a big sign saying, "This way to the egress." His notion was that many people would not know that egress meant exit and so would go to see the egress. Then, of course, they would discover themselves out on the street and have to line up and pay again if they wanted to see more.

The design of Ada's control systems for the interaction space adapted various brain models that the design team had engaged in as part of their "day job" as computational neuroscientists. These included tracking visitors both through touch (patterns of pressure on floor tiles) and through auditory cues (adapting brain models of auditory localization in mammals). More on this can be found in the overview (Eng et al., 2003). Rather than discuss these particular models further, I will present Ada's pavilion at the Swiss Expo and then introduce the sense in which Ada pursued "happiness" and expressed "emotions."

A pavilion for Ada

Complementing the particularly neuromorphic challenges in the design of Ada, there were more conventional architectural challenges that had to be met in designing the pavilion in which Ada was housed. It was clear that designing a building for an Expo would require a thoughtful strategy for controlling visitor flow. Complementing this, a crucial design phase was to test how people would react to Ada's attempts at fostering interaction. This made clear the need to educate visitors before they entered the interaction space on the sequences of cues whereby Ada would signal her "intentions." This led to the decision to employ human guides to actively inform Ada's visitors as much as possible about what they would see in the exhibit.

Such considerations further resulted in the design of the spaces that led from outside the pavilion to the space where the visitors interact with Ada, and then out again. The arrows (Figure 7.3) indicate the route taken by visitors: The visitor waiting area served as the "conditioning tunnel" where visitors received a staged introduction to the components of Ada. They were next led through the "voyeur area," where they could observe the interaction space through semitransparent mirrors before entering the octagonal room where all interaction with Ada occurs. Thereafter, visitors could see real-time graphical displays of the current dynamics in Ada's control system in the Brainarium, as well as views back into the interaction space. The last stop before the Egress was the Explanatorium, where

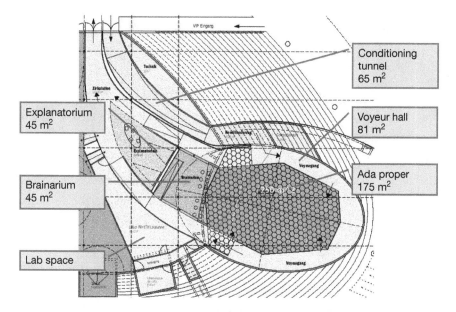

Figure 7.3 "Ada proper" is the actual interactive space of Ada. This is complemented by a number of spaces designed to orient visitors and manage visitor flow, as well as a range of service areas. In addition, human guides were available at various stations. (Diagram courtesy of Rodney Douglas and Paul Verschure.)

visitors so inclined could find information about the key technologies behind Ada. In addition, the building included service areas and working rooms for computers and their operators.

During normal operation, the main space received about 25 visitors at a time, with each group spending 5 minutes in the interactive space, giving a maximal throughput of about 300 visitors per hour.

Ada's "happiness" and "emotions"

Let's return to Le Corbusier:

The happy towns are those that have an architecture. Architecture can be found in the telephone and in the Parthenon. How easily could it be at home in our houses! Houses make the street and the street makes the town and the town is a personality which takes to itself a soul, which can feel, suffer and wonder.

What can such fanciful language mean? I would suggest that it means that there are cities and towns that elicit certain emotions in us that lead us to call one care-free but another somber—not because they have emotions, but because they elicit these moods and emotions in us. Even readers who dislike the term "smart architecture" have, I suspect, allowed themselves to call a room "cheerful." Perhaps in the same way we can ascribe a personality to a building or a town—as a reflection of the changes it elicits in our own personality. Such issues resonate with our discussions of atmosphere in Chapter 4 and Einfühlung in Chapter 5. An area of town (even a non-cybernetic one) might be cheerful on a sunny day, yet frightening at night. But isn't it going too far to say that a town can "feel, suffer, and wonder"? Perhaps. But when a building or city is a cybernetic machine, perhaps these terms become more applicable, and it may indeed have "emotions" that change with its interactions with those around and within it. To this end, let's here consider the way in which Ada has "wants" and "emotions" in some sense.

Ada continually evaluated the results of her actions, expressed emotional states accordingly, and tried to regulate the distribution and flow of visitors. In describing the computations involved, we use terminology that we would apply to a human and, with a little more trepidation, to an animal. In some sense, Ada "wanted" to interact with people. When people participated, she was "happy." When they did not, she was "frustrated." Ada's level of overall happiness is translated into the soundscape and the visual environment in which the visitors are immersed, establishing a closed loop between environment and visitors.

Ada's mood system was defined by the two parameters of arousal and valence. The current behavior mode set the arousal parameter, resulting in low arousal for sleep and high arousal for play. The valence parameter represented the status of Ada's happiness (H). Low happiness led to low valence, and high happiness resulted in high valence.

Ada's overall goal is to maximize happiness (H), and this (in the computational scheme indicated by Figure 7.4) increases with survival, recognition, and interaction. A crucial part of the design of the system was thus to instrument how these three values could be computed by Ada.

- *Survival* for a space like Ada is, of course, very different from survival for an animal, and so "survival" for her was characterized as maintaining a flow of visitors—for which a better term might be simply "throughput." However, if all Ada did was encourage people to move through as quickly as possible, you could replace all her sophisticated sensors, effectors, and computations by a chute, and there would be no time or need for the interactions that Ada was designed for. Survival thus had to be balanced by two other criteria.
- *Recognition* is related to the identification of interesting visitors, those who respond to stimuli provided by Ada and can be formed into a group. Ada probed single visitors for attention and

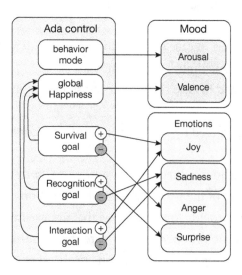

Figure 7.4 An overview of Ada's emotion system, linked to Roboser's composition of the soundscape. (Figure courtesy of Rodney Douglas and Paul Verschure.)

compliance by generating visual cues using the floor tile lights. "Recognition" measures how well Ada can track and collect data about people as a precondition for more advanced interactions.

- *Interaction* measures the extent of Ada's successful human interactions, with more complex interactions weighted more highly. In play mode, the system deployed a game in which visitors were invited to participate. Cue compliance and game participation were quantified to set the interaction parameter value.

The actual computation of H occurs in multiple ways: an explicit top-level calculation is performed using simulated neurons, and in parallel individual behavioral processes calculate their own contributions to the components of H.

The system synthesized Ada's emotions by combining the current values of the three high-level goals of survival, recognition, and interaction as follows:

- *Joy* was set by the goals of survival and interaction in the sense that joy was high if survival or interaction approached maximum achievement.
- *Sadness* was raised in case either recognition or interaction decreased from maximum achievement.
- *Anger* was excited in case survival decreased from maximum achievement.
- *Surprise* was triggered by a sudden increase in recognition.

The versions of joy, sadness, anger, and surprise in Figure 7.4 are not interiorized as part of the way Ada controls her actions in relation to visitors. Rather, they provide four measures that are used by Roboser as part of the input on which it operates to create the soundscape in a way that will convey something of these emotions to the visitors, complementing the generation of sounds as feedback to simple events detected inside the space like footsteps, whistles, or hand claps. The necessary algorithms tap into general research on how music may convey aspects of emotion to human listeners (Gabrielsson & Lindstrom, 2001), rather than attempting to get at the "inner workings" of emotion. The details are provided in "Live Soundscape Composition Based on Synthetic Emotions" (Wassermann, Eng, Verschure, & Manzolli, 2003), whose coauthors include Jônatas Manzolli, a Brazilian composer now at the University of Campinas in Brazil. Roboser composes music on up to 12 performance tracks, with the performance on each track synthesized as well as performed in real time. Musical parameters that are interactively and independently controlled in each track include those for instrument, velocity, volume, pitch bend, tempo, and articulation. During performance in Ada, the outputs of the Roboser tracks are performed using a sampler, resulting in a complex soundscape.

Following the distinction between moods (defined by the two parameters of arousal and valence) and emotions (joy, sadness, anger, and surprise) in Ada's control model, the music performance was synthesized on two separate layers: mood and emotion.

Mood layer: Two Roboser performance tracks continuously play a mood composition. The arousal parameter sets the performance's tempo, volume, and octave register. As arousal increases, the number of note onsets per second, note overlaps, and volumes increase while note pitches shift upward in octave steps. The valence parameter generates pitch material that changes from dissonance to consonance.

Emotion layer: Two performance tracks were assigned to each emotion. With the onset of an emotion, the volume of the respective two voices gradually increases from zero to maximum, fading the emotion compositions in and out on top of the mood layer composition. The musical features were based on an extension of the scheme outlined by Gabrielsson and Juslin to include the emotion of surprise and with increased contrast between the four emotions.

In the end, the key criterion for the success of a building is the experience of the visitors, so here is a fragment of an interview with Paul Verschure, one of Ada's designers (Palumbo, 2004):

MARIALUISA PALUMBO: One of the usual critics against this kind of project is that of being an always more and more perfect and intrusive control system. What do you think about this?

PAUL VERSCHURE: This is a relevant criticism of technology in general. However, Ada did not scare its visitors. We know this because we asked them. Most of them felt comfortable and happy in this space. An important contributing factor to this is that Ada was transparent; it did not only collect data and process it to decide on actions. The goals of the system were transparently communicated in Ada's language. As with a human observer, one that responds to us we can understand and accept, one that just observes without any form of feedback is threatening. Technology has so far [2004] been of the latter kind while with Ada we show that technology can and should be as our partner to help us shape and interact with a complex world.

Emotions of buildings and robots

One concern with neuromorphic architecture, or just the use of AI, is that buildings that engage in dynamic social interaction may respond in untoward ways, as exemplified in the 1962 story, "The Thousand Dreams of Stellavista" by J. G. Ballard (reprinted in 1971), with its "psychotropic" houses run amok.[2] The following quote gives some sense of Ballard's invention, but one needs to read the story for his ingenious plot, which turns on the conceit that houses may behave in ways that strongly, even alarmingly, express the emotional states of long-gone inhabitants rather than responding to the immediate needs of the current inhabitants.

As I stepped forward [the house] suddenly jerked away, almost in alarm, the entrance retracting and sending a low shudder through

---

2. I thank Branko Kolarevic for bringing this story to my attention. It stands as a fine example of "Science Fiction Prototypes as a Method for Discussing Socio-Technical Issues Within Emerging Technology" (Kymäläinen, 2016).

the rest of the spheres. It's always interesting to watch a psychotropic house try to adjust itself to strangers. . . .

The real trouble was that most of Vermilion Sands is composed of early, or primitive-fantastic psychotropic houses, when the possibilities offered by the new bio-plastic medium rather went to architects' heads. It was some years before a compromise was reached between the one hundred per cent responsive structure and the rigid non-responsive houses of the past. The first PT houses had so many senso-cells distributed over them, echoing every shift of mood and position of the occupants, that living in one was like inhabiting someone else's brain.

In Chapter 5, we discussed whether and in what sense buildings may elicit our empathy. Ballard's psychotropic houses have the opposite property—they reflect the emotions of their inhabitants. The problem is that their (fictional) expression of these emotions can last for years and have distressing expression in the dynamics of the house—a building with post-traumatic stress disorder.

If we already take care to stress that some emotions are less likely to be shared or similar in humans and other animals, then, in line with §4.2, we approach applying the term "emotion" to robots or buildings with some caution. Jean-Marc Fellous and I edited a book called *Who Needs Emotions? The Brain Meets the Robot* (Fellous & Arbib, 2005). Neuroscientists assessed the biological underpinnings of emotion, while members of the robotics and AI community reviewed computational processes that incorporated some features of emotion, including two hypotheses on hierarchies of cognitive and emotional control as seen from an AI perspective (Ortony, Norman, & Revelle, 2005; Sloman, Chrisley, & Scheutz, 2005). This encourages exploration of what might be the "emotions" of future buildings, not just the issues of atmosphere and Einfühlung, where the architect seeks to answer the question, "How can spaces be charged with the capacity to induce emotions in humans?" The "psychology" of the building, rather than the user, is under scrutiny. We asked Rodney Douglas, one of Ada's co-instigators, to consider writing an article on "Do Spaces Need Emotions?" but, unfortunately, he was too busy.

Recall the two "views" of emotion (§4.2): (a) external: emotional expression for communication and social coordination; and (b) internal: emotion for the organization of behavior. Ada's emotions seem rather disengaged from the internal role for emotion. She operates on a fixed cycle of modes of behavior, and her so-called happiness seems to play little role beyond fine adjustment of the timing of the transitions between modes within the overall 5-minute cycles. Her behavior in relation to her visitors during the various modes seems unaffected by her emotional state other than in changing the soundscape that Roboser creates—and this soundscape seems to play little or no role in communicating Ada's "emotional state" to her visitors. The one possible exception (but not realized, as far as I know, in the actual design) would be if "angry sounds" predominated if people were not leaving the room quickly enough at the end of the cycle.

Ekman's model of facial expression of emotion (Ekman, 1999), with its six basic emotional states, has been influential in work on getting robots to exhibit human-like emotional expressions. The Kismet robot (Breazeal & Scassellati, 2002), for example, can communicate an emotive state and other social cues to a human through facial expressions, gaze, and quality of voice. However, these expressions are not indicative of the robot's "inner workings." Rather, they seek to make it easier for humans to interact with the robot if it exhibits human-like responses. The computations needed to support such expressions may thus improve the way robots function in the human environment. A teaching machine coupled to a robot with a simulacrum of a face may help a student more if the student's success is rewarded by a happy, approving facial expression, while failure offers a look of try-it-again encouragement rather than sadness or anger or no response at all beyond repeating an earlier item. Note that in current systems, such facial expressions would be preprogrammed by the human who builds the system on a response-by-response basis. A far more challenging issue would be to have the machine build an individual "model" of how each student behaves and responds, and then adapt to inferring what personality type a student has and how this might affect the generation of emotional cues over hours or days or more of working with the individual. Such a system might even be trained through observation of how various excellent human teachers interact with different students. The good news is that this increases the availability to students of "individual" feedback and encouragement when human teachers have limited time available; the bad news is that the machine (like many second-rate human teachers) might ignore cumulative cues in a student's behavior, or fail to recognize when general strategies fail to meet an individual student's needs. Similar promises and pitfalls were noted in the "skippable" portion of §3.1.

The use of the term "emotion" in relation to robots or buildings should not be limited to this robotic simulation of emotional expressions. Fellous and I saw our book as part of the search for a widened cybernetic understanding that extends terms to animals and machines without implying that their use in each case must match the exact nature of human emotions. In the future, a major challenge for architects will be to assess the extent to which the "emotions" of buildings (as distinct from those of users) can play a role both in determining patterns of the building's behavior and in supporting interactions beneficial to their human users. How can specific lessons from neurobiology and ethology be generalized to apply to robots or buildings that do not share the biology of living creatures? In biology, the four Fs (feeding, fighting, fleeing, and reproducing) are paramount. However, robots and buildings will in general have access to a reliable power supply (though "low battery" may be akin to a "hunger" or "thirst" signal in a mobile robot), and autonomous reproduction will not be an issue. The key observation from our study of animals and the relation of their primordial emotions may be this: An emotion switches the modes of behavior. In anger, the interior state of an angry animal yields a switch of the body's resources to support a fighting mode. In hunger, the animal's attention becomes focused on the detection of food sources, and the related hunting or foraging strategies focus the set of available actions.

One hypothesis (Arbib & Fellous, 2004) is that this offers the key to "robot emotions" (or at least, motivational systems), by offering a higher level of control above the repertoire of generally available perceptual and motor schemas. Consider a robot (or building) with a set of basic modes, each with appropriate perceptual schemas and access to various motor schemas. The robot would continually evaluate the current state to come up with an "urgency level" for the competition and cooperation of the modes, with selection of which actions will next be performed conditioned by that mode.

Consider, for example, a neuromorphic apartment building. In its normal "emotional mode," it would simply serve the domestic needs of its inhabitants and support their movement in and out of the complex. But suppose there were a fire. It would then enter the equivalent of an animal's "fleeing" mode, with the fire alarm being, literally, the building's "alarm" call as its overall expression of "emotion," but with its sensors and effectors redirected to actions related to fire suppression, alerts to neighboring buildings, and a pattern of interaction with the users based on getting them to safety rather than supporting their normal activities. The notion is that this would not in future be a simple system whose only capability is to sound the fire alarm; rather, the building would have an elaborate system of sensors and effectors that would be deployed differently, actively interacting with the building's inhabitants, depending on the overall "mode."

The evolution of buildings would provide a greater range of responsive subsystems (the effectors) geared to this emotion-directed response, but the response would engage many functions normally involved in interaction with the building's inhabitants on a one-by-one basis in addition to those directly related to fire suppression. As noted in §2.4, we may think of the building as a set of tools for living, an assemblage of one or more *inside-out robots*. We learn to use a room or a building by adjusting our body schema not only to the tool in our hand but also to the complementary tool that is the changing interface with the building. If the building itself is endowed with a range of actions, then we may begin to learn how architecture might indeed be influenced by what we know of human interaction through social neuroscience. As suggested in §2.4, the slogan, "out from the body and in from the building," offers something deep for us to pursue and understand better. Can we speak of the body schema of the building? Only to the extent that the building has a "neural structure" that allows its actions to depend on how its physical structure is currently deployed in relation to both the external environment and the internal environment that includes the people within it.

7.4. NEUROMORPHIC ARCHITECTURE: NEURAL
AND PHYSICAL SPACES FOR BUILDINGS

Ada offers a classical example of *neuromorphic architecture*, the approach to architecture that explores the idea of "brains" for buildings (Arbib, 2012). A central aim here is to think about how buildings might interact with people—based on what we can learn from the neuroscience of the interactions of people, and other animals, with each other. I will at times use the jargon *interaction infrastructure* for the "brains" of future buildings, reserving the term *brain* (without quotes) for the brains and nervous systems of animals and humans. As noted before, neuromorphic architecture is the special case of "smart architecture" in which architects and engineers are informed by lessons from neuroscience.

From Umwelten to architecture

Neuromorphic architecture rests in great part on insights from computational modeling of brains and bodies in animals (including humans) as they interact with the physical and social environment. Figure 7.5 illustrates the distinction between animals and rooms or buildings. An animal moves around in an external environment, engaged in the action–perception cycle—its brain directing the body in such a way that it can both gain access to new information and carry out its own behaviors in

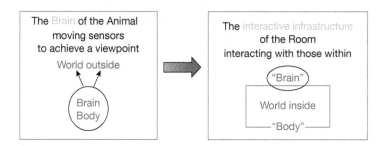

Figure 7.5 From neuroethology to neuromorphic architecture.

the world around it. For a building, we turn this inside out: the world is
inside the body, the building itself, and the brain is then monitoring the
activity inside the building (and this would extend to the courtyard and
further surroundings outside the building). Rather than a creature that
is mobile in its environment, we now consider a "creature" that is relatively static in its environment (though see Kolarevic & Parlac, 2015, on
dynamic buildings—and Jean Nouvel's Institut du Monde Arabe in Figure
7.9 later) and monitors how the world, in particular the people, move relative to it rather than how it moves relative to its external environment.

Just as humans may endow nonhumans with human characteristics—
our architecture can learn from, and extend the database for, social neuroscience. We learn to use a room or a building by adjusting our body
schema not only to our actual body or the tool in our hand, but to the
complementary "body" that is the changing interface with the building.
However, there are two further wrinkles:

- Driving a car offers an interesting pair of perspectives: as we
  approach the car and settle into the driver's seat, the car itself
  provides the environment for our actions. However, when we start
  to drive, our body schema extends to the edges of the car, and the
  environment is now provided by roads and the traffic on them.
  Similarly, we may at times see all the building as external to us,
  whereas at other times we may incorporate aspects of the building
  into our body schema.
- However, when parts of the building act somewhat autonomously, we
  may then see them as separate agents with whom we interact. To take
  a contemporary example, if we have a garage with a door that opens
  automatically as we drive toward it, we are likely to view the door
  system as a separate agent rather than an extension of ourselves.

When we study "neuroscience" of the room we may directly seek
insights from *neuroethology*—the study of how brains of diverse animals
control their behavior, ethology being the study of animal behavior. An
important notion here is that of the *Umwelt* as set forth by von Uexküll

(1957/1934): the "world" of an organism may vary from species to species as a consequence of the specialized body form with its receptors and effectors and the use made of them by the specialized nervous system. Putting this in other terms, a human's or animal's world is defined by the effectivities at their command, and the affordances they can detect that can support them. Consider, for example, a lawn as part of a creature's world. For a human, this is something to walk on or to mow, but for a mole this is a place to burrow for food and shelter. This is nicely illustrated in Figure 7.6 (Fragaszy & Mangalam, 2018).

A particularly fascinating mole, the star-nosed mole (Figure 7.7), offers a nice illustration of the fresh perspective on the co-evolution of brain and body that neuroethology provides. To dig its way through the earth, it has, like other moles, evolved especially strong forefeet with strong claws. Uniquely, though, it has an immense star-shaped structure where

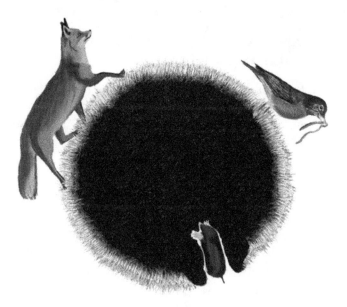

Figure 7.6 Affordances in ethological context, illustrating the different Umwelten of different species. The surface of a loamy soil affords tunneling to a mole, probing in search of prey to a bird, and walking to a fox. (Drawing by A. Osuna-Mascaró. Reprinted from Fragaszy, D. M., & Mangalam, M. [2018]. Tooling *Advances in the Study of Behavior* [Vol. 50, pp. 177–241], with permission from Elsevier.)

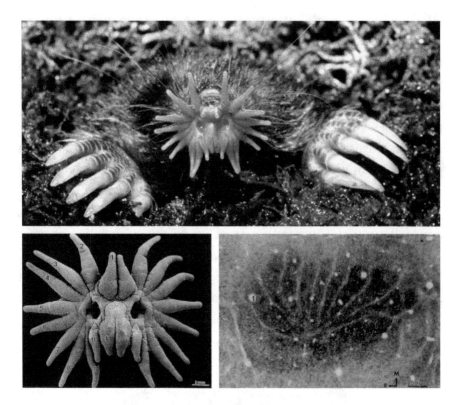

Figure 7.7 The star-nosed mole offers a novel example of the co-evolution of brain and body (including sensors and effectors). At right, we see how separate "fingers" of the apparently nose-located touch organ map to different "barrels" in the mole's cortex. (*Top*: © Kenneth Catania with permission. From Catania, K. C. [2012]. A nose for touch. *Scientist*, 26[9], 28. *Bottom*: From Catania, K. C., & Kaas, J. H. [1995]. Organization of the somatosensory cortex of the star-nosed mole. *Journal of Comparative Neurology*, 351[4], 549–567, with permission of John Wiley & Sons, Inc.)

one might expect a nose, but it is a sensitive touch and chemical organ, somewhat like two 11-fingered hands held in front of its face—if fingers were chemically sensitive. These are presumed to help the animal forage for small prey that it contacts with one or more of the "fingers," evaluating each contact by a mixture of touch and chemical analysis.

Moreover, the brain of the star-nosed mole is adapted to this sensory system. The bottom half of Figure 7.7 shows how each of the "fingers" map into its own dedicated subregion of one brain region. Then, of course, higher level processes have to figure out how to integrate the data to use it in guiding the mole's behavior. If we compare this to Ada, this is similar to having a distinct initial neural network dedicated to processing the activity from one floor tile to decide whether there is a significant signal there, but it requires further layers of neurons to integrate their outputs to infer that somebody is moving in a particular direction or that several people are converging.

Each building forms part of the Umwelt of the people within it. The "spaces" so defined within the building may differ between its various users. For example, in an art gallery the electrical outlets may be "invisible" to the art-goers, yet are crucial in different ways to the exhibition designers and to the cleaners. Of course, the experiences that can be gained within the action–perception cycle of any organism are subject to learning—and so may reflect development within a socially as well as physically constructed niche, as in shaping the different worlds of literate and illiterate humans. In airports, the electrical outlets have gone from cleaners-only to meeting a major need for travelers, and the design of waiting areas has begun to change accordingly.

In the case of neuromorphic architecture, the building too has an Umwelt, one that includes the people within it. This will depend not only on what information the building can gather but also on what actions it can perform and what interactions it can support. New goals set the search for hitherto-neglected affordances, and these change the Umwelt— the framing of which sets new challenges for the architect.

Figure 7.8 introduces some terminology. The *neural space* encompasses not only the "brain" of the building but also the whole information infrastructure that includes the sensors and the effectors. Information flow in this neural space will support the dynamic interaction of the building with its inhabitants as well as the external environment. The *physical space* is the "body" of the actual building.

The architectural design challenge as we have considered it until so far in this book has been about resolving conflicts among a building's diverse functions, including its ecological role, or its intended symbolism versus larger aesthetic intent, or the conflicts of each of those with

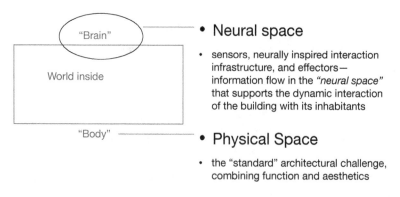

- **Neural space**
  - sensors, neurally inspired interaction infrastructure, and effectors— information flow in the *"neural space"* that supports the dynamic interaction of the building with its inhabitants

- **Physical Space**
  - the "standard" architectural challenge, combining function and aesthetics

Figure 7.8 The neural space of a building controls the physical space's dynamic interactions with the external environment and the users within it.

costs (which may require balancing initial construction costs vs. ongoing operating costs), and then combining all of the program requirements and site constraints and opportunities into a harmonious, buildable structure. Architects are very aware of this in handling clients who believe they can get everything they want in a new building for far below any realistic cost. The architect deals with compromises throughout the design process while considering various efficiencies.

Constraint satisfaction (§3.1) addresses the fact that in general one does not pick one single quantity to optimize, but (as for the three factors in Ada's "happiness"), one has to trade off between several desiderata to get good results for all these criteria even though none of them may achieve its optimum value. My suggestion is that in future it will be beneficial to think through the design of the neural space—the information flow and the action–perception cycle of the building interacting with the action–perception cycles of the inhabitants—before commitment to the final form of the physical space. Consideration of the dynamics of the building (its various effectors) will add a further dimension to the design of the "body," the physical space of the building, and this in turn will require appropriate sensors so that the "brain" can, as we shall exemplify later, serve both homeostasis and "social" interaction. Neuromorphic architecture extends the range of factors to be considered but offers the possibility that certain compromises can be avoided by letting the building's "brain" adjust interactions with the users on a dynamic basis, rather than deciding on a compromise that is fixed before construction of the building can be completed.

To return to the discussion in §7.2, it is important to understand that the AI or neural space of a house is not envisaged to be a human-like intelligence. To parody the undesirable prospect of a house that seeks to tell its users what to do, consider the following (fictional) extract from "The Hitchhiker's Guide to the Galaxy Christmas Special" by Douglas Adams[3] :

[The elevator arrives]

ELEVATOR: Hello.

MARVIN: Hello Lift.

ELEVATOR: I am to be your elevator for this trip to the floor of your choice. I have been designed by the Sirius Cybernetics Corporation to take you . . . into these, their offices. If you enjoy your ride, which will be swift and pleasurable, then you may care to experience some of the other elevators which have recently been installed. . . .

ZAPHOD: Yeah, what else do you do besides talk?

ELEVATOR: I go up or down.

ZAPHOD: Good, we're going up.

ELEVATOR: Or down.

ZAPHOD: Yeah, yeah okay. Up please.

ELEVATOR: Down's very nice. . . .

After much further wrangling, the lift does take them up to the fifth floor. The narrator comments:

It should be explained at this point that modern elevators are strange and complex entities. . . . [T]hey operate [using a] system which enables the elevator to be on the right floor to pick you up even before you knew you wanted it. . . . Not unnaturally, many

3. "The Hitchhiker's Guide to the Galaxy Christmas Special" was broadcast in the United Kingdom by BBC Radio 4 in 1978. The extract was downloaded from https://www.andreafortuna.org/2019/12/24/the-hitchhikers-guide-to-the-galaxy-the-christmas-special/.

lifts imbued with intelligence and precognition became terribly frustrated with the mindless business of going up or down . . . and, finally, took to sulking in basements. At this point a man called Gardrilla Manceframe rediscovered and patented a device he had seen in a history book called a staircase.

This example is not only amusing but also illuminating. Not that long ago , the lift in many public buildings was operated by a person who spent their working hours picking up people at one floor and taking them to the floor they requested. The lift operator may have become as bored as the fictional intelligent elevator, yet may well have been more than upset to lose their job when technology developed for the pushbutton-operated elevator. Nonetheless, most us would accept this as progress. Today, much effort in both mechanical engineering and computer technology is being exploited to make elevators in tall buildings that are not only fast but also have "intelligent controls" to optimize the scheduling of pickups and drop-offs of a bank of elevators to minimize the wait + travel time for people wanting a lift. Similarly, washing machines and dryers are among the household improvements that have replaced much human drudgery— and they have been improved by advances in electronics, mechanics, and responsive computer control.

As part of such advances in cybernetic machines, AI has developed as a technology that provides a variety of different mechanisms that function in diverse ways—some more inspired by biology, as in the control of manipulation and locomotion in robots (as reviewed by Prescott, Ayers, Grasso, & Verschure, 2016); others more akin to developments in search techniques and machine learning (the latter increasingly divorced from its biological roots as computer scientists seek fast and efficient algorithms). The early "romantic" challenge of developing a general intelligence akin to a human's has not lost its allure, but the overall focus of the field has switched to the provision of a variety of "patches of intelligence." Two examples increasingly familiar to readers will be the recommendations system of a streaming service like Netflix or a search engine such as that produced by Google. These both use AI to provide advice. The good news is that they each offer alternatives that you can choose between or reject; the bad news is that, without proper regulations, that advice may reflect financial benefit to the provider at the cost of you the consumer. Many people suffer from the unjust behavior of other people within society, and much vigilance will be required in AI-enriched society, just as it has been and continues to be in societies in which the injustice follows from human greed or ingrained prejudice.

Returning, however, to a recurrent theme: A human is a system of systems, and the nervous system has evolved to integrate specialized components of the nervous system (e.g., those involved with control of heart rate, breathing, and other homeostatic functions) and those engaged in directing the overall behavior of the body in its commitments within the action–perception cycle. As illustrated by the examples of elevators and washing machines as "intelligent" subsystems of contemporary buildings, a neuromorphic building will also be a system of systems, both human and cybernetic. The challenge for neuromorphic architecture is to design the static and cybernetic components of a building so that they work together to serve (with the usual tradeoffs) the interests of the human occupants.

When the physical space is integrated with a sophisticated neural space, we can think of buildings as (possibly simple) cognitive entities. This will be enhanced as the structure and operation of buildings becomes increasingly dynamically reconfigurable to conform itself to the needs of its users.

Kolarevic and Parlac (2015) emphasize buildings whose structure— the "effectors" rather than the "brain"—can be changed dynamically. One example was of a building that can change its shape so that the wind passing around it would cause as little damage and heat loss as possible. Their book did include some discussion of cybernetics (especially the work of Gordon Pask, e.g., Pask, Jones, & Thornley, 1962 --Pickering, 2009, has a valuable chapter on Pask's work) but did not bring in neuroscience per se. The key point for us is that a brain needs a flexible (reconfigurable, adaptive) body, not just sophisticated sensors but also diverse effectors for reconfiguration of the internal and exterior milieux . . . and for interaction.

Recent years have seen the "invasion" of the home by electronic assistants that are connected to the Internet and thus to large databases that deep learning exploits. They can use increasingly effective speech communication. Controllers can now monitor many of the appliances of the home and communicate by smartphone with absent humans, the current commercial realization of the Internet of Things for household products. Robotics may be even more relevant than general AI in neuromorphic architecture. A range of active furniture, perceiving robots that act as dedicated subsystems rather than (in general) as autonomous humanoids, would enhance this interaction, while the building itself would act as an "inside-out" robot, or even a network of such. Design would be constrained not only by the differing roles of different rooms but also by the need to support multiple users in diverse activities and their flow between the rooms.

As historical context, one may think about crowded nineteenth century tenement buildings in which there was no supply of running water and no facility for the disposal of sewage, and then consider the revolution in urban design that came when each living space could be supplied with those utilities. Similar revolutions occurred with gas and electricity and today with the Internet—and this leads directly into a smart architecture that integrates the Internet of Things with, we propose, brain operating principles gleaned from neuroethology.

Developments in AI are rooted in the study of brains and bodies because learning in real brains provided the historical basis for learning in artificial neural networks (recall §5.3), while studies of animal perception and action have helped shape robotics. Ada combined an example of ambient intelligence with lessons from neuroscience, especially the computational emulation of brain mechanisms for emotion, as well as artificial neural networks, such as those used to track people as they moved across the floor. Are there new lessons to be learned for the A↔N conversation from studying brain, body, and environment in diverse animals? The jury is still out, though I will offer certain promissory notes later.

Many have been concerned that technology will impose a "flat" global culture, but, to the contrary, modern technology can provide new forms

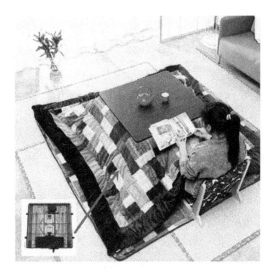

Figure 7.9 The kotatsu, a traditional Japanese household furnishing reimagined with electricity. The *inset* indicates the heater placed on the lower surface of the table top. (Image of kotatsu table heater at https://www.aliexpress.com, common domain.)

that build upon traditional cultures even while offering dramatic transformations. Here are two examples from Japan (admittedly in terms of furnishings). Traditionally, many Japanese could not afford to heat their houses. After cooking the dinner over a fire, the embers would be thrown into the pit of the *kotatsu*—a table above the pit from which extended a blanket. The family would sit with their lower bodies beneath the blanket to keep warm, and eat or socialize around the table. In today's kotatsu (Figure 7.9), the warmth is supplied by an electric heater affixed beneath the table. Again, in many Japanese homes, futons are brought out at night to convert living space into a bedroom—and technology adapts. One can now buy giant "hair dryers" that can be used to blast warm air into the bedding before one gets into it.[4]

With this, let's consider two targets for neuromorphic architecture: homeostasis and social interaction.

---

4. My thanks to Hideo and Harumi Sakata for inviting my wife Prue and me to visit their country house near Mt. Fuji. There we experienced both these examples—as well as Japanese innovations in indoor plumbing.

Homeostasis

Homeostasis refers to keeping critical bodily variables—like temperature, blood sugar, and oxygenation—in the range necessary for an animal's survival. In animals, levels of the nervous system below the cerebral cortex conduct the normal processes of homeostasis. For example, the brainstem can control breathing to maintain oxygen levels in the blood. It is only when normal breathing is disrupted that you may have to engage higher mental processes: You're suddenly in a room filling with smoke. How do you get out? You have fallen in the water. How do you struggle back to land?

One example of "exotic" homeostatic architecture may point the way to neuromorphic strategies for homeostasis in the future. In Jean Nouvel's Institut du Monde Arabe in Paris, the intriguing facade that we see from the inside contained an array of panels, as we can see in Figure 7.10.[5] In keeping with the theme of the Arab World, and as a striking example of cross-pollination of architectural traditions, each panel is based on the Islamic *mashrabiya*, walls that could break the direct impact of sunshine on people behind them. The innovation in Nouvel's structure is that all these aperures are in fact controllable. Hundreds of light-sensitive diaphragms regulate the amount of light that is allowed to enter the building. The effect is aesthetic as well as homeostatic: interior spaces are dramatically modified by these light patterns, while the exterior appearance exhibits a fluid shifting of geometric pattern. Each panel is as a beautiful piece of machinery, but it is beautiful in the way in which 18th-century clockwork was beautiful. By having such elaborate mechanisms at every scale, it was only a few years before more and

5. For more on Jean Nouvel's building, see Tim Winstanley's article online at https://www.archdaily.com/162101/ad-classics-institut-du-monde-arabe-jean-nouvel. For an account of the renovation work done on the mashrabiyas, see AMC (September 29, 2017) Les moucharabiehs de l'IMA reprennent leur danse, https://www.amc-archi.com/photos/les-moucharabiehs-de-l-ima-reprennent-leur-danse,7438/les-moucharabiehs-de-l-institu.1. The instruction "Lancer le diaporama" opens a gallery of photos by Fabrice Cateloy that show how the moving parts of the panels reconfigure the various apertures from fully open to other shapes of intermediate sizes.

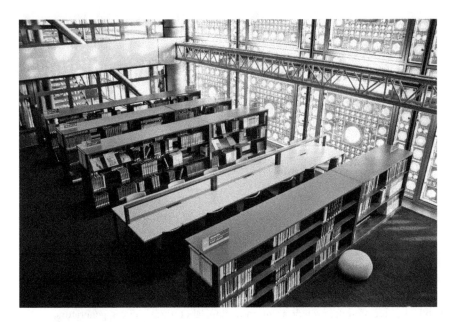

Figure 7.10 A reading room in Jean Nouvel's Institut du Monde Arabe in Paris, showing the cybernetic *mashrabiya* (brise soleil) as seen from the inside. Note that each mashrabiya contains a central aperture surrounded by a pattern of smaller apertures of two sizes, all operable. (Photo by ActuaLitté, under the Creative Commons Attribution-Share Alike 2.0 Generic license.)

more of these apertures became locked in place. Renovation work was thus undertaken to repair the system, improve the thermal insulation of the façade, and insert LEDs in every mashrabiya for a dynamic lighting display to make the building a Parisian visual landmark by night as well as by day. This emphasizes the challenge of designing a reliable "body" for a dynamic building, whether the control network is brain-inspired or not. As the star-nosed mole dramatically reminds us, the lesson of neuroethology is that the success of neuromorphic architecture will not rest on building a "brain" alone so much as in developing the neural space and the effector-equipped physical space together to close the loop in a satisfying (and readily maintainable) way for the people who experience that building.

In homeostasis, the body adjusts to the ambient conditions—in part by moving elsewhere. The latter option is less relevant for buildings, but has

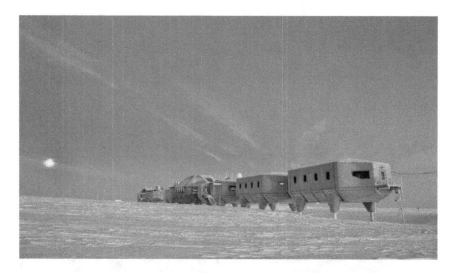

Figure 7.11 Halley VI, the relocatable research station of the British Antarctic Survey. The central red module contains the communal areas for eating and socializing, while the blue modules provide accommodation, laboratories, offices, generators, an observation platform, and other facilities. (Photo by Hugh Broughton Architects, licensed under the Creative Commons Attribution-Share Alike 4.0 International license.)

been partially realized in the Halley VI Research Station (Figure 7.11) of the British Antarctic Survey.[6] Built on a floating ice shelf in the Weddell Sea, Halley VI is the world's first relocatable research facility. It is segmented into eight modules, each sitting atop ski-fitted, hydraulic legs. These can be individually raised to overcome snow accumulation and each module towed independently to a new location. This was required during the 2016/17 Antarctic summer season, when Halley was successfully relocated to its current location. Operational teams spent 13 weeks moving each of the station's eight modules 23 km upstream of a previously dormant ice chasm. Halley VI is dynamic, but not autonomous or neuromorphic. However, it is not an unreasonable extrapolation to imagine a future version (Halley X?) that is able to accept reports about change in the ice shelf and autonomously move to a safer location while (switching

6. https://www.bas.ac.uk/polar-operations/sites-and-facilities/facility/halley/ and https://www.bas.ac.uk/project/moving-halley/

from homeostasis to social interaction) assisting its human crew in secur-
ing instruments in place and ensuring their safety during the move. Note
that, in view of the earlier suggestions that a building become a system of
systems in which some of the subsystems are indeed human, there is nothing in the previous scenario to preclude that humans would be in the loop
when such high-level decisions are being made.

Social interaction

We now move on to neuromorphic architecture for the "social interaction" of rooms or buildings with people in or near them, adapting
buildings to the needs of their inhabitants. In turning to social cognitive neuroscience for inspiration, we recall the notion of mirror neurons (§5.4). However, that inspiration may more realistically draw on
the brain's action recognition systems beyond the mirror than on mirror neurons themselves because in most cases the observed actions of
humans will not be actions in the building's own repertoire (recall the
discussion of Figure 5.6).

To illustrate this, let's consider a reactive and adaptive intelligent
kitchen that was generated by students Jacob Everist, Guang Shi, Jarugool
Tretriluxana, Gurveen Chopra, and Frank Lewis as a project in a 2003
course I gave at the University of Southern California. As this was a computer science course, the students offered only a rudimentary sketch for
the physical space. Instead, they focused on writing programs for different
components of the neural space, based on what they had learned about
modeling of systems within animal brains. The room was designed to help
a person cook food based on a recipe. All computations are conditional
on which recipe was selected. The room keeps track of progress, and helps
as needed. They envisioned the kitchen as having the layout of the type of
apartment kitchen in which cooking and eating areas are adjacent. Rather
fancifully, their design included a mechanical arm to select ingredients
from the refrigerator and place them, sequentially, on a conveyor belt joining the refrigerator and the counter. (In passing, note the benefits of that

highly specialized robot, the dishwashing machine—very helpful, even though it still requires human assistance to load and unload the dishes.)

The neural space was based on the following assumptions: Cameras were mounted on the ceiling to monitor the entrance, the dining table, the refrigerator, and the counter. The user communicated with the room via microphones on the walls. A light over the counter became active when the user began to cook. It was green while the user was following the recipe correctly but red as soon as the user made an error. Given that the cook might be too distracted to note the light changing color, we would now replace the lights with a more useful interface using spoken language to say, for example, "You need to take the saucepan off the stove before it overheats," or, "You forgot to chop the onions."

Many of the components of the room's "brain" were based on models of specific brain regions or guided by brain operation principles (Figure 7.12). The neural space included speech recognition, emotion recognition, event localization, and processing facial expressions. It also included recipe management—choosing the meal and selecting ingredients. Mirror neurons came into the mix to track the manual actions of the cook. These were integrated with systems "beyond the mirror" to keep track of the state of preparation according to a particular recipe. Iteration with design of the physical space would, for example, reassess the placement of the cameras and microphones and assess whether the use of the robot arm is the best way to provide access to ingredients. In a dynamic building, such placement would be under control of the interaction infrastructure as it learned about the person (and reconfigurable to meet the needs of different users).

If a kitchen is a "machine for cooking in" and a house is a "machine for living in," then we must ask for other typologies. For what X (or multiples X's) is each building, or each room or "subsystem" of the building, "a machine for X-ing in"? Ada is, perhaps, a "machine for being entertained in," while a school is a "machine for learning in" and a church is a "machine for worshipping in." But this raises the issue of whether such a characterization demeans architecture or enriches it. We saw that Le Corbusier's enthusiasm for an engineering aesthetics turned out to be complemented by an architectural aesthetics—and a failing of his book is that it did not

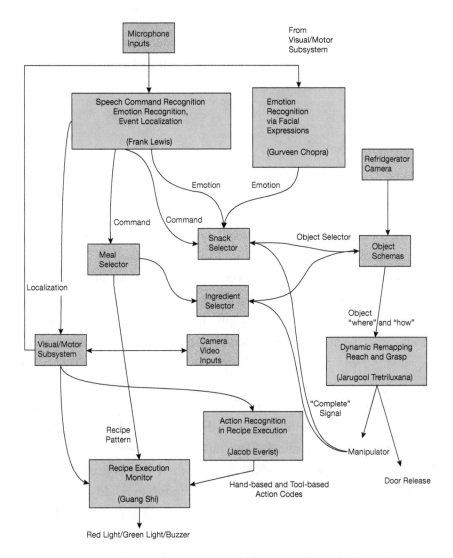

Figure 7.12 The neural space for a reactive and adaptive intelligent kitchen. The components in *blue* are labeled both with a function and the name of the student responsible for a computational model of the "brain subsystem" involved. The whole team worked together on the (unimplemented) design of the overall system of systems. The reader is invited to read the text and then map the various processes onto the modules and interactions that support them.

offer a synthesis of the two. An architectural historian could scrutinize the writings and buildings that Le Corbusier produced later in his work to assess to what extent he produced such a synthesis (see Jencks, 1973, for one such effort), but this lies outside my remit here.

Buildings that learn

Neither a colleague of mine who likes to cook nor my wife, who is a superb cook, would want a kitchen like the one designed by my students, and even a novice cook could become frustrated by a kitchen that kept offering suggestions for cooking routines that they had by now mastered. This motivates bringing in emotion and learning as crucial themes for neuromorphic architecture. Someone who cooks rarely may need a lot of assistance, and even an experienced cook may find it helpful to receive timely reminders when working with the multiple components of a complex recipe like that I use for coq au vin.[7] However, too much "help" can become intrusive. Two factors then enter. One is to use facial and vocal cues to recognize the emotional state of the user. Do they indicate frustration with excessive instruction or a measure of desperation in preparing the current dish? The room should be able to perform accordingly. And this leads into learning—about what the user can handle without assistance and where help is needed (and this changes over time), as well as how the user chooses to modify the recipe so that the room can keep track of the user's preferences.

7.5. COMMUNITY AND BIOPHILIA

Our discussion of neuromorphic architecture was informed in part by ideas from the neuroscience of social interaction. However, endowing a building with the ability to recognize the actions of its inhabitants or communicate with them through various media cannot replace the need of

---

7. https://cooking.nytimes.com/recipes/1018529-coq-au-vin

humans to interact with other humans (a sense of community). Consider the following quote from the Irish-born American architect Kevin Roche:

> The most important thing one can achieve in any building is to get people to communicate with each other. That's really essential to our lives. We are not just individuals—we are part of a community. The old-time villages did that, and then we destroyed all that in the 19th century, when we started to build these vast expansions where there was no center, there is no community.[8]

The Canadian neuroscientist turned psychologist of architecture, Colin Ellard (in his contribution to Arbib et al., 2021) expressed his concern with what Albert Borgmann (1984) calls the "device paradigm," where technology that ostensibly provides a cocoon of comfort ends up detaching us from our environment and from each other (the thermostat and central heating, which free us from chopping wood, watching the weather, etc.—some might say happily so, but still there are costs).[9] He queries the possible cocooning effect if people adapt to buildings that sense the inhabitant's physiological and emotional states and cater to them accordingly. Even E. M. Forster, the author of *A Room with a View* and *A Passage to India*, worried about this. His "The Machine Stops" (Forster, 1909) is a chilling short story about individuals cocooned by technology that includes instant messages (email!) and cinematophoes (machines that project visual images), and the total helplessness of most people that follows its breakdown. Though written over a century ago, his story is even more relevant today.

More positively, however, the present book is intended to help architects explore how cog/neuroscience, AI, and cybernetics more generally

---

8. From the interview in http://www.archnewsnow.com/features/Feature512.htm.

9. Kolarevic employs the term "device paradigm" in the context of performative architecture (see p. 12 of his Introduction to Kolarevic & Malkawi, 2005) and even cites Borgmann's book, but far from echoing Ellard and Borgmann's concerns about the cocooning effect of technology, he is simply noting the importance of taking full account of the operability of the set of devices incorporated in a building when evaluating its performance—a theme that certainly resonates with earlier sections of this chapter.

can provide some—but by no means all—the factors that make buildings that better serve people. Here's a complementary example from a very different field of the need to balance the pluses and minuses of new technology: Cars provide great convenience in personal transportation but have the three downsides of pollution, reduced exercise, and lack of community. Thus, one response in current urbanism is to emphasize walkable neighborhoods, including public transportation within walking distance of most homes for travel outside the neighborhood. But the need for travel outside the neighborhood remains, even if far less frequent.

Another dimension beyond the neuromorphic—but strongly linked to the biological—is provided by *biophilic architecture*, inspired by the biophilia hypothesis of E. O. Wilson (1986) that humans possess an innate tendency to seek connections with nature and other forms of life. However, connecting with other forms of life may be too sweeping a characterization. Architects typically address this by incorporating greenery and gardens into the design rather than, for example, spiders and mosquitoes.[10]

As an example of design with community and biophilia in mind, let's consider the Kampung Admiralty in Singapore, designed by the Singapore architecture firm WOHA, which was the 2018 World Architecture Festival Building of the Year (Figures 7.13 and 7.14). Its design stresses building a sense of community both for those who live there and for the wider neighborhood.

This is a "Vertical Kampung (village)," with a People's Plaza in the lower stratum, a Medical Centre in the mid stratum, and a Community Park with studio apartments for seniors in the upper stratum. . . . The People's Plaza is a fully public, porous and pedestrianised ground plane, designed as a community living room, within which the public can participate in organised events, join in the season's festivities, shop, or eat at the hawker centre on the 2nd storey. The breezy tropical plaza is shaded and sheltered by the Medical Centre above, allowing activities to continue regardless of rain or shine. Residents

---

10. The first draft of this section paralleled portions of the essay, "Baukultur and Subsidiarity in a Cybernetic Age" (Arbib, 2019). Further discussion of general issues of Baukultur is outside the scope of this book, but readers will also find relevant material in Arbib (2017).

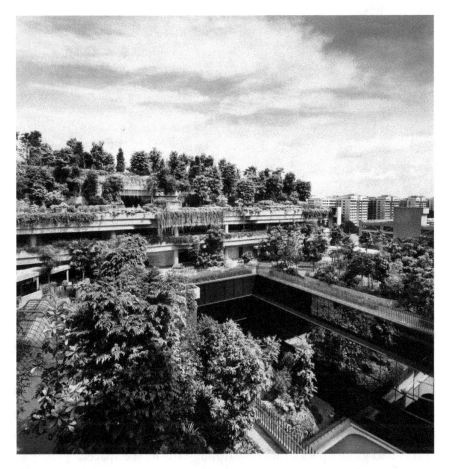

Figure 7.13 A view of WOHA's Kampung Admiralty from an interior vantage point. (Courtesy of Richard Hassell; photo credit Patrick Bingham-Hall.)

can actively come together to exercise, chat or tend community farms at the Community Park, an intimately-scaled, elevated village green. "Buddy benches" at shared entrances encourage seniors to come out of their homes and interact with their neighbors.[11]

Richard Hassell (in his contribution to Arbib et al., 2021) stresses the importance of system thinking here—a different form of cybernetics from

11. Adapted from www.woha.net/. The book *Garden City Mega City* (WOHA & Bingham-Hall, 2016) presents WOHA's approach to rethinking architecture and cities for the 21st century. Disclosure: Richard Hassell's father is a cousin of my wife. Richard is the HA of WOHA.

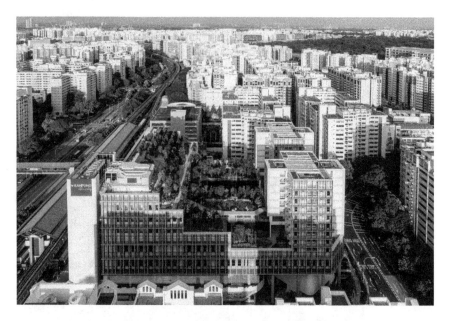

Figure 7.14 Kampung Admiralty viewed within the larger Singapore cityscape.
(Courtesy of Richard Hassell; photo credit Lim Weixiang.)

that at the heart of neuromorphic architecture. Kampung Admiralty was designed as a node within as many systems as possible. It is a gateway to the mass rapid transit system, and collects all the streets and footpaths nearby and guides pedestrian flow through the public spaces.

We are back to the important notion (§3.1) of a *system of systems*. The complex brings together old patterns, such as the hawker center, with new patterns, such as a fully covered, breezy tropical plaza, which WOHA felt were lacking in the hot tropical city. It has a public park on top designed for biodiversity. The park is also a water collector and purifier, so it inserts itself as a regenerative system between the rain and the city's water system, circulating water multiple times through reed beds and its own irrigation systems before releasing it to the city system. The medical center is a node in the national medical system, and is a new typology, a neighborhood outlet that encourages life care rather than treatment. Then the child care and elderly care are also nodes within the system, creating shared benefits through their adjacency. The elderly residents can access different urban modes on different floors—lively public space, noisy food center, caring medical center, fun activities at the center, quiet public park, community garden—all for free and without having to arrange transport.

Its residential apartments are part of the immense Singapore public housing system (not just buildings, but also political, financial, and facilities management) that houses 80% of the citizens, and so it adds a new typology to that system. It has been such a success that its design principles are being replicated in other districts.[12] It will be interesting to see other iterations by other architects now that the new typology has been defined.

In this way, Kampung Admiralty was designed from the ground up as a place for many social and infrastructural and natural systems to intersect, and through their intertwining, to create a whole greater than the sum of the parts—for social and environmental benefits to emerge. There are hints of Singapore culture here (the hawker center for food, the sensitivity to the Singapore climate), but overall it provides a general 21st-century solution for high-density housing, replacing skyscrapers in which tenants are anonymous and isolated from each other with buildings that foster both privacy and community within a green and inspiring environment.

A major challenge for urban design is that the overall city (and higher layers of government) must support, to a great extent, the particularity of each of the diverse cultures of its inhabitants while ensuring a shared framework in which the flourishing of each culture does not come at undue expense to others. (This is not to deny the possibility of conflict over achieving a stable balance between divergent interests.) Residential complexes become "nodes" linked through transit networks to those sites that give the city its culture—or, indeed, cultures. The cityscape must then preserve aspects of former glories while adding new buildings, parks, statues, and urban complexes, which in time may contribute both a shared sense of the city's history and areas where subcultures may flourish.

I write at a time when the cost of housing in California has priced too many people out of the market, creating a crisis of homelessness (intensified by the rise of Covid-19 since this section was first drafted). We see crises caused by increasing inequality of income and wealth around the world.

12. The video https://www.youtube.com/watch?v=sDjQDAad5eU&feature=youtu.be demonstrates the satisfaction of both residents and neighbors with the Kampung. However, the video is promotional rather than documenting post-occupancy evaluations.

Architecture alone cannot solve these problems, but the challenge of designing building systems that bring people together is certainly a worthy one for more architects to address. Moreover, humans are more than units in an ecologically sustainable ecosystem. We live, too, in a cultural world of language and art, of music and aesthetics, all of which combine to support a shared sense of community in no sense limited to one street or apartment building. We must work toward an architecture that does not overly cocoon us, but instead helps create an environment—the natural, the built, the social—in which each of us can thrive as social beings, not as isolated individuals.[13]

7.6. WHERE MIGHT NEUROMORPHIC ARCHITECTURE LEAD US?

As buildings become more neuromorphic, we may expect them to go from designs in which the neural space is simply an add-on for an otherwise-designed physical space to designs in which the neural space and new ideas for the physical space co-evolve to yield dramatically new designs—just as the rise of elevators made skyscrapers possible, and changed top floors of five-story apartment buildings from garrets to penthouses.

For comparison, Figure 7.15 shows a horse and carriage, the basis for the horseless carriage where the design was minimally changed—but, instead of having reins to control the horse, which then provides the appropriate gait to turn a corner, we now have a new pair of wheels that can be controlled for steering. Moreover, fundamentally, the motive power of the horse has been replaced by the motive power of the engine applied to the rear wheels. Fast-forward about 100 years, and we have today's cars, still with four wheels on the road, a steering wheel, and a motor—but so much has changed. A hidden change is that the car now has a whole range of functions controlled by a network of microcomputers. And we are now on the cusp of a dramatic further transformation, where the car becomes autonomous and there is

13. Alvaro Puertas Villavicencio (personal communication) notes that 70% of the habitations in Lima are informal (compare the favelas of Brazil or the shanty towns of South Africa). This raises important challenges concerning "urbanism without architects."

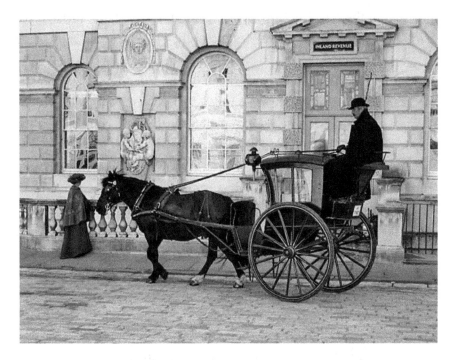

Figure 7.15 Hansom cab and driver. (HansomCab.jpg © Andrew Dunn, Creative Commons Attribution-Share Alike 2.0 Generic license.)

no longer a need for the interior to contain a space designed for a driver to control the steering wheel, brake, and accelerator.

I foresee a similar progression for neuromorphic architecture. The design of the physical space for the kitchen described earlier was conventional, with the addition of a few effectors and receptors coupled by an interaction infrastructure that could support the room's "social" interaction with the human users. After a not-too-steep learning curve, we will better understand what adaptations humans might or might not be able to make to such designs. Yes, design will be the projection of human needs, but humans still need to adapt to new circumstances—just as someone accustomed to horse and carriage would still need driving lessons before taking to the road in a motor car. To take more architectural examples, someone adept at lighting and blowing out candles still needs to adapt to learning how to turn light switches on and off appropriately; and there are a billion or more people on this planet who still do not use a flush toilet.

In future, there will be strong reconfigurations of the physical space as the constraints of the neural space and the physical space each shape the other to come up with a habitation, an office building, an entertainment space, or a recreational space that is designed to be able to exploit its interaction infrastructure, its nonhuman "brain"—or, perhaps better, its integrated network of "sub-brains"—to better enrich the experience of the people who inhabit that building.

There is nothing overtly cybernetic in the description of Kampung Admiralty, and yet the view of a building as a node in diverse urban networks complements this book's stress on networks at different levels of organization of the brain, and of each building itself as a system of systems. When we consider a building as a system of systems, we are open to a conversation about which of those subsystems may be ripe from an architectural transition to being cybernetically enabled and (possibly) to informationally coupled into a broader information infrastructure. Architecture has long counted on urban services such as the orderly treatment of garbage and, increasingly, recycling (matching the metabolism of the city to the metabolisms of its inhabitants). That late 20th-century innovation, the Internet, has spawned the Internet of Things, and is beginning to transform how a building can respond in real time to the changing needs of its inhabitants. And thus we are at the cusp of a new, transformative *neuromorphic architecture*.

In §1.3, we related lifespan architecture to Stewart Brand's (1995) *How Buildings Learn*, with its emphasis on what happens to a building as humans restructure it over time to meet different needs. In the present context, though, we can consider how the building itself may form an adaptive system, restructuring its "body" as its "brain" compiles more data. This takes us beyond the notion of "self-repair," inspired by biology, as a form of maintenance or even dramatic reinvention. This challenge is left for future A↔N conversations, but "lifelong" building information models (BIMs) may come to play an important role here (Dave, Buda, Nurminen, & Främling, 2018). We might also look ahead to where a BIM is not just keeping track of the structure of the building, but is also keeping track of how successfully it is interacting with people and how much people appreciate these interactions. Such applications certainly raise privacy issues, extending those currently under intense consideration.[14] The aim would be to come up with lessons about how the building itself might change as well as lessons that can be fed back into general practice.

REFERENCES

Arbib, M. A. (2012). Brains, machines and buildings: Towards a neuromorphic architecture. *Intelligent Buildings International*, 4(3), 4(3), 147–168. doi:110.1080/17508975.17502012.17702863

Arbib, M. A. (2017). When brains design/experience buildings: Architectural patterns for a good life. In J. W. Vasbinder & B. Z. Gulyas (Eds.), *Cultural patterns and neurocognitive circuits: East–west connections* (pp. 111–140). Singapore: World Scientific.

Arbib, M. A. (2019). Baukultur and subsidiarity in a cybernetic age. *Intertwining: Unfolding art and Science*, 2, 62–79.

Arbib, M. A., Banasiak, M., Condia, B., Ellard, C., Enns, J., Farling, M., . . . Robinson, S. (2021). Baukultur in a cybernetic age: A conversation. *The Plan Journal*, 6(1). doi:10.15274/tpj.2021.06.01.1.

Arbib, M. A., & Fellous, J. M. (2004). Emotions: From brain to robot. *Trends in Cognitive Sciences*, 8(12), 554–561.

Ashby, W. R. (1952). *Design for a brain*. London: Chapman & Hall.

Ballard, J. G. (1971). *The thousand dreams of Stellavista*. https://arl.human.cornell.edu/linked%20docs/Ballard%20Thousand%20Dreams%20of%20Stellavista.pdf)

Borgmann, A. (1984). *Technology and the character of contemporary life: A philosophical inquiry*. Chicago: University of Chicago Press.

Brand, S. (1995). *How buildings learn: What happens after they're built*. Penguin.

Breazeal, C., & Scassellati, B. (2002). Robots that imitate humans. *Trends in Cognitive Sciences*, 6, 481–487.

Dave, B., Buda, A., Nurminen, A., & Främling, K. (2018). A framework for integrating BIM and IoT through open standards. *Automation in Construction*, 95, 35–45. doi:10.1016/j.autcon.2018.07.022

Ekman, P. (1999). Basic emotions. In T. Dalgleish & M. Power (Eds.), *Handbook of cognition and emotion* (pp. 45–60). New York: John Wiley & Sons.

Eng, K., Klein, D., Babler, A., Bernardet, U., Blanchard, M., Costa, M., . . . Verschure, P. F. M. J. (2003). Design for a brain revisited: The neuromorphic design and functionality of the interactive space "Ada" *Reviews in the Neurosciences*, 14, 145.

Fellous, J.-M., & Arbib, M. A. (Eds.). (2005). *Who needs emotions: The brain meets the robot*. Oxford, New York: Oxford University Press.

14. For a range of relevant articles, see the New York Times Privacy Project, https://www.nytimes.com/series/new-york-times-privacy-project.

Forster, E. M. (1909). The machine stops. *Oxford and Cambridge Review*. https://www.ele.uri.edu/faculty/vetter/Other-stuff/The-Machine-Stops.pdf

Fragaszy, D. M., & Mangalam, M. (2018). Tooling. In M. Naguib, L. Barrett, S. D. Healy, J. Podos, L. W. Simmons, & M. Zuk (Eds.), *Advances in the Study of Behavior* (Vol. 50, pp. 177–241). Elsevier Academic Press.

Gabrielsson, A., & Lindstrom, E. (2001). The influence of musical structure on emotional expression. In P. N. Juslin & J. A. Sloboda (Eds.), *Music and emotion: Theory and research* (pp. 223–248). Oxford: Oxford University Press.

Jencks, C. (1973). *Le Corbusier and the tragic view of architecture*. Cambridge, MA: Harvard University Press.

Kolarevic, B., & Malkawi, A. M. (2005). *Performative architecture: Beyond instrumentality*. London and New York: Routledge.

Kolarevic, B., & Parlac, V. (Eds.). (2015). *Building dynamics: Exploring architecture of change*. London and New York: Routledge.

Kymäläinen, T. (2016). Science fiction prototypes as a method for discussing sociotechnical issues within emerging technology research and foresight. *Athens Journal of Technology & Engineering*, 3(4), 333–347.

Manzolli, J., & Verschure, P. F. M. J. (2005). Roboser: A real-world composition system. *Computer Music Journal*, 29, 55–74.

Ortony, A., Norman, D., & Revelle, W. (2005). Affect and proto-affect in effective functioning. In J.-M. Fellous & M. A. Arbib (Eds.), *Who needs emotions* (pp. 173–202). New York and Oxford: Oxford University Press.

Palumbo, M. (2004). Looking at the first neuromorphic space: A conversation with Paul Verschure. *ARCH'IT*. http://architettura.supereva.com/interview/20040205

Pask, G., Jones, J. C., & Thornley, D. G. (1962). *The conception of a shape and the evolution of a design*. Paper presented at the 1963 Conference on Design Methods: Papers Presented at the Conference on Systematic and Intuitive Methods in Engineering, Industrial Design, Architecture and Communications—September.

Pickering, A. (2009). *The cybernetic brain: Sketches of another future*. Chicago: University of Chicago Press.

Prescott, T. J., Ayers, J., Grasso, F. W., & Verschure, P. F. M. J. (2016). Embodied models and neurorobotics. In M. A. Arbib & J. J. Bonaiuto (Eds.), *From Neuron to Cognition via Computational Neuroscience* (pp. 483–511). Cambridge, MA: The MIT Press.

Sloman, A., Chrisley, R., & Scheutz, M. (2005). The architectural basis of affective states and processes. In J. M. Fellous & M. A. Arbib (Eds.), *Who needs emotions* (pp. 203–244). New York and Oxford: Oxford University Press.

von Uexküll, J. (1957/1934). A stroll through the worlds of animals and men: A picture book of invisible worlds. In C. H. Schiller (Ed.), *Instinctive behavior: The development of a modern concept* (pp. 5–80). New York: International Universities Press.

Wassermann, K. C., Eng, K., Verschure, P. F. M. J., & Manzolli, J. (2003). Live soundscape composition based on synthetic emotions. *Multimedia, IEEE*, 10(4), 82–90.

Wilson, E. O. (1986). *Biophilia*. Cambridge, MA: Harvard University Press.

WOHA, & Bingham-Hall, P. (2016). *Garden City mega city*. Oxford, Singapore, and Sydney: Pesaro Publishing.

Evolving the architecture-ready brain

This book has adopted the EvoDevoSocio perspective for brains in bodies in social and physical interaction with the world around them. So much of what we take to be human is not the direct expression of our genome, the result of biological evolution, but rather the shaping of that inheritance by cultural evolution to create cultural and physical environments in which today's children can develop to exhibit hitherto unimaginable capabilities.

We have seen how "the thinking hand"—the linkage of vision and touch with arm and hand via the brain—plays an important role in the A↔N conversation, grounding the case that architecture is far more than a spectator sport. In this chapter I show that the embrained hand, rather than the voice, may have been the prime mover in the early stage-setting for the emergence of language, that most distinctively human of capabilities, and that this manual foundation for "how the brain got language" offers fresh insights into our capacity for construction, drawing, and architecture. The challenge for studying cultural evolution is expressed in the hypothesis that early humans did not have language (they had "protolanguage"), and yet their brains were little different from ours—early humans had "language-ready" brains, but not "language-using" brains. Similarly, the making of stone tools, the mastery of fire, and the use of ocher in body painting are a long way from the achievements of modern technology, or of art and architecture—and so our distant ancestors also had construction-ready, drawing-ready, and even architecture-ready brains, but it required tens of millennia of cultural evolution for these latent capabilities to be realized.

In 1989, Giacomo Rizzolatti (leader of the group that discovered mirror neurons) and I published a paper called "Language Within Our Grasp," which suggested that the ability of mirror neurons to engage in both the execution and recognition of manual actions may have provided the core for the human capacity for the *parity of language*, in which the meaning of words produced by one person may be recognized by another. Subsequent work built on this to develop the *mirror system hypothesis*, tracing a path from the last common ancestor of humans and monkeys of 25 million years ago whose brain was, we suggest, equipped with mirror systems to primate ancestors with brains capable of simple imitation and more recent ancestors with brains capable of complex imitation. This in turn laid the foundation for protohumans capable of both pantomime and pedagogy, providing the basis for increasing rates of cultural innovation and their transmission. It may have required further biological evolution for the transition from the ad hoc performance of pantomime as a means of communication to the use of conventionalized protosign, with the evolution of mechanisms for vocal control that could produce protospeech scaffolded by this manual breakthrough. The further claim is that such a brain was language-ready and that cultural evolution rather than genetic change was the main supporter of the emergence of the diversity of human languages. In short, the view espoused here is that manual communication served as the key driver of the emergence of language-readiness, with vocalization playing a secondary role.

However, the importance of these considerations to the A↔N conversation lies not so much in the evolution of the language-ready brain as in the realization that such a brain was also construction-ready and drawing-ready. The commonality is that each must bring diverse elements together (whether words, building blocks, or lines and patches on a cave wall), linking mental construction with physical construction. Unlike those theories that posit a direct transition in the vocal domain from monkey-like vocalizations to speech, our approach makes the ability for drawing an immediate corollary of the ability for pantomime—when the necessary technology is available to make enduring marks on a cave wall or spatial medium. The manual gestures of pantomime translate into the manual gestures of drawing and sketching. Note that the assertion here is not that language depends on drawing or that drawing depends on language—rather, it is that early humans had brains that could (over tens of millennia) invent either, but the discovery of each was to a great extent independent. By contrast, writing depends on both as prior technologies.

These observations cohere with an important insight due to Merlin Donald: a post-biological evolutionary change that was crucial to the emergence of modern humans was the development of *external memory* as exemplified in the ability to create visual patterns that could augment internal memory mechanisms and create cohesion between members of a social group. In this chapter, such considerations provide the background for analysis of the neuropsychology of drawing, which invokes further consideration of the "what" and "how" pathways in the visuomotor brain, and reminds us of how sketching links memory and imagination.

Given the importance of sketching in both two and three dimensions (physical models) in the development of architectural designs, it is clear that our ancestors already had architecture-ready brains, though in fact the design of outdoor structures away from the safety of caves was a very late development. In addition to the reciprocal influence between culture and buildings, individual buildings can be designed that vary dramatically in their function and aesthetics and the disposition of materials to achieve them. Given this distinctive characteristic, neither mound-building termites nor nest-building birds are architecture-ready in the human sense of the term—"animal architecture" is *not* architecture in the human sense.

Finally, the linked discussion of language-readiness and architecture-readiness leads us to the question of the extent to which we may consider architecture as a language or, more appropriately, an aggregate of diverse languages. The key idea here is that a human language "in the strict sense" has both a *lexicon* (stock of words) and a relatively fixed *grammar* that provides the "constructions' that allow us to combine words and phrases into larger expressions of meaning that may be novel yet still more or less comprehensible to others. By contrast, some architects may change the "lexicon," the set of building blocks in a general sense that they bring to a project, and—to the extent that they adopt or invent novel methods of construction—they may also change what in some sense might be referred to as the "grammar" of their designs.

8.1. INTRODUCING THE X-READY BRAIN

Warren McCulloch was my strongest influence when I was a graduate student at MIT. He was an accomplished neurologist, coauthor of the foundational paper in neural network theory (McCulloch & Pitts, 1943) and a cofounder of cybernetics, and called himself an experimental epistemologist. He pondered the question: "What is a number that a man may know it and a man that he may know a number?" (McCulloch, 1961). The first part of this chapter begins to answer the question: "What are languages that humans may know them and humans that they may know languages?" This may seem widely divergent from this book's emphasis on architecture, but the second half of the chapter will provide a bridge to the design of buildings, the focus of the book's final chapters, to argue that the language-ready brain was shaped by complementary strands of cultural evolution to yield human societies that could use drawing as well as language, and that together with "the thinking hand and its brain" came to develop sophisticated construction technologies for buildings and the practices for designing them. In this way, different societies with different histories could each develop their own distinctive cultures, including different languages and different styles of architecture.

To get started, note that language has two essential properties: parity and compositional semantics. *Parity* is the key to any communication system—the receiver can make sense (more or less) of each message from a sender who employs the communication system. What *compositional semantics* adds to *language parity* is that, because of the way grammars let us combine words, the messages may convey novel meanings.

Recall the general EvoDevoSocio point that genes do not specify all the capabilities of the adult. They specify the developmental processes that will yield the adult (as well as ongoing programs for adult cells), and this development has the potential to be shaped in diverse ways by both the physical and social environment. Then, in turn, members of the group can reshape those environments (*niche construction*—they construct a new ecological niche that is both physical and cultural), thus opening new developmental pathways for future generations. Each individual engages with only certain parts of the niche and has the ability through learning to master more of it and possibly to reshape it. For this reason, a capability X may not have been part of the selection pressure that endowed a certain species with a species-specific genome, but over time groups may *construct a new niche* such that individuals raised in that niche do have the capability X. The brain was X-ready, but only though cultural evolution did a community come to invent and use such an X. In particular, this chapter will outline one account of how humans evolved to have language-ready brains, and how cultural evolution enabled much later generations, after tens of millennia, to develop languages.

The archeological record is silent about when humans first used language, but it is clear that humans and their predecessors had the ability to make stone tools. Both *Homo sapiens* and Neanderthals have left traces of engravings, statuettes, beads, and more over the past 100,000 years, with the earliest known cave paintings appearing around 40,000 years ago. Agriculture may have been invented between 20,000 and 10,000 years ago, while the oldest city may date to 4500 BCE. Which of these capabilities required genetic changes that spread to all current *Homo sapiens* and which were the product of cultural evolution building on prior capacities of brain, body, and society without a necessary change in the genome? There is consensus that the emergence of agriculture and cities falls in the latter class, while there is debate over whether the emergence of language and art required a significant change in the *Homo sapiens* genome less than 100,000 years ago. Starting in the next section, I will present the *mirror system hypothesis* (MSH) on which I have worked for the past 20 years. It is not universally accepted by researchers on language evolution, but it is one of a few leading theories, and arguments from outside language enhance its plausibility. MSH offers a hand-centered view that, unlike a voice-centered view, can explain how the human brain could also support the emergence, through cultural evolution, of drawing and model-building.

As a comparison point, consider that almost all humans can learn to read, and yet reading and writing have only existed for a few thousand years, and even today some tribes have a spoken language but no writing system. But we also know that the human brain is *reading-ready* even in illiterate societies—a child from such a society, but then raised in a literate family, has little problem learning to read—but did not evolve under any adaptive pressure to support reading. Reading is a cultural innovation. In the same way, I suggest that language is a cultural innovation. Early *Homo sapiens* had a *language-ready brain*, but only 100,000 to 50,000 years ago did humans go from having rather basic *protolanguages*—a stock of "protowords" with little or no grammar—to having flexible languages that combined a rich stock of words together with a grammar that enabled them to express novel meanings with a reasonable expectation that others in their community would comprehend them.

Given the emphasis on cultural evolution in the two or three hundred millennia in which *Homo sapiens* has existed, are the biological underpinnings still relevant to architecture? Clearly, yes. The need for places to find, store, prepare, and consume food, and the complementary places to empty the bladder and the bowels, set basic constraints, as do the need to support privacy and yet also support a sense of family and community, as well as to address aesthetic criteria that may engage biophilia or the appreciation of perceptual qualities that supported hunting and foraging. Stairs are a product of cultural evolution, but the width and height of the steps must be adjusted to serve human legs.

Yet, having noted all this, we see that so many of the architect's challenges must be met within a specific, culturally constructed niche. Focus for the moment on just the notion of "home." Consider how the demands change in the design for a cabin off the grid for a hunter living in the woods, for a self-sufficient farming family who must grow their own crops and raise their own livestock, and for a couple living in a city with food shops and restaurants nearby; and then overlay the different customs and traditions of different cultures. Note, too, that a design that makes sense in the north of Finland makes little sense in Mali unless one takes the very different ranges of temperature and humidity into account. Biology and culture are intertwined.

8.2. FROM MIRROR SYSTEMS TO COMPLEX IMITATION, PANTOMIME, AND PEDAGOGY

A couple of cautionary notes for our exploration of evolution:

1. We did not evolve from monkeys or apes—there are many different modern species of monkeys and apes, each with a long evolutionary history. Rather—and this is still a simplification—we evolved 5 to 7 million years ago from the last common ancestor we shared with great apes (LCA-c; c for chimpanzee, the great ape genetically closest to humans), which in turn evolved from the last common ancestor we shared with monkeys (LCA-m) some 25 million years ago. A further caveat is that speciation did not, in its early stage, block genetic mixing—there is no single Adam and Eve, and today's *Homo sapiens* still have a small percentage of Neanderthal genes.

2. Evolution is not directed to some end goal, such as endowing humans with language. At each time, mutations create variation on which natural selection can operate. As a result, some species go extinct and others emerge that are well-suited to some ecological niche. Moreover, some changes that initially prove beneficial by some criteria may in the long run be counterproductive—but if they were successful long enough, they establish new starting points for further change that will carry the "burden" of this maladaptation. Moreover, in *cultural* evolution, some changes will be of benefit to many members of a population, some will cater to the tastes of an elite with little impact on others, and some will involve strengthening the power of one group only at the cost of the subjugation of others. Short-term gains may breed long-term disasters.

With these caveats in mind, let us see how biocultural evolution may have created the language-ready brain, even though language-readiness was absent in LCA-m and LCA-c (Figure 8.1). The theory offered here is called the "mirror system hypothesis" (MSH) because of its roots in the study of the mirror systems in macaque monkeys and humans (Arbib & Rizzolatti, 1997; Rizzolatti & Arbib, 1998). However, "complex imitation" (described later) plays the key role in later development of the theory (Arbib, 2012).[1]

Where many approaches to language evolution emphasize a direct transition from monkey-like vocal calls to speech, MSH emphasizes our capacity shared with monkeys and apes for manual skill and the ability to learn new skills. Mirror neurons in area F5 of monkey premotor cortex contain mirror neurons. These are engaged not only in the monkey's own hand movements but also in the recognition of the manual actions of others

1. I think it fair to say that by now the theory has gained a good measure of acceptance, but it still faces competition from other theories. At a recent conference, experts from diverse disciplines evaluated its strength and weaknesses and pointed the way to further research (Arbib, 2020; Arbib et al., 2018).

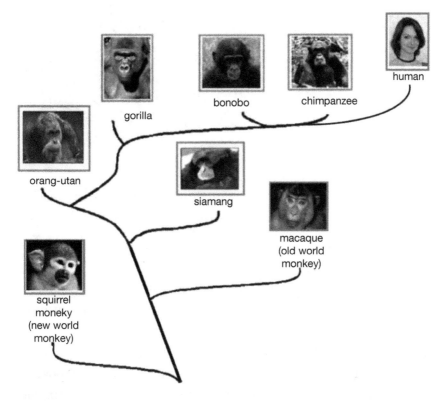

Figure 8.1 An evolutionary tree showing the last common ancestor of humans with monkeys and chimpanzees, LCA-m and LCA-c, respectively. (Adapted from Arbib, M. A. [2012]. *How the brain got language: The mirror system hypothesis.* New York and Oxford: Oxford University Press.)

(§5.3). The key observation for developing MSH was that part of Broca's area in the front of the human brain is homologous (i.e., is related through brain evolution from common ancestors; Figure 8.2) to F5 in the monkey brain, and that brain imaging of Broca's area reveals that it behaves like an area rich in mirror neurons for grasping—it is active both when somebody grasps an object and when they see somebody else grasp the object, compared to the baseline of activity for just looking at the object.

This link to hand movements might seem puzzling because, traditionally, Broca's area had been regarded as a *speech* production area. The missing link was provided by Ursula Bellugi and her husband Ed Klima, who,

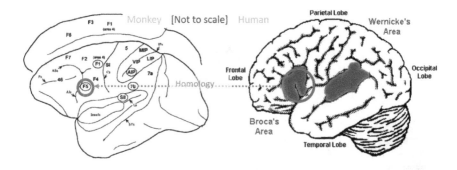

Figure 8.2 The inspiration for the mirror system hypothesis for the evolution of the language-ready brain was provided by the homology between the F5 area of macaque premotor cortex, site of the mirror neurons for manual actions, and human Broca's area, long implicated in speech production.

working with Howard Poizner (Poizner, Klima, & Bellugi, 1987), discovered that there were some deaf people who had used sign language but had had brain lesions involving Broca's area—and these people exhibited aphasia of sign language similar to aphasia of spoken language, where in each case brain damage impairs access to the words (whether spoken or signed) and, crucially, the use of grammar to combine them meaningfully. This led to the crucial insight that Broca's area is not only a *speech* production area, it is a *language* production area. Its computations can (depending on the enculturation of the language user) be equally well deployed for spoken language (audition in, vocal signals out) and signed language (vision in, manual signals out).

MSH postulates that LCA-m had a mirror system for manual actions. The challenge was to plausibly chart the transition from executing and recognizing practical actions using the hands to the use of manual gestures for communication and then (by a long and winding path) to language in both the manual and vocal domains.

A key distinction: If I say "grenting" and articulate it clearly, then, even though this is not a word of English, you would probably be able to repeat it. But that recognition of the form of a (potential) word as evidenced by your ability to repeat it even if it is a nonword is, I claim, as far as "(audio-vocal) mirror neurons evolved for language" can get you. You need brain mechanisms that support the lexicon—recognizing the word not only as a manual or vocal pattern but also as one with an associated meaning or meanings. And then, crucially, you need to master the grammar of the language. This is made up of *constructions* (in the linguists' sense) that do the following: given some words or phrases with known meaning, each construction will specify the way to combine the words in each constituent to form a new word pattern (the *syntactic* part of the construction), while at the same combining the meanings to specify a new meaning (the *semantic* part of the construction), though the interpretation of that meaning may be affected by context.

A simple example in English takes a noun phrase A, a verb V, and a second noun phrase B, and specifies that these can be combined to yield the new pattern "A V-ed B," with the meaning that "the person or object denoted by A carried out the action denoted by V on the person or object B"—so that the combination "Bill punched Bob" means something different from "Bob punched Bill." Of course, there are many subtleties that lie outside this basic process of assembling (speaking) and parsing (hearing) the resultant utterances focused on here. First, consider the parity principle: Understanding a meaning from words is not the same as empathizing with someone's mood or intentions, and paying attention to the posture and facial expression of someone may transform the meaning one extracts from words alone. Second, we know that interpretation depends on context, not just the local assemblage of words. On the page, a sentence is a visual display, but (in English) we read from left to right so that, as in speech or sign, it becomes a structure extended in time but with a particular order—unlike the ad hoc attention/task-driven sequence of fixations with which we make sense of a visual scene. But even here, our interpretation of a word may depend on more than its relation to other words in the current sentence. Consider, "They were having a terrible row." Probably you think that "row" rhymes with "cow" and that "they" were arguing or even fighting. But both interpretations may change if the next sentence is, "The waves were almost too strong for them." Now "row" rhymes with "so," and they are in a boat. Of course, the same phenomenon can occur in speech. Moreover, even if the words are unambiguous, different constructions may change the meaning. "He kicked the bucket" may be an idiom for "He died," but if the next phrase is, "and had to spend the next five minutes mopping up the water," the idiom does not apply. Just like schemas competing and cooperating in VISIONS, so too may word meanings and constructions compete and cooperate in interpreting a fragment of language, and this may involve top-down processes and extend over time in a fashion denied to the processing of a single snapshot.

From simple to complex imitation

Monkeys have manual dexterity, including a mirror system, but very little ability in the way of imitation, and their communication rests on a few innate vocal calls.

Apes have, in addition, the ability to communicate with a limited set of manual gestures, some of which are "cultural" rather than innate. They can imitate fairly well if the observed behavior is built up simply from a few familiar actions (call it *simple imitation*) but seem unable to attend to the movement details of how some overall goal is attained. A good example comes from Masako Myowa in Kyoto:

> A ball and a bowl are sitting on the floor. The human demonstrator picks up the bowl and places it over the ball, without moving the ball. The ape does not recognize that the crucial point is that the ball does not move; it just sees that the result is to have the ball in the bowl— and so it picks up both and moves them together so that the ball is covered by the bowl.

Simple imitation thus involves *attention to subgoals* more than to the details of the movements that achieve them. If the young ape sees an older ape perform a behavior of the kind, "achieve A (a subgoal), and then achieve B (the final goal)," the young ape will try to achieve A by trial and error, not paying attention to the actual hand movements the adult uses to achieve A. Similarly for B. Myowa-Yamakoshi (2018) reviews the characteristics of imitation in chimpanzees and humans, and relates her data to how these two species differ in the ways they process visuomotor information. This grounds a "developmental-comparative" approach to the development of species-specific intelligences, and shows what is shared and not shared between humans and other primates.

Unlike chimpanzees (and, presumably, LCA-c), humans can master *complex action recognition*, the ability to observe a moderately complex behavior and break it down into its constituent pieces, recognizing not only the end-states of the intermediate pieces but also some details of the pattern of movement in each one. This recognition may be an end in itself, but can also be the basis for *complex imitation*, which includes some attempt to reproduce the movement details as well as taking note of possible subgoals. This does not mean that we can imitate everything at first go, but with each attempt, we can better observe some of the details we failed to replicate earlier and in due course come to better and better approximate the observed performance.

The distinction between simple and complex imitation can be conveyed by what I call the *Ikea effect*. If you buy a furniture kit from Ikea and start assembling the item, you may see a picture of what comes next and, without bothering to look at the accompanying instructions, believe you know how to achieve the subgoal that the picture depicts. You grab a piece, you jam it in, you grab another piece, you jam it in. But the result may be quite different from what was pictured. Then you have to disassemble it and start over again, paying attention to details of the constituent movements, not just to the subgoals.[2]

---

2. For much more on this topic, see Chapter 7, "Simple and Complex Imitation," of *How the Brain Got Language* (Arbib, 2012).

"Acting" in the absence of objects: on to ad hoc pantomime

MSH posits a crucial transition in which the capacity of mirror neurons (working with systems beyond the mirror) becomes extended from the recognition of actions carried out on objects to gestures performed in the absence of objects. This supports a new, open-ended form of communication—*pantomime*. Here, the pantomime is ad hoc—repeating an action as if the object were "there," as distinct from pantomime as a set of ritualized performances in the style of Marcel Marceau. If I pantomime holding a cup and raising it to my lips (but with no cup nearby), then, depending on the context, you might see this as an invitation for you to drink or a request to you to give me a cup of coffee. The mixture of context and pantomime convey meaning.

Pantomime *as a new system of communicative action* not only rests on available brain mechanisms but also requires *cultural evolution* to exploit those mechanisms. If I had performed the absent-cup-to-lip performance in a society that did not recognize pantomime as such, it would be meaningless. This new stage (posited by MSH to occur after LCA-c) couples the extension of brain mechanisms to recognize performances in the absence of objects with the biocultural evolution that yields a culture in which protohumans could create and recognize ad hoc pantomimes and use them to communicate.[3]

Pantomime is not restricted to communicating about behaviors. It can also be based on the shape of objects with the hands "drawing contours in the air" that mimic the movements of the hand in haptically exploring the object. This observation will prove crucial in supporting the claim that the language-ready brain is also a drawing-ready brain (§8.4).

According to MSH, the capabilities for complex action recognition, complex imitation of manual skills, and pantomime all evolved long

---

3. For more on pantomime, see the first half of Chapter 8, "Via Pantomime to Protosign," of *How the Brain Got Language* (Arbib, 2012). For the debate over whether great apes can pantomime as a form of ad hoc communication that supports parity, see Russon (2018).

before the brain was language-ready. They supported the spread of new skills and tool use and manufacture. This was not "evolving toward language," though MSH can now, looking back, chart its relevance: the ability to imitate practical actions provides mechanisms that persist in the language-ready brain of *Homo sapiens*, where ability to imitate will be crucial to the child in a language-rich community building up a vocabulary, while complex action recognition will be crucial to the ability to understand what another person is saying.

8.3. FROM PANTOMIME TO PROTOLANGUAGES AND ON TO LANGUAGES

With this preparation, we can now focus on the biocultural evolution that, according to MSH, led to protolanguage and a language-ready brain, and then suggest how such a brain provided mechanisms to support the emergence of languages through cultural evolution.

From pantomime to protosign

Ad hoc pantomime has two problems. First, it is costly; it takes a long time to mime a complex behavior. Second, it is highly ambiguous. MSH thus suggests that the next cultural innovation within a community that already had pantomime was to conventionalize the pantomimes so that variants were developed that were easier to perform and less ambiguous. The downside is that one has to spend time in the community to learn how to form these new gestures and the meanings each conveys.

An anachronistic example from American Sign Language (ASL) may help. There is a handshape that is meant to indicate the shape of a plane with its wings extended. If we don't know anything about ASL and see someone move this handshape through a long trajectory, we might think they are pantomiming "plane flying." However, ASL has transformed this basic pantomime into two distinct, conventionalized signs. If you move the handshape through a long arc, it's the sign for "flying," whether or not it's a plane that is flying; but if you wiggle it in place, you get the sign for "plane." The claim, then, is that before our distant ancestors got to *signs* of a language *with a grammar*, their even earlier ancestors had *proto-signs* where conventionalization allowed them to communicate, using the hands, relatively economically *within a community*.[4]

Nonhuman apes and monkeys have little in the way of vocal control and learning, and so it required an evolutionary breakthrough to have the vocal control develop to the point where voice could be exploited as a medium for communication of novel words or protowords. MSH hypothesizes that when brain mechanisms and social structure had evolved to the point that apparently arbitrary gestures could be used to communicate new meanings, there was a new selective advantage to adapt manual control mechanisms to support vocal control as well—thus extending the ability to generate novel communicative gestures to vocal gestures. However, for too many researchers, the key feature of human language is that it is spoken, and the signed languages of the Deaf, if noted at all, are seen as a side effect of possessing spoken language. Many thus argue that vocal control emerged in humans much as it emerged in songbirds or whales, and that language emerged as vocalizations became linked to novel meanings that could then be assembled flexibly to convey novel meanings, something lacking in other species. For MSH, however, it is manual communication that first became more complex and, only later, after divergence from LCA-c, scaffolded the biological evolution of vocal control mechanisms. Vocal control did not precede the free expression of meaning.[5]

4. For more on protosign, see the second half of Chapter 8, "Via Pantomime to Protosign," of *How the Brain Got Language* (Arbib, 2012).

5. Since the focus in this chapter is on manual skills, I will not take up this debate here—it is discussed at length in Chapter 9, "Protosign and Protospeech: An Expanding Spiral," of *How the Brain Got Language* (Arbib, 2012). A fascinating question: Did the benefits of increased vocal control lead to the evolution of new brain mechanisms in protohumans in just one location and spread out from there, or was the adaptive pressure so widely shared that protohumans independently developed vocal control in diverse locations, but then migration, and interaction between different communities, finally led to such brain mechanisms dominating the human

This debate demonstrates that cog/neuroscience is by no means a closed book. Some cog/neuro topics relevant to the A↔N conversation are well established, some (as exemplified here) are open to competing interpretations, and some will not emerge until new questions are asked. Conversely, there is much neuroscience that appears irrelevant to architecture (such as the molecular biology of neurons, crucial though that may be to drug design), and much about architecture that offers no challenges of interest to the neuroscientist. But let's get back to the language-ready brain, for now.

A powerful adaptive pressure for the enrichment of protolanguages may have come from the spur to cultural evolution from being able to teach new skills to others. Patricia Zukow-Goldring (2012; Zukow-Goldring & Arbib, 2007) has shown that mothers can teach diverse skills to children too young to understand spoken instructions by using *assisted* imitation—they pantomime the constituent actions while drawing the child's attention to, for example, affordances of the objects salient for the skill. For modern adults, such early skill transfer may require at most a fragment of language, a "micro-protolanguage," to expand the range of such assistance.

Exploring the evolutionary implications of this, we may, in the spirit of Stout's technological pedagogy hypothesis (Stout, 2018), hypothesize that the diverse activities of early human groups (not just tool-making but also making a fire, child care, foraging, hunting, and much more) may have provided many protolanguage fragments. Peter Gärdenfors has developed related ideas in "The Archaeology of Teaching and the Evolution of *Homo docens* [the humans who teach]" (Gärdenfors & Högberg, 2017). He has also argued that the fundamental capacities that distinguish human teaching are demonstration and pantomime (Gärdenfors, 2017), an observation that is especially relevant to the teaching of future architects.

genome? Or did vocal control far beyond the capabilities of nonhuman primates emerge for quite separate reasons, and only later become "exapted" to support protolanguage?

Cultural evolution from protolanguages to languages

To summarize the state of play: We have summarized, briefly, the path that MSH traces from LCA-m to LCA-c and on to protohumans (perhaps early *Homo sapiens*, but perhaps even earlier ancestors, ancient enough to be the ancestors of both modern humans and Neanderthals) who had manual skills, complex action recognition, complex imitation, and protosign (both manual and spoken). Crucially, though, we have so far said nothing about grammar, and so we will not say that a band of such humans had a language, but only that they had a *protolanguage*, a system of "protowords," manual and/or spoken protosigns, but with little or nothing in the way of combining protosigns to convey new meanings beyond mere concatenation. Unlike languages with tens of thousands of words, different groups might have had different "microprotolanguages," each with just tens or a few hundreds of protowords relevant to some specific form of behavior, such as tool-making, foraging, or childrearing. Even within a single tribe, different subgroups might have had distinct microprotolanguages specialized for communication relevant to their social roles.

To complete MSH, then, the claim is that when early *Homo sapiens* emerged, they already had both manual and vocal protolanguage—an open-ended system of manual and vocal signs, but with little or no grammar. Complex action recognition supported the ability to break a pantomime or a protosign into pieces that were candidates for adding to the stock of words. The real breakthrough to grammar, though, was that the way those pieces combined could provide a basic set of simple constructions (in the linguist's sense) as the first step toward grammar.

Another anachronistic example: If I pantomime closing a door, I might mime turning a door handle as I move my hand away from my body; while if I pantomime opening a door, I might mime turning a door handle as I move my hand toward my body. What is common to the *meaning* of the two performances is that I am doing something to a *door*, yet all that is common to the *movement* is *turning the handle*. Conventionalization might then establish that the handle-turning motion is the protosign for *door*, even though it was not a pantomime of a door. The complementary parts of each pantomime might then become the protosigns for *close* and *open*. That invites you to generalize, for example *open door* to *open* X where X might be replaced by different protowords. Inserting a sign for *mouth* could convey the new meaning *open mouth*. Note that we might be tempted to call this protosign for *open* a protoverb, and these protosigns for *door* and *mouth* protonouns—but this may be getting tens of millennia ahead of the game. My hypothesis is that the first constructions were very limited—the only slot-fillers for *open* X came from a limited set of protowords for the cognitive category of "openable things," and so had very little (if anything) in common with the slot-fillers for *want* Y.

Our ancestral communities began to build such constructions as they developed new ways (whether manual, vocal, or both) of putting words together, as well as building more words (details are provided in Chapter 10 of Arbib, 2012). The result is a cognitive spiral—new words and constructions help us build new concepts of the world; we then build new ways of expressing ideas concerning those concepts, and each one feeds into the other. Co-evolution of cognitive and linguistic complexity supports the construction of new "cognitive niches." Only much later could generalization across perhaps hundreds of specialized categories of construction-specific slot-fillers have yielded what we now recognize as syntactic categories like *noun* and *verb*—though even here be warned: every modern language has both object-related words and action-related words, but how these groups of words are extended is in no way universal.

Even though some biological evolution of the human genome has continued in the past 200,000 years, cultural evolution has come to dominate the dramatic changes of the environment, both mental and physical, to which each of us adapts as we grow to become adults. We may thus talk of the *culture-ready brain* (Whitehead, 2010). But first, let's concentrate on drawing.

8.4. THE LANGUAGE-READY BRAIN IS ALSO CONSTRUCTION-READY AND DRAWING-READY

I will argue that the same properties that gave humans a language-ready brain also gave us a *construction-ready brain* and, in particular, a *drawing-ready brain*—and even an *architecture-ready brain*, thus laying the basis for discussion of the neuroscience of design in Chapter 10.

The construction-ready brain

The linguist's construction is "a tool for putting words and meanings together" but, more generally (§1.1), *construction* can be seen to include transforming and assembling objects in both mental and physical worlds. Physical construction may include subtractive construction (as in knapping to produce stone tools) as well as additive construction (the assembly of components and transforming them to fit together). Like language, human visual perception of a scene is a form of mental construction (§3.4), limited by the stock of available perceptual schemes that link visual form and meaning—but also open to the discovery or mastery of new schemas. So too for acts of imagination, including making plans for action. The work of the architect stops short of physical construction. Rather, the design process is another process of *mental* construction (though it may involve the physical construction of sketches and models), developing both general ideas and ideas focused on small parts of the building. Eventually, these become so transformed that through logic and integrative thinking they cohere into a detailed plan that can guide physical construction of the building itself. Design involves going back and forth between an emerging understanding of the whole and of the parts. Only when these are coordinated and harmonized can the design fully specify how the physical construction of the building is to proceed.

The MSH approach to the evolution of language stresses the crucial role of manual gestures. I will show how it suggests that the human brain's *readiness* to support language and sketching evolved together, even though the *cultural* evolution that developed these capabilities in human societies occurred on very different timescales. Let's focus first on drawing and then return to architecture.

External memory and the evolution of drawing

In his book, *Origins of the Modern Mind*, Merlin Donald (1991, 1993), posits three stages in the evolution of cognition and culture that separate the modern human mind from that of our common ancestor with the chimpanzees:

1. The introduction of a supramodal, motor-modeling capacity that he calls *mimesis*, and the exploitation of this capability to create representations with the critical property of voluntary retrievability.
2. The addition of a capacity for lexical invention, and a high-speed phonological apparatus, the latter being a specialized mimetic subsystem.
3. The introduction of intentional *external memory* storage and retrieval, and a new working memory architecture.

MSH is broadly consistent with this general framework, but insists that complex imitation of *hand movements* was a crucial precursor to the development of an open system of communication because pantomime provided a rich semantic range that could ground the later emergence of conventionalized communicative utterances. As for stage 2, MSH asserts that (i) protosign exploits the ability for complex imitation of hand movements to support an open system of communication; and (ii) the resulting protosign provides scaffolding for protospeech; but that (iii) protosign and protospeech develop together thereafter. The strong MSH hypothesis is that protosign is essential to this process, so that the full development of protospeech was made possible by the protosign scaffolding.

Back to Merlin Donald. He claims that, after modern humans reached their present biological form, they had a fully developed speech capacity as well as complex oral cultures. I would add the role of manual skill and gesture in these cultures. Donald's stage 3 postulates a further change: *the development of external memory*. Many actions will leave physical traces, but being able to intentionally make markings or other external reminders not only dramatically increased individual memory capacity but also created new realms of *shared* memory. Donald's hypothesis is that this transition started in the Upper Paleolithic from 50,000 to 10,000 years ago with the invention of permanent visual symbols, preceding the development of agriculture and urbanization. It is still underway.

Could such external memory systems have come about through cultural evolution exploiting the mechanisms charted in MSH, or did they require further biological evolution of brain and body? "Is the language-ready brain also drawing-ready?" The answer would seem problematic if one's theory of language origins focused only on spoken language and held that the path from monkey-like vocalizations to human vocal learning and spoken language was direct. However, if one accepts the role of complex imitation, pantomime, and manual gesture on the path to language, then the answer is, rather directly, "Yes."

The problem is that communication with spoken or signed (proto)language (as distinct from its manifestation in writing) is a social act that does not require tools. Drawing and painting do. To take the anachronistic example of a cup of coffee, we can ask: "What must be added to a brain that can lift and drink from a cup to get a brain that can draw the cup? What experience must a person with such a brain have to exhibit a capacity for drawing?"

By running my hand around the real cup, I can trace its contours in three dimensions. A skill for pantomime includes the ability to mime lifting a cup and drinking from it, but it also includes the ability to trace similar contours in midair in the absence of a cup as part of a cup-related message. The breakthrough to drawing for someone with the ability to use pantomime for communication is to go from this evanescent tracing of contours in three dimensions to the more or less enduring marking of contours on a two-dimensional (2D) surface. However, the cognitive transformation from making a mimetic gesture in midair to making an *enduring* mark on a surface *cannot occur without the availability of a supporting technology,* such as using a burnt stick to mark a cave wall.[6] Such marks can then form an external memory to aid later discussion or action. The behavior, including the relevant tool use, is clearly within the range of creatures whose brains have a flexible capacity for pantomime, yet involves cultural evolution to yield communities that can use drawings as a memory system to expand the reach of their interactions. The development of such a skill requires visuo-manual coordination as well as "surface-oriented pantomime." For a hunter, a pattern of movement in the leaves or even a piece of scat may be as clear an indication of the presence of a specific kind of animal as a clear view of the animal, and auditory cues can be just as effective. Thus, diverse perceptual experiences related to similar activities can evoke related associations even if the "reality of what the schema represents" is absent. The skill of the artist, then, may be to evoke multiple schemas beyond those elicited by direct experience (recall the discussion of "Inverting vision" in §4.4).

But there is more to visual or other perception than contours, as our appreciation of shape from shading in Figure 8.3 shows, and the extra "message" added by the color of the coffee. In the earlier discourse on visual perception (§3.2), I mentioned the work of David Hubel and Torsten Wiesel, who found neurons in visual cortex of cats and monkeys whose firing correlated best with fragments of edges. Further neural processing can integrate these fragments to extract contours. While this could help explain why you can recognize a person from a caricature, you can nonetheless distinguish between an actual face and a caricature. For this, it is crucial that higher levels of abstraction do not throw away details of color and shading but do provide a framework within which their interpretation (including implications for action) can be elaborated.

---

6. We are talking here of technologies that were needed to support, for example, the cave paintings of 30,000 or more years ago. After tens of millennia of cultural evolution, computer graphics has expanded our notion of drawing in general and sketching as part of architectural practice in particular.

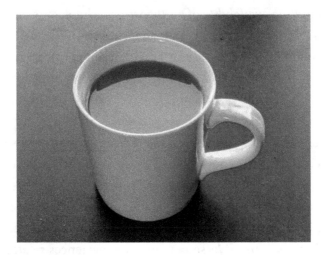

Figure 8.3 To draw this, follow the contours of the actual object—but a patch of color will help. (Author's photo.)

The knowledge of contours as a basis for action was crucial to human behavior long before there was language or drawing—knowing how to use those contours for childrearing, hunting, foraging, and taking food and exploiting it. The further cultural breakthrough was to understand ways that the contours that came from an interaction with objects could be turned into contours on a cave wall. The complementary discovery was how to use patches of color to complement those contours. This might accompany a belief system in which such depictions were understood to capture something of the spirit or soul of an animal as the basis for hunting, or for placating the spirit of the captured animal. Note, incidentally, that here—as in hunting, or tool-making, or childbearing—we see the emergence of social roles, as some develop skills that others may be able to recognize and interpret, but not to skillfully perform.

The earliest known European cave paintings use color to fill out the basic contours. This may have involved repurposing of a much older skill. We know that humans have been using ocher for perhaps 200,000 years. Dubreuil and Henshilwood (2013) discuss findings at Twin Rivers in

Zambia and at Kapthurin in Kenya that provide "convincing proof of the symbolic use of pigments during the Acheulean–Middle Stone Age transition (ca. 200 thousand years ago) associated with early *Homo sapiens*" (p. 253) and attest that "ochre pieces and bone fragments engraved with abstract patterns dated to c.75 ka . . . constitute, at present, among the most ancient persuasive evidence for symbolic behavior" (p. 254). The use of ocher to decorate the body may thus be a very ancient one, inspired perhaps by the bright plumage of birds. The huge time gap from the first known use of ocher suggests that major cultural innovation was required to master the intentional disposition of patches of color as a complement to the pantomime-derived exploitation of contours in the first known cave paintings.

Having integrated language-readiness with drawing-readiness, it is important to stress that it took different paths of cultural evolution to support the emergence of drawing and language (cave paintings are relatively recent).

The Chauvet paintings were discovered in 1994 in the Chauvet Cave located near Vallon-Pont-d'Arc in the Ardèche region of southern France and dated to 31,000 years ago (Figure 8.4). They are skillfully executed and offer an exceptionally fine and well-preserved example of early human creativity. The cave contained not only the fossilized remains of many animals, including some that are now extinct, but also extensive galleries of Paleolithic "art." I put the quotes around "art" to remind us that the creation and viewing of paintings in these caves some 30,000 years ago may well have involved psychological impulses far removed from those of the artist whose works adorn modern art galleries and the viewers who admire them. Wentzel Van Huyssteen (2006) focuses on what it must have been like to paint and view the paintings deep in the dark cave by whatever flickering light source was available at the time, and argues for the shamanic role of ancient cave paintings. However, although Chauvet shows that some humans around 30,000 years ago in what is now France were able to draw pictures of animals, we do not know how many people had this skill or to what extent it lasted for more than a generation.

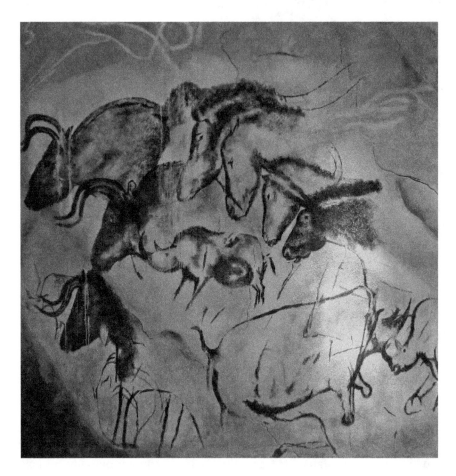

Figure 8.4 Replica of a cave painting dated to approximately 31,000 years ago in the Chauvet cave in France. As Magritte would say, "Ce n'est pas une peinture rupestre." (https://upload.wikimedia.org/wikipedia/commons/c/c0/Paintings_from_the_Chauvet_cave_%28museum_replica%29.jpg. Public domain.)

Derek Denton (personal communication) notes that the Bradshaw paintings (Gwion Gwion) in the Kimberley region of Northwest Australia[7] are painted in the open air and focus much more on the human figure (Figure 8.5). These date back perhaps 12,000 years. There

---

7. The Bradshaw paintings (known as Gwion to the Aboriginal traditional owners) in the Kimberley region of Northwest Australia were first seen by European eyes by Joseph Bradshaw in 1891 when he became lost searching for missing cattle in the million-acre lease he had been granted. Among websites with a good collection of pictures of the Bradshaw paintings are http://agricola2000.tripod.com/Kimberlies.htm and http://www.sauer-thompson.com/junkforcode/

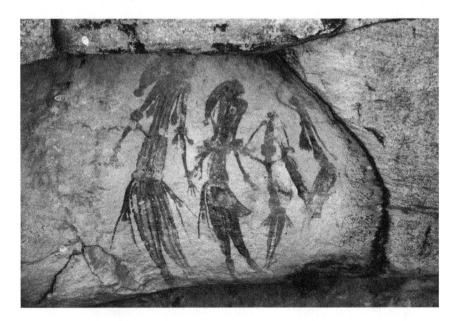

Figure 8.5 An example of the Gwion Gwion (Bradshaw) paintings. (https://upload.wikimedia.org/wikipedia/commons/4/43/Bradshaw_rock_paintings.jpg, Creative Commons Attribution-Share Alike 2.0 Generic license.)

is no single explanation for how or why (or where) humans first began to paint figures. More to the point, note the likely misapprehension in using the term "first," as if one primal discovery seeded all the others. It is far more likely that many different individuals and groups "discovered" drawing independently, at widely different times and places in human prehistory. Some such discoveries died with their discoverers, and others created new social schemas that developed across time and space for many generations, or even longer.

We still do not know what the ancient cave paintings meant to those who created them and to their contemporaries who viewed them and, perhaps, engaged in associated rituals. However, as John Onians (2007)— who established the field of "neuroarthistory" (Onians, 2008)—observes, the Chauvet paintings do provide material evidence of a crucial transition

archives/2006/09/the-bradshaw-pa.html. An intriguing novel by Nicholas Hasluck (2016) presents a modern-day law case and adventure (both fictional) focused on controversies over the provenance of the Bradshaw paintings.

from vision as a basis for interacting with the physical world to vision that can take images as their locus, with the focus on the invested meaning of those images. This brings us back to Donald's stress on the importance of intentional external memory.

Interaction with those images and the creation of new ones may thus have come to replace, or at least add symbolic meaning to, interaction with the animals these images represent. Similarly, words arranged in sentences may have an immediate relation to the demands of ongoing practical behavior or may be used within a system of references little related to such needs. All this is part of the move to symbolic systems, of which language is one, but not the only, key component—a component that includes not only drawing and painting but also the symbolism of architecture.

To further see how hand motions for a specific form of embodiment may transfer to the manual action of drawing, consider the pairing of visual and haptic affordances with the contours experienced when stroking an object, and add the ability to make sensorimotor transformations when using a tool as a possible basis for the ability to draw an object. In this case the end effector is changed from the palm of the hand to, perhaps, paint-bearing fingers or a piece of charcoal to, as technology develops, the tip of a pencil or brush.

What of the ability to draw landscapes? This would seem to rest in part on the ability to ignore size constancy, the ability to compensate for distance in estimating the true size of an object from its projection on the retinas. In general, we understand that an object is not shrinking as it moves away from us. If we see something very large in a landscape, a mountain let's say, we cannot trace the contours of the mountain directly, but we can move our hand so that it *appears* to trace the contours of the mountain, and it is these contours that allow us to transfer the object to the page. Relating a far object to possible interactions may extend to "caressing" or holding or acting upon the object "metaphorically," as in capturing the contours of a hillside or sand dunes.

But how do we get from the ability to trace a contour to artistic skill? A few brief comments will have to suffice. The key point is that mastery requires intense practice. To take an example of manual skill from another genre, in *Ways of the Hand*, Sudnow (2001) traces the process whereby he learned to become a jazz pianist from hitting the right note to "automatizing" a hierarchy from chords to varied sequences to the point that improvisation became possible. However, even the greatest pianist must practice constantly to "retune" the motor schemas in this hierarchy so that the actual performance can infuse the playing with an overall panache and emotional style.

More generally, then, to develop a creative skill, the relevant motor schemas and their perceptual tuning via available affordances must become automatized. As a result, you don't have to attend the details as you create or perform, and so can just invoke the schemas as needed and "move up a level" in thinking about the work. I have only once given a talk in Spanish. It was in Santiago de Chile, and I found it incredibly grueling because I had to concentrate on every phoneme of every word, whereas when I speak in English, the form of words needs no attention as I work at the level of overall sentences to convey my thoughts. In the Chile speech, I understood the meaning and could express the emotional shading, but not all ideas were mastered in terms of words at a production level, and thus I had to refer to a written text as I spoke.

Automatization of schemas at one level supports complex planning at higher levels—but requires knowing what can be executed successfully and with what results. Similarly, in mastering painting, one moves from thinking about brushstrokes and choosing paints to expressing one's vision of the whole. An overall image constructs a hierarchical program, but the planning is dynamic. Few details may be available at the start. Rather, the progress to date provides an unfolding context that may alter the guiding image but will certainly change the lower level actions. Creating a work of art or literature or architecture involves a process of construction whereby intermediate constructs may undergo revision and editing as we apply local criteria and better perceive patterns of the whole.

This discussion has brought manual tool use, language, and drawing together in a unified evolutionary framework that reveals that a language-ready brain is indeed culture-ready. This raises an intriguing question: "How can a brain that developed long before the dawn of cave paintings, agriculture, and cities, let alone the complexities of today's global cyber-civilization, have had the capacity to support the complex evolution of such complex systems?" One part of the answer lies in the notion that the emergence of language and of other symbolic systems such as drawing gave us the tools *to record and share memories* on a scale that kept growing, both supporting larger groups, and then further expanding as the larger group supported larger bodies of knowledge made possible by combining the growth of specialized skills with the social tools to integrate them. Another part may be that it is "easier" for a genetic change to double the size of a neural population than to add the 1% of capability that may support the immediate selective advantage. Thus, time and again, biological evolution has provided neural capabilities whose exploitation may take tens of millennia to more fully exploit. Communication *and external memory* expand this by creating communities that know how to integrate the specialized expertise of individuals in moving beyond previous capabilities, in part by developing not only external memory but also a vast repertoire of applicable technologies (Osiurak & Reynaud, 2019).

Preziosi (1979) enriches this theme by offering a semiotic perspective on the evolution of the built environment, stressing the correlations between the semiotic systems of architecture and language. We may note the open-endedness of both systems. A provocative twist on this perspective is offered by Colomina and Wigley (2016), whose notes on an archeology of design pose the question, "are we human?" to emphasize how far developments in cultural evolution, and specifically in design and technology, have indeed "redesigned the human."

8.5. THE NEUROPSYCHOLOGY OF DRAWING

The VISIONS model (§3.4) suggested that in understanding a visual scene we activate (consciously, but often subconsciously, top-down as well as bottom-up) instances of perceptual schemas, which then compete and cooperate to match some (but not all) of the details of the scene. We have considered how the sequencing of actions might have helped develop the structure of grammar in the emergence of language, but here we see how the sequencing of visual attention may have also played a role. In discussing "Inverting vision" (§4.4), I argued that in imagining a scene, we may begin to mentally assemble visual schemas, but with at best a vague specification of the details. To draw the objects and people and relations one imagines, one must refine these visual schemas to come up with the precise parameters for the motor schemas that will bring these imagined entities to the page. Then, much as the preferred schema instance for a region of a scene may change in VISIONS as new details are engaged, and newly (re)cognized context changes the dynamics of competition and cooperation top-down, the emerging patterns on the page may change the overall pattern in the imagination as well as helping to determine how motor schemas may be selected and parameterized to make the next marks on the page.

"What" versus "how" in the visuomotor brain

Given our linkage of the visual control of hand movements to both language (surprisingly) and drawing (of course), let's now return to the two visual pathways for control of the hand (§2.6): the ventral pathway is more engaged in planning a behavior; the dorsal pathway is more concerned with ensuring that motor control matches the details offered by affordances of the objects to be manipulated.

The ventral pathway is called the "what" pathway because it includes brain mechanisms to recognize objects and relationships as well as to develop plans for action, such as picking up a mug to move it to another place versus picking it up to drink from it. The ventral pathway must then coordinate with the dorsal path, the "how" pathway, to scale the various arm and hand movements to the affordances, such as size and position, of the various objects (or parts thereof, such as the handle of a mug) involved in the plan. Spatial attributes can be represented in both dorsal and ventral pathways, but the ventral representation may be more akin to verbal imprecision (e.g., "to the left but quite close"), unlike the precise metrics required to move the hand gracefully to the object.[8]

What does this distinction between "how" and "what" mean for drawing? Is there a sense in which we can talk of sketches that invoke the "how" more than the "what"?

JR, a left-handed artist, was 73 years old when he had a stroke that affected the occipital lobe, a region that contains not only primary visual cortex but also regions that transform the visual input in different ways (so that loss of blood flow in the stroke could damage various subregions, and thus affect behavior, in different ways). Despite little or no impairment in language or cognition, JR was generally unable to identify single objects on visual presentation and showed great difficulty in interpreting complex objects. Nonetheless, he retained various techniques (perspective, shading, indication of texture) that allowed him to copy the display in an *apparently* faithful fashion. One's initial impression of Figure 8.6 might be that JR had made an accurate drawing. However, rather than recognizing the rooster with a long tail, he has drawn the tail as separated from the body, and also separated the lower part of the tail, intermingling its contours with those for the feet of the stove. I suggest we might call this a "how-only" drawing, exploiting the "how" pathway to follow contours, but not the "what" pathway that characterizes what objects are represented in the picture.

Similarly, a number of autistic children may appear to be very skillful at drawing, but the skill is based on contour-by-contour copying uninfected by ideas about the nature of the objects involved. Snyder and Thomas (1997) see this as a virtue: "autistic artists make no assumptions about what is to be seen in their environment. They have not formed mental representations of what is significant and consequently perceive all details as equally important." However, a more accomplished person would use observed contours as suggestions but not as commands. If you were trying to copy the rooster from life, you would use conceptual knowledge

---

8. Note, too, the role of the cerebellum in refining the metrics of sensorimotor transformations—but this is a topic outside our present scope, though mentioned briefly in §2.2.

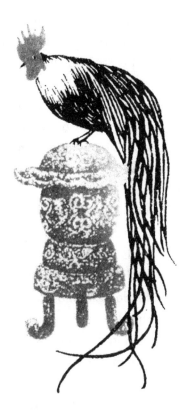
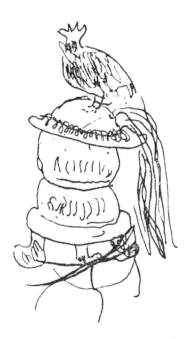

Figure 8.6 Distortions in copying of the screen print at left by JR: Contours are improperly connected due to a failure to recognize the nature of the portrayed object. (Reprinted from Wapner, W., Judd, T., & Gardner, H. [1978]. Visual agnosia in an artist. *Cortex*, 14[3], 343–364, with permission from Elsevier.)

to shape the composition to exploit and adapt, but not be limited by, observed details of form, color, and texture. All of this is not to deny that in later art forms, abstraction from the constraints of reality can constitute a valid piece of art, even one that may be highly valued. Jackson Pollock's paintings might at first seem an example of dominance of the "how" pathway, where the details in the movement replace the linkage to object contours—but here the ventral "what" of objects in the world is reassigned (as it is elsewhere in abstract art) to aesthetic consideration of placements of line and color. We also saw in §3.5 that symmetry may be one of the bases for visual aesthetics, but both in using it and departing from it—and so the present emphasis on representation of objects must be complemented by (non-Pollockian) aspects of geometric form, as highly developed, for example, in wallpaper patterns or the sacred mandalas of Tibetan Buddhism.

There are indeed "abstract paintings" made by chimpanzees,[9] and some people find some of them beautiful, but here, I suspect, the beauty is in the eye of the beholder rather than in the chimpanzee's intentions. Seghers (2014) is blunt: "little or no evidence surfaces to support the presence of intentionalist thinking and symbolic cognition among, for example, chimpanzees, in their response toward painting and drawing material. . . . The evolutionary study of art is therefore unlikely to prosper much through primatology and comparative psychological analysis of humans and their primate cousins." However, we might at least note that chimpanzee painting rests on providing them with the linked technological innovations of paints, brush, and paper. It may not be art, but they know what they like. One might thus consider the visuomotor coordination that underlies this behavior and the pleasure that chimpanzees take in this new form of play as offering new ideas about LCA-c—while recalling that ape gesture is as far from human language as, perhaps, ape "painting" is from art. It may only be the cultural evolution that the language-ready brain made possible that indeed helps us bridge both divides.

Sketching: memory and imagination

In "A System for Drawing and Drawing-Related Neuropsychology," Peter van Sommers (1989) offers a rich account of the insights into drawing one gains from neuropsychology, such as the study of JR mentioned earlier. He also offers various diagrams suggesting the flow of information engaged

9. See, for example, the video https://www.youtube.com/watch?v=GlArYBxIt4g of the chimpanzee "CHEETAH enjoying one of his favorite form of enrichment . . . Painting," and the page https://langint.pri.kyoto-u.ac.jp/ai/en/album/the_drawings_by_chimpanzees.html.

in drawing. Here, however, I want to focus on his study of sketching from memory, and extract lessons about sketching from imagination.

Having highlighted the interaction between contour information and the knowledge of objects, note too that the sound or the name of an object may initiate drawing. The *semantic system* (i.e., the system that captures meanings at an abstract level that may, for example, bridge between perception, language, and action) provides a representation of the meaning of the sound but must be elaborated into parameterized visual schemas before a drawing can be made. In drawing a bell, one goes beyond thinking of a generic bell to filling in the type of bell, its shape and its size and placement on the page—backing up to imagine a 2D or 3D scene that could satisfy the semantics.[10]

In some sense, imagination operates like this: At any time, one may already be appreciating some of the details of the emerging scene in their 2D or 3D relationship, while others may be vaguer. That's part of what the sketching is going to do by providing you with a drawing that lets you see that some aspects are not as you intuited or don't quite fit your constraints. You get a better sketch, whether you are drawing from memory or expressing your imagination, as you try to fill in the details to fit some, perhaps themselves changing, criteria for what constitutes a satisfactory sketch of a design.

When we interact with objects, they provide the affordances for our actions. After we have laid down the first part of a drawing, then different portions of that initial work provide less-constrained affordances—each group of lines or patch of color may afford different ways of continuing the process. In this process of "inverting vision," the visual working memory (as in the VISIONS model; van Sommers calls it the *visual buffer*) is extended to accommodate "top-down" imagination as well as the understanding of current visual input. In particular, working memory mediates

10. An amusing video on misinterpretation of a scene description is "The March of the Emperors," www.youtube.com/watch?v=qNd_hUqEEl4, whose title retranslates back into English the French title of the film "The March of the Penguins." The movie, unlike the video, shows the life of emperor penguins, and not Emperor Napoleons, in the Antarctic.

between a visual scene of the current environment and schemas in (visual) long-term memory to generate instances that can then be used in diverse ways, whether for describing or drawing a visual scene, or more.

Let's consider a drawing exercise as a proxy for the demands of developing a plan for a building that meets prespecified requirements. To draw "a man drinking coffee," you would have many details to work out. You need a strategy for what things are to be drawn and in what relations. Is the man standing or sitting? Where will the cup be? Will you include a bar or a table, a stool or a chair in the scene? After the basic layout is conceived (at least provisionally), will you start with a preliminary sketch to establish the overall composition, or proceed directly to drawing one object at a time? And so on. As you sketch, earlier decisions may prove mistaken, and contingent replanning of the drawing may be needed. The tentatively completed drawing may then provide the occasion for further effort, either erasing and/or modifying parts of the sketch, or by putting the drawing to one side and then repeating the process but now using the first sketch as a model for the second, and the second sketch as a model for the third, but each time changing elements in the process.

To make sense of the relationship between semantics, visual representations, and the contents of the visual buffer (including imagery), it is important to find an explanation of the gap between knowledge and graphic production that does not depend just on depiction decisions and processes, or even the structure and capacity of the imagery system. A study by van Sommers offers real insight into sketching from imagination, although here the subjects (undergraduates at Macquarie University in Sydney) were asked to draw a bicycle from memory rather than draw a newly imagined scene. Figure 8.7 shows that not only brain-impaired persons fail to produce veridical drawings! For example, we see bicycle pedals with no chain to make use of them, a chain with no pedals, and a chain that joins the front and the rear wheel.

Looking at their drawings, we might conclude that the students lacked even basic knowledge about the physical structure and appearance of common everyday objects (such as bicycles). However, van Sommers showed that the drawings were, in general, impoverished reflections of the students' knowledge. Indeed, students who produced the pictures

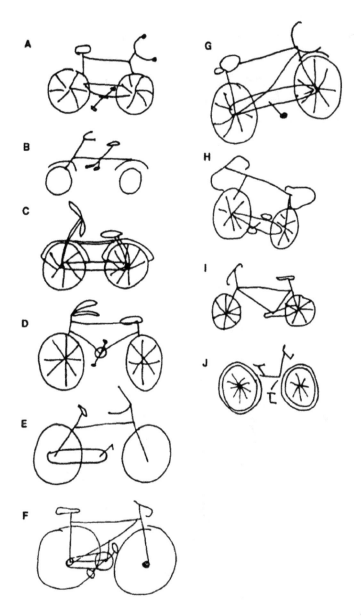

Figure 8.7 Drawings of bicycles by senior undergraduate students. (Adapted from Figure 14 in van Sommers, P. [1989]. A system for drawing and drawing-related neuropsychology. *Cognitive Neuropsychology*, 6[2], 117–164, reprinted by permission of the publisher, Taylor & Francis Ltd.)

were aware that they had it wrong. The drawings can serve as a first draft for further recall. When van Sommers asked the students to look at their sketches and try again (but with no feedback as to the drawing itself) while reflecting about what they knew or could work out about bicycles, they showed progress as typified in the drawings from a single subject shown in Figure 8.8. Subjects could often locate the area of the drawing where something was amiss before they crystallized what was wrong or missing. They might show with their hands the orientation of parts, or draw a part from a different viewpoint and then need urging to project that

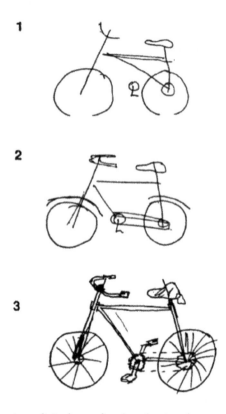

Figure 8.8 Three drawings elicited one after the other in a few minutes from a single subject without any instruction beyond asking him to try again, *reflecting carefully about what he knew or could work out* about bicycles. (From Figure 15 in van Sommers, P. [1989]. A system for drawing and drawing-related neuropsychology. *Cognitive Neuropsychology*, 6[2], 117–164, reprinted by permission of the publisher, Taylor & Francis Ltd.)

information appropriately onto the evolving drawing. Each sketch shows external memory serving not necessarily as an end in itself but also as a stimulus to further feats of (internal) memory or visualization.

Of course, in drawing something novel from imagination, you do not have a visual image that you are trying to recollect. In particular, drawing from imagination in architectural design is an emergent, integrative process. It may start with some general ideas, maybe placement in a landscape or ideas about function or atmosphere. An abstraction may serve as the nucleus of a design idea. The designer expands on this by exploiting background knowledge, constrained at certain stages (perhaps not initially) by scientific principles, material properties, and standards—and, eventually, must adapt the design to address details of the actual construction process that produces building according to the design. (More on this in discussing Frank Gehry's sketching in §9.3.) Mark Alan Hewitt (2020) adopts Merlin Donald's use of the term *exogram* for items of external memory and offers a diagram (Figure 25, p. 70) "of a mode of conception used by many contemporary architects. Exograms proceed from sketches to diagrams to plans, elevations, models, and finally to the presentation stage."

For a written work, notes that grow via successive drafts and editing can provide crucial external memory. Sketches may play a similar role in painting and in architecture, though the latter creations must take the behavior of potential users into account. For a choreographer developing new work with a group of dancers (Stevens, 2005), the use of a journal, still photos, and videos can capture the evanescent process of creating the dance. In any complex creative process, there is the risk of fleeting insights slipping away—and of other "insights," when held up for inspection, proving not so insightful after all. We again see the crucial role of memory, both in the head and external to it.

8.6. IS ARCHITECTURE A LANGUAGE FOR THE ARCHITECTURE-READY BRAIN?

What is an architecture-ready brain? It must be both drawing-ready and language-ready, and it must be able to move beyond the "here-and-next" (given the current situation, here is what to do next) to the realm of imagination, where the ability to imagine complex goals can be transmuted into the development of plans to achieve those goals. What, then, does it take for someone, endowed with such a brain, to become an architect? Briefly, it is acquiring the skills to take a novel program that describes just some of the specifications for a desired room, building, or larger environment and—in the spirit of performative architecture (Chapter 1)—develop the detailed plans that will guide construction of a structure that will perform well on (most of) the specifications for its use and its experiential quality. Clearly, many people were architects in the informal sense long before the emergence of architecture as a profession, and much of the world's built environment involves "folk architecture" even to the present day.

Animal "architecture" versus human architecture

Many of us are fascinated with "animal architecture," with examples ranging from termite mounds to bird nests and diverse other constructions.[11] Juhani Pallasmaa (2002) writes of how as a young boy he was fascinated by the constructions of animals, and then, many years later, this interest was rekindled by Karl von Frisch's 1974 book *Animal Architecture*, leading in due course to the 2002 exhibition *Eläinten Arkkitehtuuri/Animal Architecture* he curated at Suomen Rakenunustaiteen Museo/Museum of Finnish Architecture.

Termite and ant nest building (Perna & Theraulaz, 2017) is an emergent property of local behavioral rules (e.g., termites have no "mental model" of what ensures the form or "air conditioning" of a termite mound) but, turning to birds, it remains an open question as to what is needed to underwrite the ethograms of species-specific nest "designs." Peter Goodfellow

---

11. Broad overviews include *Animal Architecture* by Karl von Frisch (1974) and *Built by Animals: The Natural History of Animal Architecture* by Mike Hansell (2007). Books focused on bird nest construction include *The Origin and Evolution of Nest Building by Passerine Birds* (Collias, 1997), *Avian Architecture: How Birds Design, Engineer, and Build* (Goodfellow, 2011), and *Bird Nests and Construction Behaviour* (Hansell, 2000).

(2011) provides a detailed look at avian "architecture," with a taxonomy of bird nests—cup-shaped nests; domed nests; hanging, woven, and stitched nests; group nests; and more. What his overview makes clear is both the diversity of nest types and, in most cases, how specific the *type* of nest is for each species.

The construction of bird nests often involves long hierarchical sequences of actions even though the required behaviors involve little, if any, cultural learning. However, although the "core" combination of instructions is to a great extent "innate," the nest will vary greatly as it is adapted to the specific site and the available materials. Moreover, there is a secondary role for individual learning. For example, Bailey, Morgan, Bertin, Meddle, and Healy (2014) found that male zebra finches choose nest material based on the structural properties of the material, but that their preference is not entirely genetically predetermined. After a short period of building with relatively flexible string, the birds preferred to build with stiffer string, while those that had experienced only stiffer string were indifferent to string type. After building a complete nest with either string type, however, all birds increased their preference for stiff string when building further nests. The stiffer string appeared to be the more effective building material.

Perhaps more tellingly, animal "architecture" offers lessons to the human architect who seeks novel forms and is fascinated by the different ways in which creatures build, from termites who follow simple local rules to cooperatively construct their mounds, to birds that are individually capable of the complete process from choosing nest site to procuring materials to finishing the nest. Nonetheless, animal "architecture" offers few if any lessons relevant to our A↔N conversation. In the nonhuman case, we have animals following variations on innate blueprints to build species-specific structures, whereas humans can design and build habitats and other buildings with an immense diversity and varied complexity that reflects cumulative learning across generations and populations, with no relevant change in the genome.

We can certainly drop the quotes and talk of *animal architecture*, but only with the understanding that nonhuman creatures lack the ability of human architects for flexible designs where use and aesthetics comes into play in an explicit design process that precedes construction.

Further confounding any hope of gleaning lessons for the evolution of the human architecture-ready brain from comparative studies is the fact that nonhuman primates are lousy "architects." Chimpanzees form "nests" simply by climbing into trees and bending and breaking the smaller branches to make the place they sleep more comfortable. Fruth, Tagg, and Stewart (2018) review sleep and nesting behavior in primates, focusing on chimpanzee nests as sleeping places, noting that "an ape will usually build a new nest each evening and, despite lack of systematic investigation, is assumed to use it for rest from dusk until dawn." Placement of the nest may reflect knowledge of possible predators. Berger et al. (2010) suggest that "it is possible that early hominins continued to sleep in trees, long after becoming terrestrial, perhaps until the controlled use of fire." The implicit suggestion here is that a campfire might be a base for a camp.

Fruth et al. do suggest that "modern humans show deeply-rooted architectural preferences that likely evolved in our distant past through natural selection; for example, preference for a good view is likely related to height and an avoidance of being discovered." Refuge as well as prospect may indeed be fundamental principles of human behavior shared with distant primate ancestors and that come into play when we choose a home and homesite or "safe" place to relax: "refuge" from predators, including other humans, and "prospect" as a view allowing early discovery of opportunities or threats (on the "savannah" below), with "height" adding the implication of dominance. This preference can be seen at work in the design of offices, status and prestige, and real estate values (see, e.g., pp. 21–49 of *Origins of Architectural Pleasure*, Hildebrand, 1999; R. Kaplan & S. Kaplan, 1989; S. Kaplan, 1987; Sussman & Hollander, 2014).

Despite the relevance of such preferences to architecture, there seems little evidence from the study of human hunter-gatherers that could tie an evolutionary account of our capacity for architecture back to inferred linkages of sleep and nesting in our last common ancestor with chimpanzees. Instead, I suggest that the path to architecture is indirect—rooted in manual dexterity and the motivation to communicate. Specifically,

I argued in §8.4 that the language-ready brain was also drawing-ready, and now conclude that the neural underpinnings were thus in place for the eventual emergence of varied buildings and their conscious design by humans.

Jaubert et al. (2016)—in line with the realization that we must assess Neanderthal culture in exploring the cultural evolution of modern humans—report the dating of Neanderthal constructions found deep in Bruniquel Cave in southwest France. Broken stalagmites were arranged in regular circles, and associated traces of fire demonstrate the human origin of these constructions. Jaubert et al. were able to date the circles as having been formed around 175,000 years ago, "making these edifices among the oldest known well-dated constructions made by humans. Their presence at 336 meters from the entrance of the cave indicates that humans from this period had already mastered the underground environment, which can be considered a major step in human modernity."

Alas, further exploration of this theme lies outside the scope of this book. But one thing is clear: Neither mound-building termites nor nest-building birds are architecture-ready in the human sense of the term.

Languages reconsidered

Given my argument that the evolutionary process that yielded a language-ready brain gave humans the capacity to develop various approaches to architecture through cultural evolution, I need to address directly the question, "Is architecture a language?" My unequivocal answer is "no" . . . and also "sort of."

In the strict sense of human languages like Chinese and Warlpiri and ASL, a language contains a stock of *words* (the *lexicon*) and a stock of *constructions* for modifying and combining them hierarchically (the grammar). The words and their construction-based combinations (let's call them *utterances*) have both a form and a meaning, and when someone generates an utterance to convey a meaning, they expect the receiver of that utterance to be able to understand much of that intended meaning.

The lexicon of a language changes slowly—some words shift meaning, other ones become used less often, and new ones will be coined to link to changes in the language community's world—and the grammar changes even more slowly.

A common extension of the use of the term "language" is in the term *body language*, which has no clear lexicon and no formalizable grammar, but nonetheless plays a crucial role in human interaction. The way architecture "in general" communicates is like a body language—unwritten, and communicating via atmosphere, forms, and affordances. The meanings communicated through our body's behavioral and emotional responses might be construed as our responses to the meanings conveyed by the architect's "utterances in the language of architectural space." Here, though, I want to assess such notions as "the language of architectural space" more rigorously in relation to the linguist's notions of "lexicon" and "grammar," especially as these correspond to aspects of distinctive styles of architecture.

Does architecture have an overall lexicon or grammar? No. We build up an appreciation not just for buildings in general but also for the works of a particular architect—with a sense of their "vocabulary" and of their style of construction. Then our experience of a new work exploits that understanding, and we in part judge the work on the extent to which the new composition overly resembles prior work or finds new ways of exploiting the architect's style. Moreover, if the architect changes style, we may at first react negatively because it fails to "make sense" in terms of the previous style, though in time we may come to master the elements of the new style and the works that are now built upon it.

Perhaps, then, we might want to say that architects who belong to the same "school" share an architectural language, but that the more creative artists may change their personal "dialects" as they mature, or as they work on different types of building. We are again at the point where we accept that our terminology takes on new or extended meetings, as in our earlier acceptance of the terms *artificial intelligence, smart architecture,* and *animal architecture.* We may talk of words as being the "building blocks" of human languages, but the "language" of architects is not a language in the same sense as a spoken or signed human language. Nonetheless, we can get a deeper understanding of humans if we look more deeply at the claims that the "language-ready brain" is "construction-ready" and, indeed, "architecture-ready."

A key to this discussion is the essential "aboutness" of language. In this book, I talk *about* brains and buildings, using the English language. To do this, I have had to slightly modify your idiolect, your own personal variation of English. There may be nouns like *hippocampus* or names like *Pallasmaa* that you have not used before, but I am unlikely to change your grammar or have any need to do so. Importantly, the first time I use a new word, you get only a fragment of its meaning, a meaning that becomes extended, modified, and corrected, as you experience it in new contexts within the book or through associations with your own lived experience— and the latter may shade that meaning in ways that, to some extent, may not match my own intentions. If I mention the name of an architect whom I admire but whose works leave you cold, then this may change the way you read a paragraph from trusting what I say to questioning or even rejecting it. At times, you may smile at an intended, or even an unintended, joke and at other times miss a joke entirely. You may find most of my sentences clear, yet some may seem ill-constructed or ambiguous—and I hope that every now and again you will "step back" from a sentence's meaning to take pleasure in an unusually well-crafted arrangement of the words.

Crucially, language changes in part because what we talk about changes, and indeed language itself can help bring about those changes. For two recent examples, a whole series of technological advances is encapsulated in the word "smartphone," and then one simple behavior using smart-phones is captured in the word "selfie." The availability of these two words then allows us to exploit a realm of shared knowledge to talk about both personal experience and social trends.

What I am trying to say here is that English (and all other rich human languages) are both languages and meta-languages—they enable us to talk (and sign, and write) about the external world, about mental worlds, about imagined worlds—and even about language itself. "Architecture as a language" conflates "language" with "what language is about"—the construction of descriptions, the design of buildings, and the buildings themselves. And there is yet another "language" involved, the "language" of experience, contrasting the static form of a building with the diversity of dynamic behaviors based on the scripts it offers that can be followed, adapted, or rejected. If the building is frozen music, the behavior it supports is the interweaving dynamics in space and time of an opera (to offer a new variant on our Chapter 4 discussion of stage-setting).

Within the richness of a language like English, we can extend our general vocabulary with specialized vocabularies that let us talk knowledgeably *about* architecture, but this is different from the languages (in the extended sense) *of* architecture that address the construction of architectural forms, expressed in the various component forms and their modes of composition that may distinguish one architect or group of architects from another (and may vary for them across time, and for different types of project). In the distinction offered here, *atmosphere* is part of the former but not the latter—and so each architect employs both languages in the successful completion of a project.

There are at least three "levels" to consider:

1. The spatial arrangement of those features that will affect the users and inhabitants of the building, both for their utility and for their aesthetic impact

2. The details that are crucial to the physical process of construction: For example, the user may experience a hallway with a solid wall on one side and a wall with a number of windows on the other. The construction details must relate the framing of the wall to the foundations and to the covering of, let's say, sheets of plywood with "mud" to create a smooth uninterrupted surface that is in turn to be painted. Here, we might speak of a "construction language," embracing all the components of the building, how they are formed, what materials are used, and how they are combined. This engages a 2D description language based, for example, on construction drawings.

3. The construction "script" that includes timing so that the
   electrician's work coheres with that of the carpenters, plasterers,
   and painters

Level 1 is probably the level at which we might seek the "language" of
the architect (or at least the "dialect" specific to this and related buildings), with just enough of level 2 to ensure that what is specified in level
1 is indeed buildable. Level 2 uses a language of construction drawings employing a "vocabulary" and "grammar" of great complexity, but
made readily available in a manipulable external memory by systems for
computer-aided design. The details here are seldom part of the "language"
in which the architect thinks about the building and develops its design,
but they must be meaningful to those who do the actual building, and may
well rely on their knowledge and skill to achieve what is at best explicit in
the construction drawings. Architects will rarely be concerned with level
3 (though they may visit the site from time to time to check that construction is proceeding according to the design). This is more the domain of
the building contractor, who must convert the construction drawings into
a detailed script that extends to the procurement and storage of materials,
but may need to engage engineers to provide specialized techniques to
provide novel "building blocks" and the tools to assemble them.

With this, I turn to Christopher Jencks's discussion of Le Corbusier's
"languages" to exemplify some of the points made earlier. Jencks (1973,
p. 54) notes Le Corbusier's search for a "universal language" that would
be trans-historical and nonconventional. This quest is reminiscent of the
search for a universal language by Leibnitz and others (Knowlson, 1975),
and like them is doomed to failure. More relevant to our present discussion is the "language" of basic forms associated with the villa at Garches
and the Villa Savoie (Jencks, pp. 85–87) that can be seen as abstract cubes
of space in which various geometric elements are freely disposed according to Le Corbusier's "Five Points of a New Architecture": the house on
stilts or *pilotis*, which frees the ground for circulation; the roof garden
allowed by the flat roof; the free plan and facade allowed by the independent frame structure; the curtain wall system that liberates the façade

from the entanglement of load-bearing elements; and the ribbon window, which gives more light than that possible in a load-bearing wall. To these, Jencks adds the ramp or bridge, the double-height space, the scissor and spiral staircase, and the curved bathroom or solarium. Jencks sees these as "invented for both their technological and aesthetic potential and then used as fixed words in an abstract system of Cartesian space." As for "grammar," Jencks notes that

> Corbusier smashes his elements into and through each other to produce [what Jencks would call] "compaction composition" . . . holes of space are cut violently through floors, columns are placed very close to walls, curved partitions jut into rectangular rooms, etc. Compaction composition is very close, as a method, to *collage*, inasmuch as the superimposition of elements obscures parts, instead of allowing them to be seen through (except in the unique case of glass). Hence when one wanders through a Le Corbusier building one finds a succession of elements partly hidden and partly revealed. This accounts for their excitement and suspense.

Here, we are far from the hierarchical combination of words and phrases that is tightly specified by the constructions of a natural language's grammar. There is a freedom of distortion of the elements and the ways their placement may penetrate and directly transform other elements. Nonetheless, the way we have discussed the language-ready brain in relation to the development and imitation of complex manual skills and external memory clarifies why such a brain might, through cultural evolution, become capable of entertaining such ways of imagining and specifying new constructs and linking them to more detailed specification of how to construct buildings that may conform with this abstract "architectural language."[12]

---

12. Jencks devotes a whole section of his book to "Other Languages of Architecture 1946–65." Note the plural, and all this within the oeuvre of one architect, Le Corbusier. The

Consider Jencks's comments that "the succession of elements partly hidden and partly revealed . . . accounts for their excitement and suspense." Here, we may consider the analogy with poetry—the poetics of architecture, if you will. The core of language, characterized by the lexicon and grammar, is the ability to find forms that convey certain types of meaning: "This is what the sentence means." But just as the architect's specification of the elements of a building and their combination does not exhaust its aesthetic impact or eventual use, so does language offer a field for invention. After our distant ancestors built up a stock of words with a well-defined phonology, they could discover alliteration and rhyme and could begin to put words together that exploited these effects, giving the listener a pleasure that another choice of words would lack. Assuming that language, song, and dance evolved together (though not necessarily in tightly synchronized stages), certain word patterns might be chosen more for their rhythmic qualities than their meaning.

Adding another dimension: As language fluency increased, lengthy narratives could be spoken, memorized, understood. And then conventions could arise for what constitutes successful storytelling—creating suspense, leaving out some extraneous details, and adding others that are not necessary to the eventual denouement but add "richness" and "color" and thus may better engage the attention of the audience. The narrative not only builds up a "word picture" for the listeners but may also engage their emotions.

Here, we see that the use of language in the word- and sentence-based sense of the term provides just the foundation (another metaphor creeping back from architecture) for many dimensions beyond the way in which lexicon and grammar combine to convey novel meanings. The previous discussion suggests that they are as relevant to architecture and art as they are to language—language-readiness in the narrow sense now

section (especially pp. 157–162) contains interesting and relevant material, but his discussion of Le Corbusier's early "language" will suffice for our present assessment of the claim that architecture—or, at least, each architectural "style"—is "sort of" a language, but only in a way informed by a very general flexibility of construction.

stands revealed as also being "language"-readiness in a broad sense that extends to architecture and other domains of culture.[13]

For the *languages of architecture*, one might say that "each building is a narrative, while the parts of the building and their relationships constitute the utterances from which that narrative is formed."

This suggests another dimension for the future richness of the A↔N conversation as we seek to better understand the diverse cognitive processes that are engaged in architectural design and experience and how the brain supports the diverse interactions between them. The study of architecture (as well as poetry!) can enrich the study of the brain in ways that extend far beyond the laboratory.

REFERENCES

Arbib, M. A. (2012). *How the brain got language: The mirror system hypothesis*. New York and Oxford: Oxford University Press.

Arbib, M. A. (Ed.). (2013). *Language, music and the brain, a mysterious relationship. Strüngmann forum reports* (Vol. 10). Cambridge, MA: MIT Press.

Arbib, M. A. (Ed.). (2020). *How the brain got language: Towards a new road map.* Amsterdam and Philadelphia: Johns Benjamins.

Arbib, M. A., Aboitiz, F., Burkart, J., Corballis, M., Coudé, G., Hecht, E., . . . Wilson, B. (2018). The Comparative Neuroprimatology 2018 (CNP-2018) road map for research on how the brain got language. *Interaction Studies*, 19(1–2), 370–387.

Arbib, M. A., & Rizzolatti, G. (1997). Neural expectations: A possible evolutionary path from manual skills to language. *Communication and Cognition*, 29, 393–424.

Bailey, I. E., Morgan, K. V., Bertin, M., Meddle, S. L., & Healy, S. D. (2014). Physical cognition: Birds learn the structural efficacy of nest. *Proceedings of the Royal Society B: Biological Sciences*, 281, 20133225.

Berger, L. R., De Ruiter, D. J., Churchill, S. E., Schmid, P., Carlson, K. J., Dirks, P. H., & Kibii, J. M. (2010). Australopithecus sediba: A new species of Homo-like australopith from South Africa. *Science*, 328, 195–204.

13. Another general question, but one outside our present scope, is to what extent music is a "language." Certainly, language in the strict sense can convey propositional meaning in ways that music cannot, while music may have a more direct impact on the emotions than language—though language can be employed to construct emotionally charged narratives and poems. The book, *Language, Music and the Brain: A Mysterious Relationship* (Arbib, 2013), brings together diverse scholars to explore these issues.

Collias, N. E. (1997). The origin and evolution of nest building by passerine birds. *Condor, 99*, 253–269.

Colomina, B., & Wigley, M. (2016). *Are we human? Notes on an archaeology of design*: Zürich, Switzerland: Lars Müller Publishers.

Donald, M. (1991). *Origins of the modern mind: Three stages in the evolution of culture and cognition*. Cambridge, MA: Harvard University Press.

Donald, M. (1993). Precis of origins of the modern mind: Three stages in the evolution of culture and cognition. *Behavioral and Brain Sciences, 16*, 737–791.

Dubreuil, B., & Henshilwood, C. S. (2013). Archeology and the language-ready brain. *Language and Cognition, 5*(2–3), 251–260.

Fruth, B., Tagg, N., & Stewart, F. (2018). Sleep and nesting behavior in primates: A review. *American Journal of Physical Anthropology, 166*(3), 499–509. doi:doi:10.1002/ajpa.23373

Gärdenfors, P. (2017). Demonstration and pantomime in the evolution of teaching. *Frontiers in Psychology, 8*(415). doi:10.3389/fpsyg.2017.00415

Gärdenfors, P., & Högberg, A. (2017). The archaeology of teaching and the evolution of Homo docens. *Current Anthropology, 58*(2), 188–208. doi:10.1086/691178

Goodfellow, P. (2011). *Avian architecture: How birds design, engineer, and build*. Princeton, NJ: Princeton University Press.

Hansell, M. (2000). *Bird nests and construction behavior*. Cambridge, UK: Cambridge University Press.

Hansell, M. (2007). *Built by animals: The natural history of animal architecture*. Oxford: Oxford University Press.

Hasluck, N. (2016). *The Bradshaw case*. Melbourne: Australian Scholarly Publishing.

Hewitt, M. A. (2020). *Draw in order to see: A cognitive history of architectural design*. San Francisco: ORO Editions.

Hildebrand, G. (1999). *Origins of architectural pleasure*. Berkeley, CA: University of California Press.

Jaubert, J., Verheyden, S., Genty, D., Soulier, M., Cheng, H., Blamart, D., . . . Santos, F. (2016). Early Neanderthal constructions deep in Bruniquel Cave in southwestern France. *Nature, 534*, 111–114. doi:10.1038/nature18291; https://www.nature.com/articles/nature18291#supplementary-information

Kaplan, R., & Kaplan, S. (1989). *The experience of nature: A psychological perspective*. Cambridge, UK: Cambridge University Press.

Kaplan, S. (1987). Aesthetics, affect, and cognition: Environmental preference from an evolutionary perspective. *Environment and Behavior, 19*(1), 3–32. doi:10.1177/0013916587191001

Knowlson, J. (1975). *Universal language schemes in England and France 1600–1800*. Toronto and Buffalo: University of Toronto Press.

McCulloch, W. S. (1961). What is a number, that a man may know it, and a man, that he may know a number. *General Semantics Bulletin, 26*(27), 7–18.

McCulloch, W. S., & Pitts, W. H. (1943). A logical calculus of the ideas immanent in nervous activity. *Bulletin of Mathematical Biophysics, 5*, 115–133.

Myowa-Yamakoshi, M. (2018). The evolutionary roots of human imitation, action understanding and symbols. *Interaction Studies, 19*(1–2), 183–199.

Onians, J. (2007). Neuroarchaeology: The Chauvet Cave and the origins of representation. In C. Renfrew & I. Morley (Eds.), *Image and imagination. A global history of figurative representation* (pp. 307–320). Cambridge, UK: Cambridge University Press.

Onians, J. (2008). Neuroarthistory: From Aristotle and Pliny to Baxandall and Zeki. New Haven, CT: Yale University Press.

Osiurak, F., & Reynaud, E. (2019). The elephant in the room: What matters cognitively in cumulative technological culture. *Behavioral and Brain Sciences.* doi:10.1017/S0140525X19003236; https://doi.org/10.1017/S0140525X19003236

Pallasmaa, J. (Ed.). (2002). *Eläinten Arkkitehtuuri/animal architecture.* Helsinki: Suomen Rakenunustaiteen Museo/Museum of Finnish Architecture.

Perna, A., & Theraulaz, G. (2017). When social behaviour is moulded in clay: On growth and form of social insect nests. *Journal of Experimental Biology*, 220(1), 83–91. doi:10.1242/jeb.143347

Poizner, H., Klima, E. S., & Bellugi, U. (1987). *What the hands reveal about the brain.* Cambridge, MA: MIT Press.

Preziosi, D. (1979). *Architecture, language, and meaning.* The Hague, Paris, and New York: Mouton Publishers.

Rizzolatti, G., & Arbib, M. A. (1998). Language within our grasp. *Trends in Neurosciences*, 21(5), 188–194.

Russon, A. E. (2018). Pantomime and imitation in great apes: Implications for reconstructing the evolution of language. *Interaction Studies*, 19(1–2), 200–215.

Seghers, E. (2014). Cross-species comparison in the evolutionary study of art: A cognitive approach to the ape art debate. *Review of General Psychology*, 18(4), 263–272. doi:10.1037/gpr0000015

Snyder, A. W., & Thomas, M. (1997). Autistic artists give clues to cognition. *Perception*, 26(1), 93–96.

Stevens, C. (2005). Chronology of creating a dance: Anna Smith's red rain. In R. Grove, C. Stevens, & S. McKechnie (Eds.), *Thinking in four dimensions: Creativity and cognition in contemporary dance* (pp. 169–187). Melbourne: Melbourne University Press.

Stout, D. (2018). Archaeology and the evolutionary neuroscience of language: The technological pedagogy hypothesis. *Interaction Studies*, 19(1–2).

Sudnow, D. (2001). *Ways of the hand: A rewritten account.* Cambridge, MA: MIT Press.

Sussman, A., & Hollander, J. B. (2014). *Cognitive architecture: Designing for how we respond to the built environment.* New York: Routledge.

Van Huyssteen, J. W. (2006). *Alone in the world? Human uniqueness in science and theology.* Grand Rapids, MI: Eerdmans.

van Sommers, P. (1989). A system for drawing and drawing-related neuropsychology. *Cognitive Neuropsychology*, 6(2), 117–164. doi:10.1080/02643298908253416

von Frisch, K. (1974). *Animal architecture.* New York: Harcourt Brace Jovanovich.

Whitehead, C. (2010). The culture ready brain. *Social Cognitive and Affective Neuroscience*, 5(2–3), 168–179. doi:10.1093/scan/nsq036

Zukow-Goldring, P. (2012). Assisted imitation: First steps in the seed model of language development. *Language Sciences*, 34(5), 569–582. doi:10.1016/j.langsci.2012.03.012

Zukow-Goldring, P., & Arbib, M. A. (2007). Affordances, effectivities, and assisted imitation: Caregivers and the directing of attention. *Neurocomputing*, 70, 2181–2193.

Experience and design:
Case studies

Much of this book has emphasized the cog/neuroscience of the experience of architecture, gleaning ideas for design but giving little or no attention to the mechanisms, whether at the level of schemas or neural networks, that make the design of architecture possible. In this chapter and the next, we shift the focus onto the design processes. The present chapter offers two case studies; the next develops a preliminary conceptual model for the neuroscience of the design of architecture that builds strongly upon insights developed cumulatively through the preceding chapters. The general framework is to understand design as an exercise of the imagination, but then to see the way in which that imagination is rooted in memories .

The first case study is devoted to Jørn Utzon's design of the Sydney Opera House. We will see how his experience in both

boat-building and as a yachtsman offered him a new perspective lacking to other architects of how to develop the site on
Bennelong Point on Sydney Harbour. Other inspiration came
from Mayan and Chinese temples, in which a building was erected
above a pedestal, and clouds or the roof in some sense floated
above the building. The case study both extracts a number of basic
principles from Utzon's process of designing (as distinct from
the final design itself) and provides some sense of the triumphs
and tragedy of the historical events that led to Utzon's resignation
before the building had been completed.

The second case study focuses on Frank Gehry's design of the
Guggenheim Museum Bilbao. This study will emphasize how
sketching and model-making make intuitions explicit in a way that
can be the basis both for self-discovery and for teamwork. Crucially,
the current sketch may not only provide ideas for further development but also reveal quirks that had not been consciously derived
but that nonetheless suggest ideas to enrich or modify the design.

Although we will not pursue this observation further, it is striking that
both projects involved dramatic changes in the "language" of each architect
and required novel design methods linked to innovations in construction
techniques. Instead, we will turn in the next chapter to a cog/neuroscience
analysis of the design process that addresses certain aspects of the two
case studies, but also leaves much untouched as a basis for future A↔N
conversations.

These last two chapters do not offer advice on "how to be a better
designer." Nor is my aim to privilege Utzon or Gehry above all others or to
suggest that the creativity of architects can be reduced to neuroscience formulas. The case studies emphasize how their specific memories influenced
the creativity of Utzon and Gehry in very different ways. *Neuroscience does
not limit the styles of different designers.* Rather, we seek to understand how
the mechanisms that make possible action, skill, memory, imagination,
and more, which can act more or less in concert for coming up with solutions to the new challenges we face from day to day, may also provide the

mechanisms employed in design by *all* architects. Architecture remains our focus as we advance our A↔N conversation.

This chapter owes a special debt to conversations with two men and the books of two women. The men are both architects: Richard Leplastrier,[1] who was a young colleague of Utzon's during construction of the Sydney Opera House, and Edwin Chan, who was a key collaborator of Gehry during the design of the Guggenheim Museum Bilbao. The two women wrote the books that provided prime references for enriching my understanding of the designing of these buildings: Francoise Fromonot's *Jørn Utzon: Architect of the Sydney Opera House*, and Coosje van Bruggen's *Frank O. Gehry: Guggenheim Museum Bilbao*.

9.1. IMAGINATION AND DESIGN: OUR INITIAL FRAMEWORK

When discussing Zumthor's design of the Therme at Vals (§1.1), I suggested that

> there is a dynamic interaction of considerations of form and function as design proceeds. In the end, the Therme is a great success because it blends with the landscape, it is beautiful, and it works well as a place to experience the different springs. All this suggests issues that a cognitive neuroscience of design must face. How does form get represented? How does function get represented? How do the two interact as design proceeds? And what happens when the design is carried out by a team?

1. When I saw "Sydney Opera House: Man-Made Marvels" (7Mate, 2008?) for the first time, I learned that one of the then-young architects who had worked with Utzon, and who was interviewed extensively in the video, was Richard Leplastrier, a high school classmate from my Sydney days, and now one of Australia's leading architects. As a result of this, we met for the first time in more than 50 years. Richard also appears in a beautiful film on Utzon, *The Man and the Architect Jørn Utzon*, a 2018 Nordisk film made by Lene Borsch Hansen. This gives a broad view of Utzon's life and varied career. One comes to appreciate him not just as an architect but also as an exceptional human being.

For Juhani Pallasmaa (personal communication):

A great architect imagines and designs the experiences, existential and aesthetic values of a piece of architecture before giving them material shape and aesthetic articulation. In the process of making, the experiential and the material, the image and the form, the structure and its existential meaning arise together and cannot be separated from each other.

My challenge, however, is to dig beneath this holistic view to understand something of the underlying cognitive processes. Even if "the structure and its existential meaning . . . cannot be separated from each other," our cog/neuro analysis must illuminate how the brain serves these different aspects and mediates between them. Each decision on one aspect may feed back, whether consciously or unconsciously, to change decisions on another.

Each of us has (some would say "is") a brain in a body in a social and physical environment, shaped by the surrounding culture as well as individual experience. The particularities of genetic happenstance, development, environment, and learning combine to give each of us a singular brain that forms and supports a singular personality, a singular mind. Nonetheless, we must not forget the key notion that the successful architect succeeds in part through his or her ability to anticipate the experience of those who will use the building, and here generalities about groups of users must predominate over the singular, save, for example, in homes defined for particular clients.

One more point: In general, architecture involves what Loukissas (2012) calls *co-designers*. On a large project, many people collaborate and then share their ideas to invite more elaborations of one part or another. This implies that in some cases the term "the architect" should be understood as shorthand for "the architectural team." Indeed, our discussion of the Sydney Opera House will remind us of the fact that although we credit Jørn Utzon as the designer, it took the creativity of others to work with him to determine how to construct his initial, but tragically incomplete, design. However, in this case, the overall shape of the design was Utzon's, and Utzon's alone. In other cases, we may see that even the overall design emerges as the product of interaction between two or more architects and other collaborators.

9.2. JØRN UTZON'S EXPERIENCE AND DESIGN: THE SYDNEY OPERA HOUSE

When we talk of "experience and design" together, we are considering two different forms of experience: the experience of the architect that informs the design, and the experiences that users will have in and around the building. In particular, the architect's experience will guide projections of the user's experience, but many other factors enter the design process.

Jørn Utzon (Figure 9.1) created a landmark on Sydney Harbour, the Sydney Opera House (Figure 9.2), and I will use a number of key elements of his individual design process to provide "data points" for assessing the neurocognitive theory of design presented in Chapter 10.

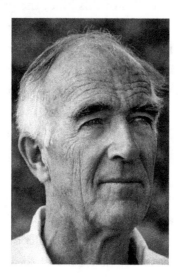

Figure 9.1 Jørn Utzon (Photo: Utzonphotos, courtesy of Flemming Bo Andersen.)

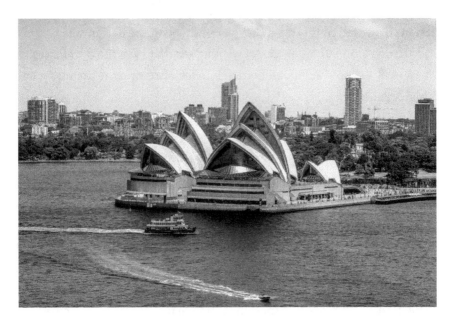

Figure 9.2 The Sydney Opera House as seen from the Sydney Harbour Bridge. (https://commons.wikimedia.org/wiki/File:SydneyOperaHouse20182.jp. Solvarsity, CC BY-SA 4.0, via Wikimedia Commons.)

As more architects and neuroscientists work together to develop more clearly articulated case studies of this kind, the process will yield more insight into architectural design, and more challenges for basic research on the underlying cognitive and neural mechanisms.

A key advocate for a Sydney Opera House was Eugene Goossens, conductor of the Sydney Symphony Orchestra, who asserted that Sydney should have a fine concert hall and a home for an opera company and chamber music. Joe Cahill, who became New South Wales Premier in 1952, convened a conference in 1954 to build support for an opera house for Sydney. He said, "This State cannot go on without proper facilities for the expression of talent and the staging of the highest forms of artistic entertainment which add grace and charm to living and which help to develop and mold a better, more enlightened community. . . . Surely it is proper in establishing an opera house that it should not be a 'shadygaff'

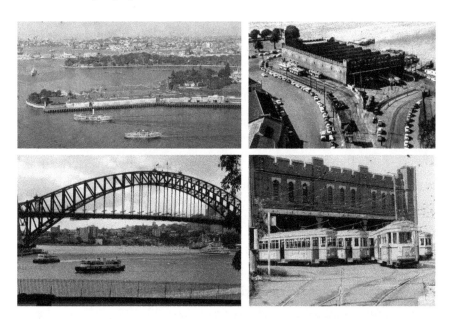

Figure 9.3 Bennelong Point, circa 1955. (*Top*) Two views of the point. The one at l*eft* shows the view from the Sydney Harbour Bridge. (*Bottom left*) Sydney Harbour Bridge as seen from Bennelong Point. (*Bottom right*) The tram shed on Bennelong Point. (*Top left*: https://historyinorbit.com/content/73890/1a6934850399207ebcce3244b34c1ffb. jpg. *Top right*: https://upload.wikimedia.org/wikipedia/commons/3/33/NSWGT_ Fort_Macquarie_Tranways_Depot.jpg. Public domain. *Bottom left*: http://sydney-eye. blogspot.com/2015/03/tarpeian-way-parade-of-icons.html. *Bottom right*: http://www. visitsydneyaustralia.com.au/images/Bennelong-Pt-Tram-Depot1.jpg)

place but an edifice that will be a credit to the State not only today but also for hundreds of years."[2]

The competition for the Opera House was internationally advertised in December 1955 with the deadline for registration set for March 15, 1956 and submissions required by December 3, 1956 (the month I completed high school in Sydney). The site chosen was Bennelong Point, on the opposite side of Circular Quay, Sydney's downtown ferry terminal, from the Sydney Harbour Bridge. Figure 9.3 shows several views of Bennelong

2. https://www.sydneyoperahouse.com/our-story/sydney-opera-house-history/the-competition.html

Point and one of the Harbour Bridge at the time of the competition. The Point was no longer important as a dock then, but served as a large tram depot.

The competition had a simple program (in the architect's sense of the general specification of what the building was to accomplish). It stated that the site, Bennelong Point, "is probably without equal in the world . . . one that fulfills all the requirements—dimensions, space and beauty—essential for the type of building that should be constructed." The program called for two auditoriums, with additional space for rehearsal rooms, a broadcasting center, a restaurant, and two meeting rooms as well as bars and foyers for the various halls. To simplify matters, the competition brief specified that only line drawings were to be submitted—the use of color and models was forbidden.

Joe Cahill announced the results on January 29, 1957. We met the top three entries, briefly, in §3.1, and revisit them in Figure 9.4. There, we noted how the practical demands of the program were met by divergent designs that involved both bold decisions as to the overall form (easily captured in a sentence or two) and then the sculpting of the forms in a way that would also meet the various utilitarian demands on the buildings. We saw the various tradeoffs between diverse design considerations involving both utility and aesthetics. The third-place entry put the auditoriums in two separate buildings, and the design did not respond to the site other than in the size of the bounding rectangle. Had the second design been built, it would, I think, have been a success. A central core housed the stage machinery for both auditoriums, and the auditoriums and other venues were wrapped around this central core. Moreover, the form of the building is distinctive and interesting.

But site analysis is at the heart of the initial design process. Utzon made three crucial decisions: He put the auditoriums side-by-side with the footprint of the building strongly linked to that of Bennelong Point. He stressed the special vantage for the site afforded from the Sydney Harbour Bridge, offering a "fifth façade." And he had each auditorium building ascend to a lobby with a glass wall to provide a

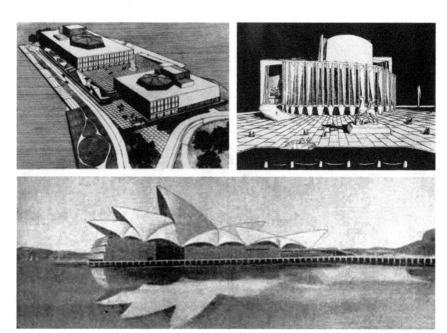

Figure 9.4 (A repeat of Figure 3.1). The front page of *The Sydney Morning Herald* of January 30, 1957 announced the top three place-getters in the competition to design the Sydney Opera House. (*Top left*) The third place entry. (*Top right*) The second place entry. (*Bottom*) Utzon's winning entry. "Ironically, the perspective of Utzon's scheme was not drawn by him. It had been commissioned from local architect Arthur Baldwinson" (Watson, 2006, p. 50). Presumably, this is because Utzon's freeform sketch (see Figure 9.5) might have caused the public to question the committee's choice. (© *The Sydney Morning Herald.*)

superb viewpoint for appreciating the beauty of the harbor (Figures 9.5 and 9.6).

All three designs addressed the requirements of the program, but each architect had a distinctive "big idea" that became the nucleus for the initiation of creative form-making and overall formal design. Having said this, there is no necessary strict ordering of these design processes. For example, varied sketches might be made before the "big idea" crystallizes, perhaps establishing just one of these sketches as an island of reliability for further development.

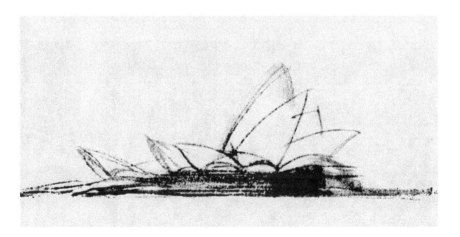

Figure 9.5 Utzon's winning entry. His freeform sketch of the Opera House from the "Red Book," the first presentation document prepared for the New South Wales (NSW) government in 1958. (Department of Public Works; NRS-12707, "Sydney National Opera House" ("Red Book"), March 1958. Sketch Sydney Opera House Red Book. By courtesy of NSW State Archives and Records, custodian of the Materials.)

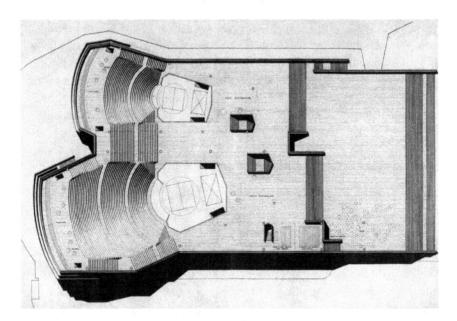

Figure 9.6 A plan showing not only how Utzon's design conforms to the shape of the site but also the way in which Utzon envisioned the stairs and the auditoriums incised into the platform. This is one of the floor plans on page 5 of Jørn Utzon's Competition Entry. (Department of Public Works; NRS-12825 Competition drawings submitted by Jørn Utzon to the Opera House Committee, 1956. NRS-12825-1-[SZ112]-[7] | West elevation National Opera House, Sydney, Australia, 1956. By courtesy of NSW State Archives and Records, custodian of the Materials.)

Utzon's design, while initially overlooked, eventually caught the imagination of the jury (thanks in part to Eero Saarinen, whom we will meet again, and Leslie Martin[3]) and won the competition. Robert Geddes (2006), a member of the Philadelphia Group that placed second, said, "We almost won but we didn't. Why? Because Jørn Utzon's design was a masterpiece." Utzon excelled in addressing the unique contextual and ecological elements of the site.

We now assess some aspects of the creation of this masterpiece. Of course, designing a building of this magnitude would require multiple iterations, and the more we know of these, the better might we be able to characterize the mental processes of the architects. My challenge to historians of architecture, then, is to fill in the gaps to create more specific data on the stages of design to ground and challenge (neuro)cognitive theories.

Design of a distinctive building may require immersing oneself in the site, seeing the landscape in terms of its growth, its light, its impact, its form, and how it works. Richard Leplastrier (personal communication) speaks of developing this in terms of a connoisseurship of place/nature/culture and the need for the human condition to be inspired by life. Such a mixture of previous understanding and immersive experience of the site can develop an intuitive sense of place as a basis for imagining what the place could become. Yet, amazingly, Utzon was able to get his exceptional feel for the site without visiting Sydney before or during the competition. He had to gather his own documentation to complement the photographs and the two plans reproduced in the competition handbook. He watched a film on Sydney at the Australian Embassy in Copenhagen, and obtained maritime charts from which he, as an experienced sailor, "could measure distances and form a judgement of heights, the importance of the color of the sea [and] the shades of light." Utzon's understanding of the forms of

---

3. https://www.pidgeondigital.com/talks/sydney-opera-house/ includes a discussion between Henry Ashworth (Professor of Architecture at the University of Sydney and Chairman of the Opera House competition jury) and his fellow assessors Eero Saarinen and Sir Leslie Martin (Professor of Architecture at Cambridge University), on January 29, 1957.

the land and the underwater contours enabled him to see how to rebuild the headland of Bennelong Point.

In awarding first place to Utzon, the jury said, "The unity of its structural expression creates a striking architectural composition admirably suited to Bennelong Point. The white sail-like forms of the shell vaults relate as naturally to the harbor as sails to yachts." However, Figure 9.7 emphasizes that sails and the Opera House shells have quite different forms. When Utzon watched that film in Copenhagen, he observed the clouds that lingered over the harbor. He later said (Utzon, 1962) that these clouds had inspired him to think of white roofs floating over the platform. Recall the discussion in §1.1 of Zumthor's images coming to mind (though they need not be half-forgotten): new ideas may involve the melding of diverse aspects of very different sources of inspiration, a theme whose (neuro)cognitive elaboration will be a key aspect of Chapter 10.

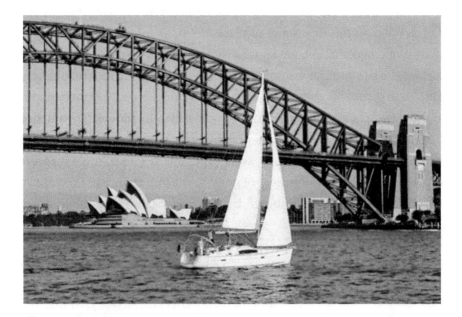

Figure 9.7 Those aren't sails on the Opera House! (© onboat.com, with permission.)

When ideas are coming to mind, they are based not only on what the architect has experienced directly but also on an understanding and experience of the work of other architects—whether it provides inspiration, or helps define a road one declines to travel. Mies van der Rohe was a master of modernism, and when I visited Manhattan in January 1961 (on my way to graduate school at MIT), I thought his Seagram Building one of the finest skyscrapers in Manhattan, yet at the same time I was stunned (in a positive sense!) by Frank Lloyd Wright's Guggenheim Museum (Figure 9.8) which, opened in 1959, is amazing for the way in which the gallery swirls downward. However, the very success of buildings in the Miesian style invited too many less successful variations:

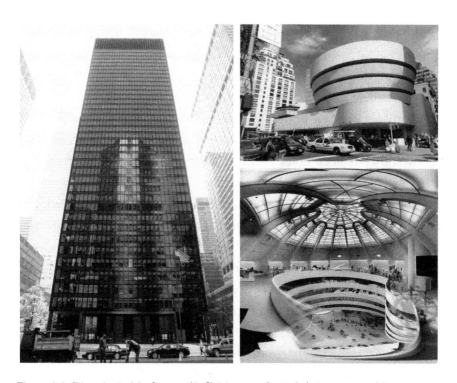

Figure 9.8 Diversity in Manhattan. (*Left*) Mies van der Rohe's Seagram Building (completed in 1958). (*Right*) Frank Lloyd Wright's Solomon R. Guggenheim Museum (opened in 1959). (*Left*: Noroton, May 1, 2008, public domain, via Wikimedia Commons. *Top right*: Jean-Christophe Benoist, CC BY 3.0, via Wikimedia Commons. *Bottom right*: https://delectant.com/frank-lloyd-wright-organic-architecture/)

At the beginning of the 1950s there was a marked loss of momentum in the heroic ideals of modernism. The dominant architecture of the time was drifting in two directions: the international standardisation of Miesian sublimity and its calcification in the prismatic buildings of corporate America; and a search for greater individual expression inspired by forms and references, long since sidelined. If Mies had realised the Seagram Building, then Le Corbusier had just built the Ronchamp Chapel, Wright the Guggenheim Museum and Aalto had begun his work on the Imatra Church. . . . The issue is not that Mies was tapped out (though his imitators might have been) so much as Utzon's inspiration was to be found elsewhere. (Fromonot, 1998, p. 55)

The early work of Le Corbusier was much more one of straight lines, but in 1954 he created the Ronchamp Chapel with its curved roof suggestive of the wimple of a nun, the curling headgear of her traditional garb. Le Corbusier, who learned much from other cultures, was also influenced by the mosque of Sidi Brahim at El Ateuf in Southern Algeria. This provided one of the images that came to Le Corbusier's mind in conceiving the windows as deep holes punched in thick walls, very different from other mosques or chapels (Figure 9.9, *top*). Alvar Aalto was an important influence on Utzon's development (Aalto in Finland; Utzon in Denmark and Sweden) and in his Imatra Church we again see the movement away from the straight line and toward the curve (Figure 9.9, *bottom*). To use our language analogy (§8.6), we can see the beginning of a new "vocabulary"—but, to stretch the analogy, what arose was not a small fixed stock of "words" but rather the opening up of a new way to create "words," to invent forms for architecture. These new ideas did not provide the specific form of the Sydney Opera House, but did encourage Utzon to explore the use of dramatically curved forms, rather than rectilinear ones.

While meditating on Zumthor's essay, I not only invoked half-forgotten ideas, but also quoted him as writing, "Construction is the art of making a meaningful whole out of many parts. . . . I feel respect for the art of joining. . . ." Intriguingly, though, this same period was one

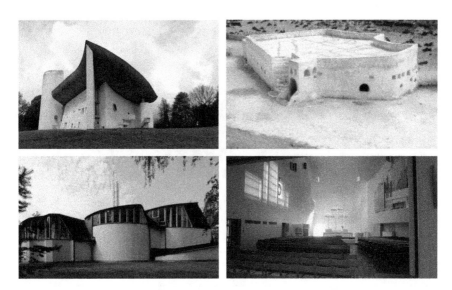

Figure 9.9 (*Top*) Le Corbusier's Ronchamp Chapel (built in 1954) and the Mosque of Sidi Brahim (constructed in 1155). (*Bottom*) Alvar Aalto's Imatra Church (completed in 1958). (*Top left*: Public domain. *Top right*: https://www.euratlas.net/photos/time/12th_century/el_ateuf.html, © Christos Nüssli 1981—euratlas.org. *Bottom left*: Daniel McCarthy Architect LLC. *Bottom right*: By Mikkoau, CC BY-SA 4.0 via Wikimedia Commons.)

in which new methods of construction were coming into play *which did not rest on joining*, but instead allowed vast structures to be cast in concrete. To push our language analogy even further, we can say that the new vocabulary was complemented by a new grammar of construction. Wooden frames would be built, and then the concrete would be formed atop them. Although not completed at the start of the Sydney competition (it opened in 1957), the general plan of Eero Saarinen's TWA Terminal at Idlewild Airport (now JFK) in New York was already known to architects including Utzon (I assume). Figure 9.10 shows exterior and interior views. Having flown in and out of this terminal several times in the early years, I can attest to the playfulness of the interior design as well as the amazing swoops of the exterior. This was indeed an influential masterpiece, though for many years it was left derelict and has now been repurposed as a hotel.

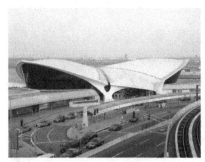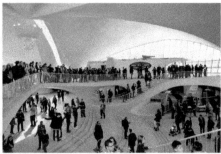

Figure 9.10 Eero Saarinen's TWA Terminal at Idlewild Airport, New York (1957). (*Left*) Exterior view, whose curved forms express the "big idea" of wings and flight. (*Right*) Interior view after repurposing. (*Left*: Dmitry Avdeev, CC BY-SA 3.0 GFDL 1.2, via Wikimedia Commons. *Right*: Bogframe, CC BY-SA 4.0, https://creativecommons.org/licenses/by-sa/4.0, via Wikimedia Commons.)

With this, let's try to probe Utzon's imagination, seeking insights based on specific experiences. In discussing his father, Aage Utzon, Jørn Utzon wrote:

> I have benefited greatly from the many hours I have spent with my father. . . . attached to a large shipyard, where all trades were represented, and large-scale work was carried out.
>
> When I was about to draw the Opera House in Sydney, I was not really worried that I had to convert sketches into curved surfaces towering 60 meters, define them geometrically and have them constructed. As a child I had seen huge ship-hulls.
>
> My father helped me construct the large-scale models required. Without any specific agreement he made the wooden models. After a couple of days the delicate forms were in the drawing room.[4]

For me, looking at the curves on either side of the hull of Aage Utzon's yacht with the keel dividing the two halves brings us much closer to the

---

4. From the Guide to Utzon website: http://www.utzonphotos.com/about-utzon/curriculum-vitae-and-biography/biography/aage-utzon-father/

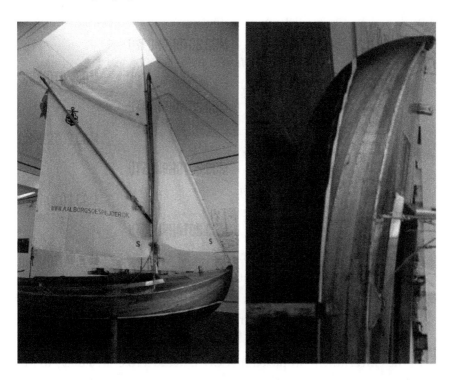

Figure 9.11 (*Left*) A yacht designed by Aage Utzon. (*Right*). Making the case for ship hulls (this one rotated from the yacht at left) as a major source of inspiration for the shape of the shells of the Sydney Opera House roof. (Photo: Utzonphotos, courtesy of Flemming Bo Andersen.)

shells of the Sydney Opera House, each with its well-defined ridge line, than a sail or a cloud does, though each of them may well have been part of the subliminal images that influenced the final design (Figure 9.11).

Utzon's "big ideas"—the shape of the shells, and the side-by-side placement of the two auditoriums—provide the basis for many further decisions. Each decision, once made, could then provide a target for further elaboration, lead to reconsidering earlier decisions, or be set aside until later becoming the focus of the architect's attention.

Utzon's tragedy was that even though he shared Zumthor's respect for "the art of joining, the ability of craftsmen and engineers . . . ," he had not, at the time of the competition, thought through the challenges of going from wooden ship shapes to massive concrete shells. This failure contributed to the escalating costs that were in part the cause for his removal before completion of the building. Anne Watson's book, *Building a Masterpiece: the Sydney Opera House* (Watson, 2006, pp. 8–9) contains a detailed timeline for Utzon's career and for the Sydney Opera House. Here are some relevant dates:

September 1961: Utzon develops spherical scheme as final solution for shell design.

March 1962: Utzon and Arup's Jack Zunz present new spherical scheme in Sydney.

November 1963: Commencement of erection of first precast rib vault.

1965: Utzon's request for funding for construction of plywood mock-ups for stage 3 [the interior] not met. Utzon makes repeated claims to State Government for fees owing to him.

1966: Hoping that it will elicit movement on funding from the State Government, Utzon submits letter of withdrawal on February 28. The Government proposed that Utzon takes a role subsidiary to the State Government Architect.

"Utzon-in-charge" protests and demonstrations followed, but the Government did not respond. Utzon and his family left Australia on April 28, 1965. Peter Hall was appointed to lead the local team charged with finishing the job. The team had to master every detail before moving forward.

To supplement this, here are excerpts from the TV documentary *Sydney Opera House: Man-Made Marvels* (7Mate, 2008?). In addition to reviewing the design of the Opera House, the video demonstrated that Utzon's winning proposal lacked details needed to carry construction through to completion.

John Nutt, Structural Engineer: The radical shape's construction bordered on the near impossible 50 years ago. The sails curve up to 20 stories tall, and each must hold its own weight. The ridge lines posed another problem: concrete shells don't like sharp ridge lines. For 3 years, various solutions failed.

A further problem was that the acute angle of the leading shells (Figures 9.4 and 9.5) caused a considerable horizontal thrust that was removed in the final design by making the shells more upright. However, Joe Cahill insisted that construction start before these problems were solved. He was up for re-election in 1958, and his party was likely to lose, so he wanted to ensure that the project could not be cancelled by his opponents.

> **Malcolm Nicklin**, Construction Engineer: Need a carefully planned base designed to support the sails, yet only freehand sketches of the sails were available. Yet on March 2, 1959 construction started before the plans were final. Design developed as they were building.
> **Ian Mackenzie**, Site Engineer: Late 1962, construction was well under way but behind schedule and over budget—and still no final design. "A fair bit of trial and error."

The challenge was to build multiple shells of different-looking shape and size. The engineering firm Arup had the task of figuring out how to construct the shells, but years of effort proved fruitless. But then Utzon had an "aha experience" while peeling an orange and realized that different shapes could be obtained from the surface of the same sphere, not even needing different diameters. But how could these "spherical triangles" be built, and how could they be arrayed to defy the force of gravity? The shape of the shells ruled out pouring them in situ. The solution was to divide the shells into identical ribs and then break each rib into smaller segments. Larger shells had more segments and longer ribs. The solution further involved designing an ingenious assembly method.

> **John Kuner**, Construction Engineer: The concrete segments were cast on site. A special crane was designed to lift the segments to be attached in place, constructing each shell one rib at a time [to "grow" the shells from the closed to the open end].

Over 6 years, the shells at last took shape. They were covered with tiles "like a mountain capped in glistening snow." To achieve this effect, the tiles were mounted on sheets in a complex diagonal pattern that were then affixed to the shells.

> **Michael Tomaszewski**, Architect: "The most exciting building in the world at that time." Utzon wanted to create a new design, but the quest for perfection takes time and money. You need prototypes. But the government held back the needed funds.

This emphasizes the importance of a team effort, whether several architects, or architects and engineers working together.[5] Here, Utzon is clearly the sole creator of the overall shape of the shells and their size, placement, and covering in white tiles, but their realization required immense effort by the engineers. Understanding the final totality requires us to enquire who is responsible for what, and how the participants could communicate so that, between them, they come up with the final coherent design.

Here are further recollections from the documentary:

> **Rick Leplastrier**: Who would dare complete an unfinished painting by Matisse? "It would have been a bloody disaster."

Utzon's plans for the interior were scrapped and purpose-designed stage machinery demolished.

> **Ian Mackenzie**, Site Engineer: "If I've got a regret, it's that the building wasn't left there then . . . a 21 million dollar sculpture, and they took the 80 million dollars they still needed to complete and put up a totally functional building elsewhere . . . so you had an opera house *and* a sculpture."

---

5. The chapter "Reconciliation" of *Architect and Engineer: A Study in Sibling Rivalry* (Saint, 2007) sees problems with Saarinen's TWA terminal as foreshadowing Utzon's (though, in fact, the engineering solutions are completely different). Saint also discusses the work of architect Louis Kahn with the engineer August Komendant (both of them Estonian).

In what follows, let's extract several design decisions *specific* to Utzon. Our task in Chapter 10 will be to descry *general* principles for the underlying cognitive and neural mechanisms that support design. Rather than starting with vague ideas and finally filling in details, Utzon made some very clear, symbolically precise decisions early on, with the sketching and the working out of details firmly constrained by these decisions. Note that the ordering of the decisions below has no necessary relation to the order in which they occurred to Utzon. Indeed, any one of them may have influenced the working out of others.

A building to be seen from all sides

Unlike the other competitors, Utzon thought through how the Opera House would be seen from different perspectives—on the harbor, from the Botanical Gardens, and looking down from the Sydney Harbour Bridge. In thinking about the view from the harbor, Utzon was greatly influenced by his experience as a lad sailing near Helsingør (the area where Shakespeare placed Hamlet's castle). He was struck by similarities with Helsingør peninsula on which Kronborg Castle sits "where the forms stand out in a horizontal line, the sea and the clouds without a single vertical line" (Figure 9.12)[6]—an evocation of familiar places "charged with poetic memory." Yet the view from the Harbour Bridge that is so important in assessing Bennelong Point is missing in the flat surroundings of Helsingør. Combining old memories of sailing around Helsingør with imagination of the fifth façade observed from the Harbour Bridge provided Utzon with a new framework for his design.

6. For Leplastrier, what is most significant about this photo is the yacht! He thinks it may be a two-ended yacht, a spidsgatter designed by Aage Utzon, Jørn's father, "a beautiful and radical design."

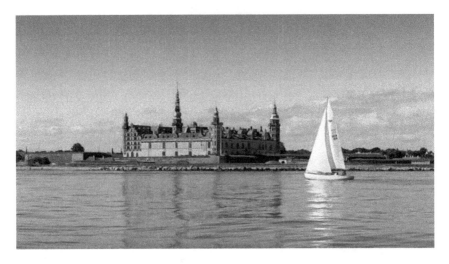

Figure 9.12 A view of Kronborg Castle on the peninsula at Helsingør. (Credit: Thomas Rahbek, Agency for Culture and Palaces, Denmark.)

Placing the auditoriums

Placing the auditoriums side by side: The competition brief called for two auditoriums. Utzon's solution was unique among the entries in putting them side-by-side.

Conforming the design to the contour of the site: Moreover, Utzon housed all the functional activities within a stone-clad platform and married it to the contours of the site. With this base he reconstructed the headland of Bennelong Point so that it became integrated with the two auditoriums (Figure 9.13).

Emphasizing a secondary function: Utzon realized that the further end of Bennelong Point afforded a spectacular view of the harbor. As a result, his design not only provided the auditoriums but also added a new *aesthetic function*—not of the building as such, but in providing visitors with a special vantage point. Each auditorium has the stage at the "landward" end, from which the seats slope up in the direction of the far end of the Point. Lobbies at the upper end behind each auditorium offer a grand view of Sydney Harbour, complementing the functionality of the auditoriums.

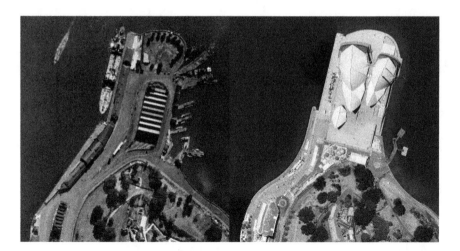

Figure 9.13 Conforming the design to the contour of the site. At *left* we see Bennelong Point back in 1943 in its tram-shed days; at *right* a 2012 view of the placement of the Sydney Opera House with the broad ends of the auditoriums looking across the Harbour. Both panels show the Botanical Gardens abutting the Point. (https://twitter. com/sydthenandnow/status/579935802630619136. From Six Maps/by Phil Harvey. Public domain.)

Three layers

The Opera House shells bear little relation to the structure of the auditoriums that they cover. The design principle here was to build three separate layers:

- A platform containing the hidden workings of the opera house
- The performance space above this
- The roof as the shelter

The performance space and the roof constrain each other—the low points of the roof must remain high enough to accommodate the heights of the performance space, but the latter did not match the shape of the former. The roofs became a fifth façade, the building a sculpture. However, Utzon was fired before he actually got to exploit his ideas about the auditoriums, and their interior design was left in the hands of local architects.

What images had come to Utzon's mind in coming up with this tripartite structure? Certainly, the building elevated on a platform is a trope of Western architecture since at least the days of Classical Greek temples, but non-European examples had a greater personal impact (Figure 9.14). In

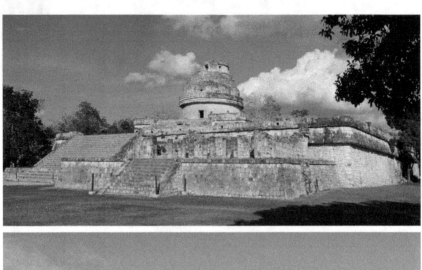

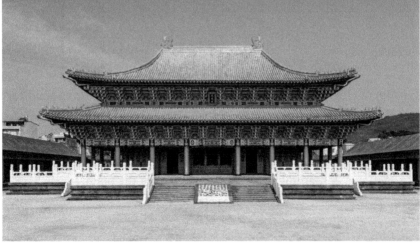

Figure 9.14 Mayan and Chinese Influences—platforms, "floating" roof, a grand sweep of stairs. (*Top*) Clouds floating above the Observatory, part of the pre-Columbian Mayan site Chichén-Itzá, Yucatan, Mexico. (*Bottom*) Temple of Confucius, Kaohsiung, Taiwan. (*Top*: https://upload.wikimedia.org/wikipedia/commons/8/8f/Chichen_Itza_ Observatory_2_1.jpg, Creative Commons Attribution-Share Alike 3.0 Unported license. *Bottom*: © CEphoto, Uwe Aranas, https://commons.wikimedia.org/wiki/File:Kaohsiung_ Taiwan_Kaohsiung-Confucius-Temple-01.jpg)

"Platforms and Plateaus," published in the year the spherical scheme for constructing the shells was presented, Utzon (1962) wrote:

> The platform as an architectural element is a fascinating feature. I first fell in love with it in Mexico on a study trip in 1949, where I found many variations, both in size and idea of the platform, and where many of the platforms are alone without anything but the surrounding nature.
>
> Yucatan is a flat lowland covered with an inaccessible jungle, which grows to a certain uniform defined height. In this jungle the Mayas lived in their villages with small pieces of land cleared for cultivation, and their surrounding, background as well as roof, was the hot, damp, green jungle. No large views, no up and down movements.
>
> By introducing the platform with its level at the same height as the jungle top, these people had suddenly obtained a new dimension of life, worthy of their devotion to their Gods. On these high platforms, many of them as long as 100 meters, they built their temples.
>
> They had from here the sky, the clouds and the breeze, and suddenly the jungle roof had been converted into a great, open plain. (Utzon, 1962)

Of course, Sydneysiders do not live submerged in the Harbour as Mayans lived submerged in the jungle. For the Sydney Opera House, the platform lifted the building to a commanding view—but above the ever-changing colors of the waters of Sydney Harbour, not across the treetops.

For Utzon, human activities such as the religious practices of the Chinese had to unfold on an artificial plane, raised above ground, dissociating them from the earth. There, "the spectators receive the completed work of art." In line with these observations, Utzon noted the importance of the stairs leading to these plateaus as well as the contrast between the massive base and the floating roof above them (Fromonot, 1998, p. 49; commenting on Utzon, 1962, "Platforms and Plateaus: Ideas of A Danish Architect"). Utzon further comments:

In the Sydney Opera House scheme, the idea has been to let the platform cut through like a knife and separate primary and secondary functions completely. On top of the platform the spectators receive the completed work of art and beneath the platform every preparation for it takes place.

To express the platform and avoid destroying it is a very important thing, when you start building on top of it. A flat roof does not express the flatness of the platform. [My italics. Presumably Utzon's point is that the flatness is emphasized only if the structure atop contrasts with that flatness, rather than blending in with it.]

Utzon presents a number of sketches—a platform in the Yucatan, providing a vantage above the trees of the forest; the roof of a Chinese temple or Japanese house "floating" above a platform; and so-called "schemes for the Sydney Opera House" that bear no obvious relation to the distinctive shells of the actual building (copies are available at http://www.transfer-arch.com/monograph/platforms-and-plateaus/). Utzon further remarks:

As shown here . . . you can see roofs, curved forms, hanging higher or lower over the plateau. The contrast of forms and the constantly changing heights between these two elements result in spaces of great architectural force made possible by the modern structural approach to concrete construction, which has given so many beautiful tools into the hands of the architect.

The shapes of the roofs

It is the design of the shells that people most think of when they ponder Utzon's design. In his submission, Utzon stated, "Light suspended concrete shells accentuate the plateau effect and the character of the staircase constructions. . . . The whole exterior radiates lightness and festivity." This was the crucial feature that has made the Sydney Opera House an icon of world architecture. But in the end the shells were not "light suspended concrete shells" after all.

With variations in size, the basic shell design is repeated. This would seem to be a strong example of Utzon's interest in additive architecture, but no mention of the Opera House appears in Volume V of Utzon's Logbook, *Additive Architecture* (Utzon, 2009).

The two-fold access

In his submission, Utzon explained:

> The architecture emphasises the character of Bennelong Point and takes the greatest advantage of the view. The approach of the audience is easy and as distinctly pronounced as in Grecian theatres by uncomplicated staircase constructions. The audience is assembled from cars, trains and ferries and led like a festive procession into the respective halls, thanks to the pure staircase solution.

Here we see another architectural "memory," the Greek amphitheater, as Utzon designs the staircases that first bring the public from their cars and taxis and strolls from Circular Quay up a broad staircase to the lobby at the landward end of the building. Utzon provides further affordances, easily preparing the visitor both to climb up to the auditorium and then, at intermission, to climb further to the upper lobbies with their sweeping views of the Harbour.

I don't know in what order these realizations came to Utzon, but what I want to stress is that there may be "aha" moments that yield precise but high-level descriptions, and these are interleaved with exploration of form and function via diverse sketches. These (and later) design features could "talk to each other" to eventually provide a stable base for relatively independent efforts at design refinement. Design is not a linear process from vague to precise. Rather, it involves a back-and-forth approach that, during this process, integrates layers of information, goals, and values to ultimately yield the fully realized building.

9.3. SKETCHING AND MODEL-MAKING: FRANK GEHRY'S BILBAO GUGGENHEIM

We now turn to the work of Frank Gehry in the design of the Guggenheim Museum in Bilbao to exemplify the interplay of sketching using drawings and physical three-dimensional (3D) models, as well as examining the utility of computers and the role of collaboration in architecture.

There is a well-known sketch of Frank Gehry's (for a similar sketch, see van Bruggen, p. 84, top), which has the property that, without foreknowledge, one would be unlikely to guess it relates to the Bilbao Museum. However, when we have a view of the building as shown in Figure 9.15, we find that the sketch contains a preview of the massing of structure at the right, as well as the upward sweep at the left. The sketch also includes a vertical structure that does not appear in this photo of the finished building, but presumably refers to the tower on the other side of the bridge hinted at by the diagonal "rectangle" in front of it. The question before us is this: How do such sketches fit into Gehry's design process?[7]

---

7. Why don't I show the sketch described here and those mentioned in what follows? When I requested permission from Gehry Partners to reproduce images for which they hold copyright, I was asked for the then current draft of the section. In due course, partner Meaghan Lloyd wrote to say that, "There is a fair amount in what you've written that doesn't reflect the realities of our practice. Mr Chan's memories, in particular, are not in synch with those of other architects in the practice who were working with frank [*sic*] and the team in the same timeframe that Mr. Chan references. . . . It does not therefore make sense for us to give you permission to use the requested images/illustrations for this piece." I replied in detail the next day to express my willingness to attend to any corrections to my account she or her colleagues might offer. *No reply.* I then followed through with a revised draft with a cover email to Ms. Lloyd stating that "Edwin Chan . . . suggested that, because I had discussed Bilbao with him, my notes over-emphasized his role in the project. He has thus graciously agreed to let me remove his name from description of the work of Gehry and the team. . . . He also corrected a few errors I had made. . . . It is my hope that with these changes, [the new version] is now (or soon will be, with further changes the Gehry team may wish to suggest) in a form that allows you to provide the requested permission for the figures. . . ." *Again, no reply.* And, despite two further enquiries,

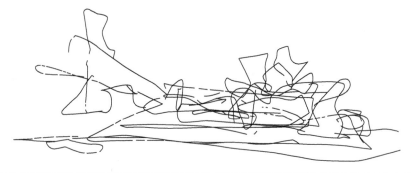

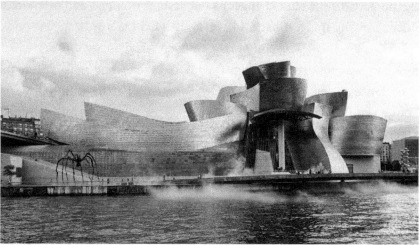

Figure 9.15 The Guggenheim Museum in Bilbao (bottom). (https://commons.
wikimedia.org/wiki/File:Bilbao_-_Guggenheim_aurore.jpg, PA, CC BY-SA 4.0, via
Wikimedia Commons.)

What is the cognitive status of Gehry's sketch? We need a sense of how
scribbled shapes, and not just carefully shaded regions bounded by precise contours, can be configured together to suggest the overall shape of
an imagined structure or scene. The actual building is prefigured in the
drawing, but its construction can only be specified when the whole is

Ms. Lloyd has still not replied. I have thus had to strip out the images. Fortunately, however,
they are available in Coosje van Bruggen's book, and so I can at least refer you there to see the
figures—and a wealth of further material that will let you decide whether what I have written
does indeed distort the realities of Gehry's practice.

decomposed into large components, with further elaboration required to determine how the metal plates, glass, columns, and so on are assembled to make the final form.

In commenting on an earlier draft of this section, the cognitive scientist (and 2021-22 ANFA President) David Kirsh asked: "What is Gehry hoping to remember when he looks at the sketch again? The sketch itself is the tip of the iceberg compared to the cognitive processing that went into its production. What does he rule out by the choices he makes? And how does this prepare for the later changes as the design is refined and extended?" Since receiving this feedback, I have studied Coosje van Bruggen's book, *Frank O. Gehry: Guggenheim Museum Bilbao* (van Bruggen, 1997), which goes part way toward answering David's questions, and makes clear the importance of detailed analysis of development of architectural projects. Coosje van Bruggen (June 6, 1942—January 10, 2009) was a Dutch-born American sculptor, art historian, and critic who collaborated extensively with her husband, Claes Oldenburg. Her book provides an invaluable reference for understanding the design of the museum, and includes extracts from her conversations with Frank Gehry, Edwin Chan, and Thomas Krens. My contribution in this section developed from reflections on a reading of van Bruggen's book, conversations with Chan, a visit to the museum in 1999, the LACMA exhibition of models of Gehry's work, twice viewing Sydney Pollack's 2005 movie, *Sketches of Frank Gehry*, and further reading.

As in the previous section, my aim is to hypothesize a variety of particulars about the decisions made in a design project to provide a touchstone for the beginnings of a cognitive neuroscience of architectural design that is offered in Chapter 10. The neuroscience does not explain the *particulars* of these examples of the creativity of individual architects; rather, it helps us develop some understanding of general processes that underlie the particularities of the design, and thus helps us develop a more hypothesis-driven approach to investigation of further case studies from a cog/neuro perspective.

Gehry's creation of semiautomatic drawings alternated with the development of carefully crafted 3D physical models as well as rapidly assembled and modified 3D physical "sketches." Note that computers were not involved in the design phase of this project, but only in the final phase of developing specifications for construction. Thus, in what follows (except right at the end), the 3D models referred to are physical models, not CAD models. Van Bruggen's book shows how pliable the design is at its early stages, where one sketch may "contradict" another. But, most helpfully, her book offers written interpretations without which it is often impossible for outsiders to make sense of the sketches. However, they functioned well as part of the design process not only (a) as a basis for Gehry's own development (he certainly knew *at a general level* what he had in mind as he drew the sketches, even though he made new "discoveries" as he later reviewed those sketches) but, further and crucially, (2) he could share these interpretations with his colleagues as the actual design began to take shape. In particular, he could transfer his understanding of the sketches to his team, who could then turn these sketchy sketches into 3D models where the relative sizes and more specific forms of the sketched volumes could be given a tentative specification. Notably, this could not involve simply transcribing the sketch into a model but required lengthy discussion with Gehry, clarifying and in some cases modifying what was implicit in the sketch. The physical model could then form the basis for further consideration, elaboration, and modification.

A complementary point is that a number of design elements here had already developed in some form in other Gehry buildings, so that we see the development of a "vocabulary" and also the way in which with each building the elements of that vocabulary and the "grammar" of their composition may develop. As before, the "vocabulary" is not a set of rigid structures to be put together, but rather a sense of plastic forms that the imagination can play with, modifying them and assembling them in new combinations.

Whereas Utzon won the Sydney competition without having ever visited Sydney, Gehry was invited to Bilbao by Thomas Krens, director of the Solomon R. Guggenheim Foundation, to discuss a proposal by the Basque Administration for a partnership with the Foundation even before the design competition. The Administration had proposed to convert the

Alhóndiga, a former wine storage warehouse, into a cultural facility. But when Gehry visited Bilbao on May 20, 1991,[8] he found the Alhóndiga unworkable as a museum. Subsequent discussion led to selection of a new site that, unlike the Alhóndiga, was at the side of the river, and included areas on both sides of a prominent bridge. Gehry analyzed three directions from which the site could be viewed. I am reminded here of Utzon's realization that the Sydney Opera House would be viewed not only from the ferries and yachts passing on the harbor but also from the vantage point of the Sydney Harbour Bridge. However, the fifth façade, the view from the hills across the river, is little seen by visitors.

For the Basque administration, the main programmatic requirement was the design of an art museum that would not only serve as a showcase for art but also have a strong iconic identity to attract visitors to the building for itself—to do for Bilbao what Jørn Utzon's Sydney Opera House had done for Sydney. The Guggenheim Foundation, as represented by Krens, had requirements about the nature of the galleries, given that they wanted different Guggenheim museums to emphasize different aspects of their international collection. They required an extremely large gallery to house large, complex pieces from the Guggenheim collection such as, it later turned out, the 172-ton steel sculpture by Richard Serra, entitled *Snake*, built specifically for the space.

Going beyond this program, Gehry established a set of five "design principles" after the site visit (Chan, personal communication):

1. An entry plaza that addresses the city, welcoming people as they approach the museum from the city side
2. The museum to serve as a region of transition from the level of the city to the level of river, adapting to the local topography
3. A river garden offering another zone of transition, reinforcing the relation of the museum to the river
4. Integrating the bridge into the scope of the museum, an urbanistic decision

8. All these precise dates are based on van Bruggen's book.

5. At the bend in the river, constructing a highreader (that is, a structure of notable height) visible from the old town (this was before deciding on a tower as the highreader)

None of these would apply had the original plan to repurpose the Alhóndiga been preserved. However, after these choices are made, they constrain—but are also open to modification by—the architect's design process. Perhaps the general point is that as the program is elaborated, both before and after the project is placed in the architect's hands, certain high-level components, both of the building and concerning the building and its surrounds begin to emerge, and analysis then involves a sort of elastic matching of these to each other and to loci on the site.

After the Basque Administration cleared the purchase of the new river location, a brief competition was held between Gehry, the Viennese team Coop Himmelblau, and Arata Isozaki from Japan. The selection committee was interested only in getting an impression of the overall vision of each architect—with the explicit design process starting only after the selection was made. Gehry's proposal was selected during meetings on July 20 and 21, 1991.[9]

Van Bruggen's chapter, "The Origins of the Bilbao Guggenheim" (van Bruggen, pp. 30–93), presents "the story of the architect's initial sketches, how they were programmatically translated, sculpturally defined, sometimes creatively misinterpreted, and shifted toward the building of a rough model, all within a span of less than two weeks [in July 1991, prior to submission of the competition entry]." I won't repeat the details (she provides a broad selection of photos and Gehry's sketches along with her text) but rather focus on the role of sketching, model-making, and interaction that was involved.

The first step was for Gehry to tour the site, and then sketch how the building might relate to it, with respect both to the program requirements and to establishing a strong identity for the museum in its context: "he began to

9. See van Bruggen (1997, pp. 26–29) for details "On the Architect's Selection Process and Preliminary Program Statement."

sketch his first impressions on the front and back of the hotel stationery; in these fast scrawls and mere annotations, the hand functions as an immediate tool of the mind. Moving the pen to occupy space on the paper, Gehry began to explore and familiarize himself with the site" (van Bruggen, p. 31). What is worth repeating is that the sketches would be unintelligible (to me at least) without van Bruggen's text and—crucially—bore no apparent relation to the sketch discussed at the start of this section. Gehry, of course, would generally use these rough sketches as a form of external memory to anchor his own growing understanding of the site and the emerging ideas for the building. The two-dimensional (2D) sketches anchor a 3D imagination in which, as the work progresses, some aspects become well-defined "islands of reliability" (to recall a term from §3.4), while others remain fluid, imagined in vague visual or sculptural terms, or anchored by a verbal expression.

Van Bruggen proposes that the sloping space underneath the bridge, with its road deck stretching over it like a roof, suggests an outdoor amphitheater, with overtones of an earlier proposal by Gehry for a temporary amphitheater built for the 1984 World's Fair in New Orleans, Louisiana. In response, Gehry stated:

> I was not as conscious that it had something to do with what I did before until later because . . . I'm just looking at what I see. I tend to live in the present, and what I see is what I do. And what I do is I react. Then I realize that I did it before. I think it is like that because you can't escape your own language. How many things can you really invent in your lifetime? You bring to the table certain things. What's exciting, you tweak them based on the context and the people. . . . (Gehry, quoted in van Bruggen, p. 33)

Here, we see again the idea of the architect having his own "language" that develops with each project, and which may "come to mind" whether consciously deployed or not.[10] A crucial discussion point for Chapter 10

---

10. Van Bruggen discusses the Winton guesthouse, Wayzata, Minnesota, and the American Center, Paris, as exemplifying the way in which Gehry's prior buildings may yield quotes for the

will be that the memories that come to mind may involve particular episodes, or may be part of semantic or procedural memory (§3.3). How Gehry sees the site depends on his choice of viewpoints and the relation to existing buildings and on conversations about what people want for their building. Later, the unfolding design will be affected by further conversations (but not, in this case, A↔N conversations).

Such conversations include, in part, the use of sketches as the basis for interaction with his team to yield formal models formalizing a range of decisions and sketches; Gehry would be the critic; and his further sketches might be his response to the models. For example, a Polaroid showing placement of the boot-like shape on the north façade (van Bruggen, p. 82) suggests how the model of which this is one view was, presumably, the basis for the rather detailed and structured sketch of the west elevation of July 13, 1991 (van Bruggen, p. 86), as well as the less structured sketch of the west elevation 2 days later (van Bruggen, p. 87). Presumably, the less structured sketching here frees Gehry from the details to develop new ideas that can then be subjected to the interaction with others that formalizes them for further consideration.

The result was a dialectic as each interpreted the productions of the other. The formal models in turn were the basis for extended discussions that include "sketchy" 3D modeling—some of these models could use crumpled paper to explore changes in the roofline; others could look more polished—to try out various forms as modifications of the current model, and to gain new understandings of the developing design. These 3D sketches could be very rough and swiftly varied to address diverse issues as the design was iterated. They provided a means to aid and assess progress and evolving ideas for refining the program and functionality while revealing flaws that needed to be further addressed. At later stages, the elaboration could respond to, and inform, interaction with the structural engineers. The models could also aid communication with the clients,

---

design of new buildings, even though the new building in no way replicates the earlier building in its overall design.

allowing the architects to assess their responses and the scope for new ideas—and then the process resumes.

Together, these 3D structures *and the mental structures that form while constructing them and then while contemplating them afterward* become the basis for further sketching, modifying old ideas and developing new ones. As for the drawing, Gehry commented:

> It's just the way I draw when I'm thinking. I think that way. I'm just moving the pen. I'm thinking about what I'm doing, but I'm sort of not thinking about my hands. . . . I'm looking through the paper to try to pull out the formal idea. . . . And that's why I never think of them as drawing. . . .

This is reminiscent of how tool use changes the body schema so that the hands are no longer the end effector; instead, the body ends at the tip of the tool, and this evokes a new range of affordances and effectivities. However, Gehry's semiautomatic sketching subsequently yields to careful inspection—which may bring subconscious ideas to the surface, where they can be discussed and developed—or he may see patterns that (perhaps) were not part of his original intention, but which can be folded into the ongoing design process.

Forms may appear and disappear, some never to return, others to resurface but perhaps modified to adapt to the emerging spaces of another part of the building. Gehry would take Polaroid photos to record views of his 3D models as they were repeatedly changed. One may compare this with the use of videos in a case study in choreography (mentioned in passing in §8.5) where Kate Stevens (in the book evocatively titled *Thinking in Four Dimensions: Creativity and Cognition in Contemporary Dance*; Grove, Stevens, & McKechnie, 2005) described a collaborative process between the choreographer Anna Smith and her group of dancers in the creation of a new dance, *Red Rain*. The videos were used to provide an external record of an even more dynamic design process than the architect's—where the form itself is coordinated movement rather than a structure that will provide an arena for the manifold movements of its visitors in relation both to the building and to each other.

Rather than verbalizing his intentions and then seeking a formal drawing to realize them, Gehry lets the emerging disposition of lines on paper begin to establish relationships, with hand and eye coordinated in the production of new forms. There is a form of automatization (§8.4) here. In many cases, these subconscious productions will later yield new explicit ideas as they are consciously considered and reviewed with others. We see (hear?) echoes of Pallasmaa's *Thinking Hand*.

> In the first sketch I put a bunch of principles down. Then I become self-critical of those images and those principles, and they evoke the next set of responses. And as each piece unfolds, I make the models bigger, and bigger, bringing into focus more elements and more pieces of the puzzle. And once I have the beginning, a toehold into where I'm going, then I want to examine the parts in more detail . . . and at some point I stop, because that's it. . . . (Gehry, quoted by van Bruggen, p. 130; see also p. 71.)

This exemplifies a notion that we will develop in §10.3, inspired by the view of perception as a process of mental construction offered by the VISIONS model of §3.4: imagination can retrieve multiple memories-as-constructs, tear them apart, and then transform and assemble various pieces to construct something new. External memory (sketches and models) can support the iteration of this process.

> *From time to-time, misinterpretations produced by the design team in the translation of Gehry's directions and annotated sketches into architectural elements even trigger new departures. . . .* [My italics.] (van Bruggen, p. 71.)

In the end, selected ideas that emerge from the varied sketches and models must coalesce to yield the construction plans. There, each detail

has meaning for the construction process that yields the actual building—
yet these construction drawings may express little of the myriad meanings
the building will gain through the diverse ways it performs for its visitors
and its workers.

A detour into symbolism and form

Let's leave Bilbao for the moment, and see how fish and snakes entered
Gehry's vocabulary.

> [Gehry] attributes his fascination with the fish form to a vivid
> childhood recollection involving his grandmother, with whom he
> went to the market on Thursdays: "We'd go to the Jewish market, we'd
> buy a live carp, we'd take it home to her house in Toronto, we'd put it
> in the bathtub and I would play with this goddamn fish for a day until
> the next day she'd kill it and make gefilte fish." (van Bruggen, p. 49)

By contrast, the snake form first occurred in Gehry's work in a 1981
project for which the sculptor Richard Serra was thinking about a coiling
snake in tile next to a fish shape Gehry wanted to explore. (The figures
on van Bruggen, p. 42, show Gehry's fish and Serra's snake as designed
for *Follies: Architecture for the Late Twentieth-Century Landscape* at Leo
Castelli Gallery, New York, 1983.) During the process of executing a small
model of the fish, Gehry realized that by making the fish scales out of overlapping glass tiles, rounded along one edge, *he had inadvertently hit on a
method of shingling adaptable to structures of any size.* This presaged the
construction method that, after major technical breakthroughs, became a
key to the distinctive use of titanium in the Bilbao project.

Based on the motif developed with Serra, Gehry proposed in 1983 a
prison in which he put the snake and the fish together.

> In describing the project, [Gehry] stated, "I think that the primitive
> beginnings of architecture come from zoomorphic yearnings and

skeletal images." Next to a glass pavilion in the form of the fish was a coiling snake, which was to be constructed of brick in order to give the building "the physical solidity associated with the word 'prison.'" Gehry deemed the snake a fitting emblem . . . as it evokes fear. . . . (van Bruggen, p. 45)

Here, we see a zoomorphic form providing explicit symbolism for a building, the snake symbolizing the fear of the criminal associated with incarceration (or the fear others associate with criminal acts?). However, while *zoomorphic* architecture does indeed give buildings a zoologically inspired form, our *neuromorphic* architecture (Chapter 7) is designed to endow buildings with brain-like functions, not brain-like forms. By contrast, Foster's Philological Library (Figure 6.4) is *not* neuromorphic in my sense. I distinguish the *shape* of the brain as adapted by Foster from the *information-processing capabilities* of the brain as adapted in neuromorphic architecture.

But sometimes a fish is just a fish, while a snake is just a spiral. Gehry's 1987 Fishdance restaurant on the waterfront in Kobe, Japan, contained a huge fish sculpture made of chain-link mesh alongside the actual restaurant building designed as a copper-clad spiraling angular snake form. As an example of how shapes at one stage of the design become transformed over the course of several projects, consider that the snake as symbol (for fear, in the prison concept) was at odds with the idea of a restaurant concept. Manipulating the snake in this new context required ridding it of its past associations, and in time it becomes replaced by a single "ziggurat." The snake keeps its skin but sheds its symbolism. One wonders whether the spiraling form of Wright's New York Guggenheim was just as powerful an influence as Serra's snake. Que Serra sera.

In 1991–1992, Gehry designed a highly abstracted, floating-fish sculpture, which functioned as a shading device for a retail court along a waterfront promenade in Barcelona. As Lundgren (2018) says, "the Kobe fish and the [Barcelona] fish structures are also designed to bring curious people into the attached buildings and restaurants. . . . [They] are not only beautiful zoomorphic structures but clever advertising."

Both these fish are made of mesh, rather than overlapping scales, so the inspiration from working on the fish design with Serra has yielded both a form to employ and a separable method of construction. There are echoes here of the process we posited in language evolution (§8.3) where an overall pantomime or conventionalized protosign could be fractionated both to yield new words and to yield new constructions in the linguist's sense.

Moreover, sometimes a fish is no longer a fish. The iridescent, overlapping shards in Formica or glass of the 1981 project with Serra led him to focus on the fish's skin. Subsequently, he derived an abstract shape from the fish image by cutting off its head and tail. For example, a truncated "fish-shape" provided an enclosure to exhibit small objects in a 1986 retrospective of Gehry's work at the Walker Art Center. The fish image yields both an innovative idea for a building's skin, and insight into how to make double curves in buildings. In the Bilbao Guggenheim, truncated "fish-forms" became transformed into leaf- or boat-like shapes and applied in some of the side galleries. Thus, the fish becomes endowed with a more elusive metaphorical quality, signifying fluid, continuous motion as a sculptural abstraction vivifying the building (van Bruggen, pp. 55–57).

"Mere building" versus "sculptural architecture": seeking a synthesis

Although Gehry's sketches may give the impression of an artist sketching the exterior form, he does not design projects from the outside in. Indeed, collaboration with the Guggenheim team on, for example, the requirements for the galleries played a crucial role, with Krens being an exceptional client with whom to work. For Bilbao, the design process following the competition took 3 years until the start of construction. At each stage, the process always involved a team, even at the competition stage. During the project, perhaps 30 to 40 architects were involved overall. Throughout, Gehry provided the guiding vision, while others served both to provoke Gehry's thinking and convert his ideas into physical form. The client also had a team, including curators working with Krens to ensure that the design matched their vision for the various galleries. Of course, each team's work responded to the progress of the other, in a beneficial interaction toward the shared goals. Many focused studies were needed.

Contrast the Sydney Opera House competition that Utzon won in great part based on the envelope—although we saw in §9.2 that certain key decisions were made as the basis for determining what would be enveloped. In each case, then, we see design as a back-and-forth, inside-out, and outside-in process that integrates diverse ideas and diverse external constraints at many levels of detail.

Functional problems of the building were worked out in schematic models in which pragmatic solutions to the building prevail over aesthetic decisions, followed by sculptural study models to and fro leading up to the final scheme. Krens had insisted upon different types of galleries, some sculptural, with six more classical, rectilinear ones. Gehry responded to this, while holding firm to the aesthetic principle that the classical white box housing these galleries had to become part of the building as a whole, seamlessly interwoven and juxtaposed with the sculpturally shaped galleries, resulting in a unity of opposites, the rigor of the geometric combined with the fluidity of the organic (van Bruggen, p. 112).

Van Bruggen titles her final chapter, "Toward a Unity of Opposites: A Mere Building Versus Sculptural Architecture." However, as we have seen throughout the book, "mere building" and "sculptural architecture" are at two ends of a continuum, with many architects working out a balance between the functional demands of each project and its sculptural qualities. Indeed, her chapter opens (p. 95) with a quote from Frank Gehry that reminds us of our discussion of architecture in relation to sculpture in Chapter 1:

I have been fortunate to have had support from living painters and sculptors. I have never felt that what artists are doing is very different. I have always felt there is a moment of truth when you decide: what color, what size, what composition? How you get to that moment of truth is different and the end result is different.

Solving all the functional problems is an intellectual exercise. That is a different part of my brain. It's not less important, it's just different. And I make a value out of solving all those problems, dealing with the context and the client and finding my moment of truth after I understand the problem.

But recall our insistence on the experience of someone acting and interacting within the building as a marker of the challenges that distinguish architecture from many other forms of art. However, apart from the discussion of the need for both the large gallery that would house Serra's *Snake* (echoes of their earlier partnership?) and various smaller more conventional galleries, van Bruggen tells us rather little about the functional considerations that constrained the development of the museum's dramatic forms and their relation to city and waterfront. One exception:

In the atrium design, Gehry started out with the complexities inherent in architecture of what functionally had to be: two elevators and two stair banks, mechanical shafts and catwalks. . . . from a distance, the Guggenheim Bilbao [had to] blend into the urban landscape, even though close up it would feel larger than life. Thinking about the mechanics of how to direct the flow of people to and from the galleries, and envisioning at the end of the gallery space on the second-floor level a balcony as a lookout on the city, evoked visionary urban designs. . . . Gehry liked the idea of creating a central place indoors as a metaphor for the ideal modern city, into which artists could put pieces and capture the space, an impossibility if situated in the actual cityscape, where outdoor sculpture always is dwarfed by the environment. (van Bruggen, p. 116)

When I visited the museum in 1999, I was disappointed by the way art was displayed in the smaller galleries, but captivated by the way views shifted as I walked around the public spaces. Van Bruggen captures something of this on pages 119 and 121:

For instance, standing inside the atrium space, one can see oneself in relation to a fraction of the huge skylight on top of the boat gallery, and a piece of the Puente de la Salve all at once. Turning around, one catches a glimpse through the entry of the buildings along the Alameda de Mazarredo; in the opposite direction one overlooks a corner of the Universidad de Deusto across the Nervión River. At the same time, the interstitial curtain-wall glazings function as negatives of sculptural elements disposed vertically around the periphery of the atrium's interior, such as three rectangular twisted limestone obelisks housing mechanical equipment; [and] two elevator towers. . . .

The computer, at last

For many architects today, the computer is integrated into even the conceptual stages of developing a design (whether or not accompanying hand-sketching and 3D model-making). In the Bilbao project, however, the computer played an essential role only after the design of the building's form had been completed. CATIA, software developed for the aerospace industry, was used to take measurements from a metrically accurate physical model, to compute the curvature of various surfaces, and to use that analysis to make explicit the size and shape of large titanium panels for areas of low curvature and small panels for areas of high curvature.[11] This was then converted into shop drawings to specify in great detail the framing that was needed, details of the pieces that had to be fabricated, and even the detailed instructions to the construction workers for assembling these walls, and so on. Figure 9.16 illustrates seven stages in the process:

11. For further perspective see van Bruggen's two Appendixes: Appendix I, "On the Use of the Computer," including discussions with Jim Glymph who traces the use of CATIA forward from the challenge of creating a realization of Gehry's design of a large-scale fish sculpture for the Villa Olimpica complex (1989-92) in Barcelona. Appendix II, "Gehry on Titanium," details the challenges of getting the titanium "right" for the project.

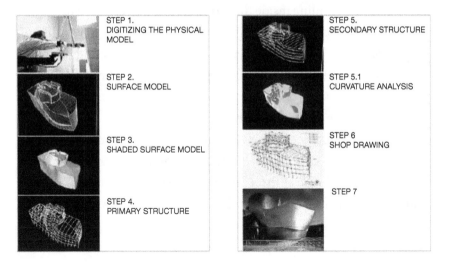

Figure 9.16 From physical model to specifying metal plates. CATIA, a 3D computer modeling program originally designed for the aerospace industry, is supplemented by more traditional 2D CAD programs. (Adapted from a no-longer-available webpage at www.arcspace.com.)

Step 1.   Digitizing the physical model produces a series of points encoded in the computer, which together represent a shape that roughly resembles the shape of the physical model.

Step 2.   The surface so defined is then manipulated, cleaned up, and smoothed out to yield the surface model.

Step 3.   The shaded surface model may be useful as a visual display, perhaps, but is inessential to the ongoing computations.

Step 4.   For Bilbao, the primary structure of the building represents the steel skeleton of the building.

Step 5.   The curvature analysis determines whether the metal panels will need to be pressed to adhere to a certain curve. Because pressed metal panels are more expensive, this analysis seeks to assess how to specify panels in a way that keeps costs low. For Bilbao, the secondary structure is part of the structure that supports the galvanized steel underlayer of the cladding system.

Step 6.   The CATIA computer model is used to generate the steel-
shop drawings.

Step 7.   The finished building.

Here is a strong parallel between the practice of architecture and science, complementing the observations in §2.7. Most work employs well-
established methods, but occasionally someone recognizes that a pressing
problem requires a new technology. Much research is then required to
bring that technology to a form where others can use it—consider the
role of functional magnetic resonance imaging (fMRI) in imaging human
brain function in relation to neuroanatomy, or the incorporation of elevators into the design of tall buildings—but the result can be transformative. Another parallel is that, just as the architect may gain an overarching
concept and be able to maintain it, with variations, throughout the working out of details of the design (but sometimes the original idea must
be changed or rejected), so may scientists gain an immense insight that
gives them the faith (yes, faith) to invest years, even decades of effort, into
the mix of experiments and theoretical analysis to prove the hypothesis
correct—even while understanding (§4.3) that.

> [w]hen preparing construction drawings, the architect may employ
> the precise distances and angles of Euclidean space as the frame in
> which the building is located. However, our experience of the spaces
> the architect designs are, instead, in terms of how the surfaces are
> shaped that enclose or confront us, including those that we readily
> perceive from the current vantage point, and different neural systems
> will accept diverse invitations of the affordances for exploration and
> action, as well as the atmosphere that shapes our mood, or offers
> opportunities for aesthetic experience. There is a real value to
> architects if they think in terms of the "unfolding" and changing
> of all these varied affordances as we spend time within a building,
> acting, interacting, or contemplating.

I would not presume to claim that, had Zumthor or Utzon or Gehry
talked more to neuroscientists, their design of the Vals Therme, the

Sydney Opera House, and the Guggenheim Museum Bilbao would have been improved. But I do presume to claim that our A↔N conversation allows us to step back from their work and make explicit various conscious and unconscious processes to provide observations that can indeed enrich architectural education in the future.

REFERENCES

7Mate. (2008?). Sydney Opera House: Man-made marvels. https://www.youtube.com/watch?v=oOCFj5CkOdk

Fromonot, F. (1998). *Jørn Utzon: Architect of the Sydney Opera House* (C. Thompson, Trans.). Milan: Electa.

Geddes, R. (2006). Second thoughts: Reflections on winning second prize. In A. Watson (Ed.), *Building a Masterpiece: the Sydney Opera House* (pp. 56–67). Haymarket, Sydney: Powerhouse Publishing/Aldershot, UK: Lund Humphries Publishers.

Grove, R., Stevens, C., & McKechnie, S. (Eds.). (2005). *Thinking in four dimensions: Creativity and cognition in contemporary dance.* Carlton: Melbourne University Press.

Loukissas, Y. (2012). *Co-designers: Cultures of computer simulation in architecture.* New York: Routledge.

Lundgren, N. (2018). *From elephants to skyscrapers: Zoomorphic architecture.* Leander, TX: Fulton Books.

Saint, A. (2007). *Architect and engineer: A study in sibling rivalry.* New Haven, CT: Yale Univ Press.

Utzon, J. (1962). Platforms and plateaus: Ideas of a Danish architect. *Zodiac*, 10, 114. http://www.transfer-arch.com/monograph/platforms-and-plateaus/

Utzon, J. (2009). *Additive architecture: Logbook* (Vol. V). Copenhagen: Edition Bløndal.

van Bruggen, C. (1997). *Frank O. Gehry: Guggenheim Museum Bilbao.* New York: Guggenheim Museum Publications.

Watson, A. (Ed.). (2006). *Building a masterpiece: The Sydney Opera House.* Sydney: Powerhouse Publishing.

Experience and design: Bringing in the brain

Long before architecture, protohumans could scan a landscape. In part, this would be to find "landmarks" for places known to reward foraging or hunting, places to avoid because of encounters there with dangerous predators, or places of refuge, whether already established or as a new place to spend the coming night. The landscape would also provide opportunities for exploration to establish new "landmarks"—and yet the broad vistas might offer aesthetic satisfactions of their own, in part genetically based yet further tuned by prior experience. But, of course, the brain had evolved to do more than recognize and establish landmarks. Building a cognitive map is important, but the affordances for which the brain is adapted go beyond those afforded by the landscape. During the course of the day, a person may encounter other people, predators, prey, and animals and plants that were unexpected and may elicit interest or action or simply be ignored. If the world is a stage, then the other players may be many and unexpected, and each "player" may have to repeatedly revise the "script" they are following.

Going beyond this, though, we must consider how this ancestral brain with its capabilities for survival in a "natural environment" could, in due course and via cultural evolution, come to support the construction of dwellings and, even later, the ability of architects to create and restructure built environments that users could then explore to build their cognitive maps, maps in many cases approximating those imagined by the architect in planning the building. Such considerations have been implicit throughout the book, and briefly surfaced in our evolutionary account of the "construction-ready brain" and "architecture-ready brain" in Chapter 8. They moved to center stage with our exploration of cognitive processes engaged in Jørn Utzon's designing the Sydney Opera House and Frank Gehry's designing the Guggenheim Museum Bilbao. These case studies could only hint at the richness of their designs and the complex memories they evoked, but they did show how deeply the specific experiences of each architect informed what is distinctive about their designs. They brought to the forefront certain processes crucial to design.

Sections 10.1 through 10.4 brings these ideas together in offering a first pass on characterizing a conceptual model, IBSEN (a model of *Imagination in Brain Systems for Episodes and Navigation*), for integrating cognitive neuroscience into the analysis of architectural design. Finally, §10.5 signals the end of the book but, hopefully, the beginning of many further A↔N conversations. This book has offered an overall framework for linking the experience and the design of architecture to cognitive science and neuroscience, and reflects my own experience as a neuroscientist who develops computational and conceptual models as a way to understand, in part within an EvoDevoSocio framework, how the brain supports and integrates such phenomena as action, perception, emotion, memory, and language. The final section encourages future collaborations between architects and scientists that will address specific problems (whether or not they modify this overall framework), developing and analyzing cog/neuro data relevant to specific architectural challenges and taking cog/neuroscience out of the lab and into the building and the street.

10.1. TOWARD IBSEN: MODELING IMAGINATION IN BRAIN SYSTEMS FOR EPISODES AND NAVIGATION

This final chapter has been the hardest to write, in part because it tries to make sense of the current, early, stages of my effort to develop a cognitive neuroscience of architectural design. It will also prove, in some ways, the hardest to read—not just because you are being asked to share in this effort, but also because this is the least self-contained chapter of the book because IBSEN builds on a range of ideas from earlier chapters.

This chapter will synthesize much of what we have learned from developing cog/neuro models of diverse aspects of the *user's* experience of architecture. In relating the design process of the architect to the user's projected experience of the building, we will build on the discussion of the artist's creation of a painting as in some (carefully analyzed) sense being the "inverse" of visual perception (§4.4). Just as a set of key buildings may provide reference points for architectural discussion, so does a set of computational models engaging cooperative computation at the level of schemas and neural networks anchor IBSEN. The chapter brings together the notion of scripts as framing general patterns of behavior, lessons from the VISIONS model of understanding a visual scene, ideas about the scheduling and control of actions, and the taxon affordance/world graph model (TAM-WGM) of navigation, enriched by much we have learned from focused studies of action-oriented perception. Central to our linkage of scripts and world graphs (WGs) is a new perspective on locomotion and navigation: they serve not merely a way of getting from place A to another place B, but as a way of getting to a *sequence* of places that may satisfy the affordances for performing the actions of some intended behavior, whether or not it is closely constrained by a script.

To ease the burden of reading this material, I have structured it in four sections. The present section summarizes some of the key background from earlier chapters in a form that stresses their relevance to the current conceptual sketch of IBSEN, and §10.4 sets out how these ideas are factored into IBSEN. Together, these two sections will provide many readers a satisfying understanding of the status of this approach to the cognitive neuroscience of design for architecture. The intervening sections then provide optional reading:

§10.2 shows how lessons from the VISIONS model for visual perception considered as a process of mental construction (§3.4) and its extension to multimodal perception within the action perception cycle (MULTIMODES, §3.6) may be exploited for imagination when fragments of diverse memories are transformed and assembled to create new multimodal images that extend in time—in other words, to imagine new episodes that might inform the architect's creation of a building that will support diverse user experiences (both practical and contemplative).

§10.3 links this material to neurobiology by sampling brain imaging studies that look at the hippocampus not only for its long-understood role in episodic memory (§3.3) but also for its role in episodic imagination, as well as studies that view the role of hippocampus in memory to be to index fragments of that memory distributed across cerebral cortex. I will also stress the importance for imagination of other memory systems that complement episodic memory.

Our aim in this chapter is neither to specify the particularities of any one architect nor to offer a straitjacket for the design processes of all architects. Rather, IBSEN explores how imagination exploits the individual memories of each architect in addressing the particularities of program and site to design buildings that support diverse scripts for the practical and contemplative behavior of its users. It thus provides a framework for *myriad* future A↔N conversations that focus on particular aspects of the design process and their neurocognitive implementation.

The spaces of architecture are defined by a disposition of surfaces in relation to each other that support not only our actions, whether praxic or social, but also our contemplation of the building from within, or as viewed from the outside, or the vistas that the building frames of the landscape or townscape beyond. We distinguished (§2.2) *effective* space and *affective* space—of space as structured by the behaviors we can effect with the building, and the affects that the building can engender in us. However, the architect's work does not end until all the surfaces that define the effective and affective spaces of the building are fully specified in terms of the three-dimensional (3D) space around and including the site where the building will be constructed. Virtually all works of architectural theory, from Vitruvius onward, discuss part–whole relationships. What this book adds is that the notion of systems of systems—and not just wholes and parts—applies to both buildings and brains, so that we emphasize dynamic relations between brains and buildings, not just the static forms of buildings.[1]

Multimodal perception within the action–perception cycle

Recalling (from §1.1) Zumthor's claim that "When I think about architecture, images come into my mind. . . . When I design, I frequently find myself sinking into old, half-forgotten memories . . . . Yet, at the same time, I know that all is new . . . ," our challenge is to stress that the relevant "images" for the experience, and thus the design, of architecture are not limited to static visual images but must also include images of *episodes* linking multimodal experience and action extended over some period of time.

The VISIONS model provided our paradigmatic example of "competition and cooperation as the style of the brain," in this case with this "cooperative computation" at the level of schema instances. It offered an account of how an assemblage of schema instances (a *schema assemblage*, for short) might emerge that provided a coherent interpretation of the scene—while noting that this interpretation might depend in great part on the current task and motivation of the viewer. Within VISIONS, working memory is

---

1. For a broad architectural perspective on design, see *Draw in Order to See: A Cognitive History of Architectural Design*. As the title suggests, Mark Alan Hewitt (2020) offers a perspective that is enriched by varied linkages to cognitive (neuro)science, including the view of design as a process of cumulative extension and refinement of exograms noted in the discussion of "Sketching: memory and imagination" in our §8.5. As such it provides a worthy sequel to the pathbreaking, *The Architect's Brain: Neuroscience, Creativity, and Architecture*, by Harry Francis Mallgrave (2009).

a dynamic system in which the interaction of top-down and bottom-up processes converges on the coherent schema assemblage that interprets the bottom-up data from visual input. With continued contemplation of the static scene, further details may come to enrich the assemblage, and aspects of the initial interpretation may change.

Our conceptual extension of these insights begins by extrapolating these mechanisms from the interpretation of a static visual scene to episodes (moving from the implemented computational model VISIONS to the conceptual MULTIMODES model). Working memory then extends beyond the immediate present within a time course that includes aspects of past experience with goals and expectations. As a basic example, consider looking for your car in a parking garage (or substitute a comparable example specific to your culture) where your current perception is goal-directed while also activating some knowledge of the layout of the garage and (possibly fallible) working memory of where you had parked the car that morning. We talk here, almost paradoxically, of *long-term working memory*.[2] Note that the car and garage memories may not have come to mind at all between leaving the garage that morning and deciding it was time to get the car. What is fascinating as we ponder architectural design (and many other complex activities) is how memories that have long resided outside consciousness become somehow promoted to be held in readiness as we work on one project rather than another, but can also enter into subconscious processes that will bring other memories into play for promotion into this long-term working memory. Moreover, the development of external memory and team efforts serve both to enrich the extent of relevant memories and to make more complex the process of winnowing these memories to determine (both consciously and

---

2. Ericsson and Kintsch (1995) provide a classic account of *long-term working memory*, and thousands of subsequent papers have explored the phenomenon at all levels from molecular mechanisms in neurons to psychological studies in diverse domains. I will not review this literature (it even includes papers on architectural design), but mention it here for those who wish to pursue A↔N conversations on the cognitive processes underlying design.

subconsciously) which ones, at least for now, should be transformed to become part of the emerging design.

Not all ideas that "come to mind" during design need be new or personal—indeed, a team of architects may place pictures of previous designs (whether by themselves or others) on a storyboard to provide reference points for their own imaginations. Parts of an old "vocabulary" may be rejected while aspects of a new vocabulary may begin to arise. In general, a single overall image cannot provide the key to construction, but it may spark a cascade of further design ideas. Several ideas may occur to the architect at around the same time, and any one of them may influence the working out of others. The order in which the different challenges are attacked may be arbitrary, or there may be clear dependencies that constrain the ordering. Whatever is done earlier sets the boundary conditions for what comes later; but later decisions may require reconsideration of design aspects established earlier.

According to VISIONS, what we see depends not only "bottom-up" on the pattern of light hitting the retina but also "top-down" on our stock of visual memories and our current concerns. However, design is dominated by top-down constraints set by the program for the building rather than the demands of sensory input—even though we have seen how visual attention, and thus scene interpretation, may be strongly influenced by the demands of a current task. In balancing top-down and bottom-up processes, *islands of reliability* will emerge that endure for a certain period in the design, allowing the individual or team to focus on a subproblem without (for the moment) worrying about other subproblems. We used this term in describing assemblages in the understanding of a visual scene (§3.4) that proved stable enough to anchor further considerations for the ensuing period, even though later processing might lead to its rejection as other considerations came into play. Similarly, in the design process, the solution may in some cases lead to a change in the specification of the subproblem, and this may disrupt some of the "contracts" or consistency conditions with other pieces of the puzzle, leading to some renegotiation of specifications before work on the other subproblems can proceed.

As design proceeds, the emerging "schema assemblage" is not limited to images that have come to mind. As humans, we find it hard to separate our conscious memories from verbal descriptions that may enrich those memories or may bleach them of their particularity. "Aha" moments may yield precise but high-level descriptions before exploration via diverse sketches has begun, but others will emerge as design continues, with partially realized design ideas and attendant challenges creating the cues for activation of memories that had long remained dormant (whether these constitute complex images that can be conformed to the current problem, or cues to seek specific data and ideas that had been hitherto ignored). Moreover, the "aha" moments may be triggered by conversations with others as well as one's own ruminations. For one dramatic example, Kahn had imagined the courtyard of the Salk Institute landscaped with trees—but a discussion with the Mexican architect Barragán (Louis meets Luis) catalyzed a transition to the bare design that yielded the iconic courtyard we know today (Amado Lorenzo, 2012). Moreover (recall the discussion of Le Corbusier's Carpenter Center for the Visual Arts at Harvard University in §3.5), the design may converge on "what" to place and *approximately* where to place it, but may require (non-verbal fine-tuning to determine "how" to place the various elements to achieve a harmonious balance—transferring to the design side the perceptual capabilities of the "what" and "how" visual pathways in the guidance of hand movements (§2.6). This type of "balance" feeds into a more general aesthetic sense, invoking emotional tone and atmosphere.

The architect must imagine the experiences and action–perception cycles of users of yet-to-be-designed spaces, and then extend this to imagine new spaces in which these experiences and behaviors may unfold. Certain precise verbal decisions may be made (as in Utzon's decision to place the auditoriums side by side) at any stage of design, with the sketching and the working out of details firmly constrained by these decisions. Within these and surrounding these are vague ideas whose details are to be filled in as design progresses. Note how the competition and cooperation that frames the integration of cognitive and neural processes at different levels may extend from the lone individual's introspection and weighing of alternatives to the social interactions within a group of people and their artifacts.

 A major step towards IBSEN is to extend our account of perception from the analysis of a visual scene (VISIONS) to the multimodal action-oriented perception of ongoing episodes (MULTIMODES). Let's develop the general motivation for this here, leaving the (optional) details for §10.2. Staircases provide a fine example of an architect offering users an essential invitation to action. The approach to the staircase, the effort of ascending it, and the vista when you look back from the top step or look ahead at the new level you have reached are all grist for the memory mill. Stairs can remain in memory for diverse reasons, whether positive (a notable sculptural look, a way to swiftly move from floor to floor) or negative (inconvenient access, uncomfortable steps).

Each staircase provides a special kind of transition, from one level to another (Figure 10.1). It will have a visual appearance, but a handrail, once grasped, will appeal to the sense of touch. The tread of the steps may make locomotion effortless or require attention to proprioception to gain a firm footing for each step. What, then, are the images that come to the architect's mind? For one thing, the architect must share the sculptor's skill for imagination in the round. An initial image of the staircase may see it from one perspective, but further design must realize it as a 3D object. In one design, the form may take precedence in imagination; in another, it may be the practical problem of getting from one floor to another that provides the associative trigger for evoking images of diverse staircases—both as observed from different vantage points and as experienced while ascending or descending. Further imagination may be stimulated depending on whether the spatial relation of these floors to the site has already been established. If not, the staircase itself may be the anchoring factor that helps shape that relationship. Moreover, the stairway may have symbolic or atmospheric value that helps determine its width, height, and form (recall the ascents to knowledge in our discussion of libraries in §6.1).

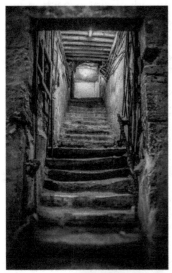

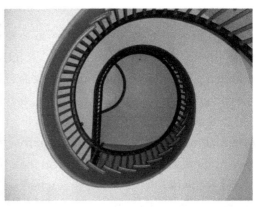

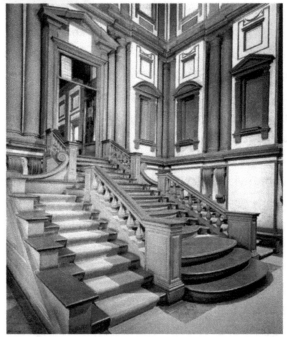

Figure 10.1 A potpourri of staircases. (*Top left*) Old stone stairs. (*Top right*) Spiral staircase in the Trustees House at Shaker Village at Pleasant Hill, Kentucky. (*Bottom*) Michelangelo's stairs ascending to the Laurentian Library in Florence. Compare the ascending library staircases in §6.1. (*Top left*: old-house-stairs-cellar-basement-1201552. jpg. Public domain. *Top right*: https://commons.wikimedia.org/wiki/File:Shakertown_ Staircase_2005-05-27.jpeg, Creative Commons Attribution-Share Alike 2.0 Generic license. *Bottom*: From *Biografías y Vidas. La enciclopedia biográfica en línea*, www. biografiasyvidas.com, with permission.)

"What" and "how" revisited

Within our framework of action-oriented perception, then, we require that regions of a building be assessed not simply in terms of "what" they are but also in terms of "how" we might interact with them, their affordances—and this includes recognizing movements around us, some of which may alert us to actions by (not necessarily human) others. In some cases, the details of these movements may be crucial to our ongoing behavior (consider catching a ball, for instance). This recalls the dichotomy in analysis of visuomotor coordination (Figure 2.16, updated as Figure 10.2) of a *ventral "what" pathway*, making a conscious evaluation of the overall disposition of components of a scene as a basis for planning action, and a *dorsal "how" pathway* that analyzes fine details of affordances as a basis for tuning the parameters of motor schemas.

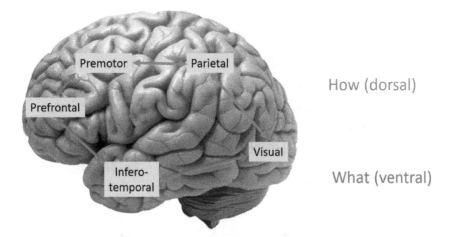

Figure 10.2 This embellishes Figure 2.16 in two ways. (1) It extends consideration from hand actions to the control of actions more generally. The ventral pathway analyzes the scene to establish the objects, agents, actions, and other relations of interest. This enables the prefrontal cortex—taking task, working memory, motivation, and emotion into account—to plan "what" to do. The dorsal pathway then fills in the details of "how to do it," passing affordance parameters forward to adjust motor schemas for the selected actions. (2) The coupling between dorsal and ventral paths is now shown to be bidirectional, so that dorsal details can modify ventral decision-making.

We can caricature this by saying that

- the ventral pathway encodes both semantic memory and procedural memory that supports sequencing the actions needed for some behavior), while
- the dorsal pathway encodes the sensorimotor fine-tuning to support graceful execution of each action as well as transition to the next.

The cortex works in collaboration with the basal ganglia and cerebellum to achieve such scheduling successfully and gracefully.[3]

Extending these observations:

- The dorsal path is closely coupled with the ventral path so that, when particular actions are scheduled for execution, the dorsal path can pass detailed parameters concerning affordances to tune the motor schemas that execute the action.
- However, there is another factor that we have not considered until now, signaled by the bidirectional arrows of Figure 10.2. *The coupling between dorsal and ventral paths can go both ways.* In particular, in assessing the relative executability of two actions (now taking into account the relative effort and chance of success of the two actions, rather than the binary data on whether or not they have an affordance), the ventral path may require dorsal input on fine parameters of motor schema tuning to choose the next action.

Top-down considerations of creating atmosphere and setting an emotional "tone" may modulate the balance between variation of design features within the building and the unity of its architectural expression—in

3. Analysis of the basal ganglia and cerebellum lies, for the most part, outside the current scope of our A↔N conversation. However, if you want to learn more, you can read Chapters 9 and 10 of Arbib, Érdi, and Szentágothai (1998) or Chapters 42 and 43 (and many others!) of Kandel, Schwartz, Jessell, Siegelbaum, and Hudspeth (2013). A relevant model of learning is supplied by "The Super-Learning Hypothesis: Integrating Learning Processes Across Cortex, Cerebellum and Basal Ganglia" (Caligiore, Arbib, Miall, & Baldassarre, 2019).

relation to blend of form and functionality in both its exterior and interior forms.

Extending our meditation on Figure 10.2 in MULTIMODES fashion, there would be a number of ventral paths originating from the primary cortices for different sensory modalities, activating instances of perceptual schemas for actions as well as objects and agents, and the relation between them, so that prefrontal cortex could plan an appropriate course of action.[4] Next, let's recall certain ideas on action sequencing (§5.4). We saw that assessment of the scene could invoke both the *desirability* of possible actions (not those perceived in the scene, but those possible within the scene), based on current needs and tasks related to expected reward, and their *executability*, based on available affordances, including the scheduling of actions to make affordances available for highly desirable actions:

Desirability is in some sense need-, task-, or script-specific—in general, a script is invoked to satisfy some need, and that need may be very general, "quell hunger," or very specific, "get to see that painting by Rembrandt." The design of a building (or its current embellishments) may offer what might be called *incentives* designed to catch the user's attention and then raise the motivational level for activating a particular script, perhaps by the aromas wafting from a food stand in the former case, or a bold poster, "Rembrandt Returns!" outside the art gallery.

Executability reminds us that a building may be designed to meet very special needs, such as door handles and furniture adjusted to the dimensions of small children in a kindergarten, or wheelchair access in public (and other) buildings. Neuromorphic architecture explores ways a building might respond in dynamically adapting to meet the needs and abilities of users and changing our behaviors accordingly—as in recognizing whether or not a door will open automatically.

In the augmented competitive queuing (ACQ) model of flexible action scheduling, the highest priority action gets scheduled next, with priority combining executability and desirability. However, we also saw that

---

4. For example, papers by Rauschecker, Romanski, and others (e.g., Rauschecker & Tian, 2000; Romanski et al., 1999) initiated the study of ventral versus dorsal paths in the auditory system.

habitual behaviors may be constrained by scripts that may be fairly rigid (following a route) or fairly flexible (how to behave at a birthday party). Let's add here that the effort of "setting it up" can factor into the assessment of the executability of the action to be carried out there. Consider, for example, that you develop a sudden craving for ice cream. You go to the fridge to get the ice cream, and then you eat it. But suppose you find that there is no ice cream in the fridge, but there is an apple. In your current state, eating an apple is somewhat desirable—somewhat sweet and ready to eat—and it is readily executable. If your craving is not so strong, you may choose not to eat at all, and simply put ice cream on your shopping list. But if that craving is really intense and ice cream–specific, then you may find going to the store to buy ice cream of higher priority than the stay-at-home alternatives despite its much higher executability-cost.

As we turn from the user to the architect, recall that ACQ also models the learning of the desirability and executability of actions in different situations, and employs mirror neurons as an aid to improving one's own actions rather than assessing the actions of others. This involves a mixture of semantic and procedural memory in learning how to recognize an affordance and how to use it in executing a desired action. But note, too, questions concerning the imagination of users and designers that lie beyond the scope of ACQ. How does the user exploit prior knowledge to recognize that a novel object provides a sought-for affordance, or that a familiar object can be used in a novel way? How does the designer endow an object or a space with the means for a user to recognize and exploit its affordances?

Linking memory and imagination as processes of mental construction

We have already discussed the importance of the hippocampus in navigation at some length (Chapter 6), and have shown that there are modes of navigation that do, and others that do not, engage the hippocampus, with the former requiring the interaction of multiple brain regions to support the development and use of cognitive maps. To complement this, §10.3 will look in more detail at the role of the hippocampus in episodic memory, and sample brain imaging data showing that it also forms part of larger systems engaged in imagination. However, just as there are processes of navigation that do not involve the hippocampus, so we shall see that memory and imagination are not just episodic and that they can be supported by brain regions interacting without the hippocampus.

We have seen that VISIONS models our perception of a scene as resulting from a process of mental construction that assembles schema instances that have been modulated to accommodate some of the details of the observed scene. In this spirit, we stress that imagination is not the invocation of a specific prior (episodic or other) memory, but rather develops new schema assemblages, exploiting fragments of prior memories that over time can come together to yield a novel design that meets the challenges of a new program for a new building on a new site. §10.3 will cite studies of the hippocampus concordant with that view. It will also look at data on the organization of hippocampus along the dorsal-ventral axis that raises important neuroscience challenges about the encoding of WGs and locometric maps in diverse brain regions, including but not limited to the hippocampus.

Linking scripts and cognitive maps

How, then, does the architect go from imagining the experience and behavior of users to designing a building that will support them? Top-down considerations of creating atmosphere and setting an emotional "tone" may modulate the balance between variation of design features within the building and the unity of its architectural expression. However, the architect does far more than create visual forms. Not only may the architect's images be multisensory, in which vision, hearing, and other senses combine with action, but they also may extend in time, invoking "scripts" for possible behaviors of the eventual users in the building being designed, although the final design may provide opportunities for exploration and for the user's development of new scripts.

Bear in mind that "scripts" here are not written prescriptions for exact behaviors, but rather express general patterns of lived experience of a particular kind. The design process must thus address the integration within a building of scripts with places (where are various affordances to be provided?) and navigation (how will users move through the spaces provided in developing their current variations on the general script?).

Each script involves (whether quite specifically or with great flexibility) the exploiting of affordances—whether Gibsonian or non-Gibsonian—at different places in and around the building. An affordance is a perceptual cue that an action may be possible at a particular place or using a particular action. However, one may recognize a door and plan to go through it but find it is locked or, on coming close, see a small sign "staff only" that "cancels" the other affordance. Recall, too, our distinction (Figure 10.2) between an affordance that invites one to an action and the "parameterized affordances" that (often subconsciously) tune motor schemas to execute that action gracefully. Contrast recognizing a ball coming toward you, and the eye-body-hand coordination that yields a successful catch (and that involves optic flow supplying, again subconsciously, time-until-contact information).

Moreover, the scripts may be unconventional so long as users can accommodate to them—consider the "script-bending" of Lina Bo Bardi's Sao Paulo Art Museum. This exemplifies the distinction between designs that exploit the ability of users to activate widely held scripts, and design that builds on the architect's own lived experience *and imagination* to create designs that encourage the formation of new episodic memories and scripts by creating memorable settings for behavior and experience.

We introduced WGs to formalize the notion of cognitive maps in terms of *significant* places (nodes) and the relations between them (edges) but, as noted earlier, we now stress that cognitive maps serve more than navigation—and §10.4 will complete our sketch of IBSEN by extending the insights of TAM-WGM to better understand how we use and experience buildings, and the implications this has for the design process. When we perform a script within a building, we are developing and exploiting cognitive maps to proceed from place to place within the satisfaction of that script, rather than simply seeking a locomotor path from start point to goal. Thus, as we further consider what it means for the designer to some-how imagine and then "invert" the experiences and behaviors of users of the forthcoming building, we must assess the process whereby each user will form their own cognitive maps (note the plural) of the building not just for navigation but also for the efficient—or leisurely—satisfaction of a range of scripts, and as the basis for forming new scripts for their own exploration and enjoyment of the building.

An important reminder: Despite the name, we do not have a single WG; we do not live in a single "world." Rather, our brain encodes diverse WGs at different levels of detail so that, for example, we may have a fairly sparse WG for finding our way from one room to another in a building, and fairly detailed WGs for each of one or more rooms to support our behav-ior there. With this in mind, let's consider some relevant aspects of the WGs that may be associated with a building:

> A building on an urban thoroughfare may be visible only from just along that street, or there may also be aerial views from other, taller buildings nearby—and the architect must decide whether to ignore these viewpoints or take them into account in explicitly designing the "fifth façade." Thus, some of the WG nodes will be outside the building. A building on a corner, or set aside on its own land, may offer further "faces" to challenge design. The façade may offer affor-dances for the passersby (what does it add to their experience of the street or neighborhood?), for those planning to enter (are there parking places nearby; are there different entrances for different purposes?), and for those inside (exits, windows). What atmosphere is suggested on approaching and entering the building?
>
> When the building exists, it provides the affordances that each inhab-itant may explore to create their own "meanings." Indeed, as in the pleasures of waylosing in Venice, a successful design for some typologies of building or urban scene may go beyond provision

of intended functions (as captured in the various scripts) to also
allow the pleasure of exploration, or discovering new details, or
personalization.

The nodes and edges of a WG developed during design must in the
end be linked to their specific placement and realization in 3D
space, and such placement will in turn provide new challenges in
detailing and choice of materials. Additionally, a building will have
to satisfy diverse scripts and that, in general, many places in the
building will serve multiple scripts. This sets the challenging of har-
monizing diverse scripts as "nodes" in their WGs are merged.

To provide further motivation for this perspective and to prepare for
the fuller development in §10.4, let's consider a particular example,
blurring any line between architecture and interior design. A building
can have a range of WGs at different scales. This reflects the hierarchical nature of our action-oriented spatial cognition, attending to details
in relation to the current task. In one WG, each room is indeed a node.
If it's dinner time and dinner has already been prepared, I may simply
find a path from my study to the dining room, perhaps with a detour
to the bathroom to wash my hands. But if I need to prepare or help
prepare the meal, my path must lead to the kitchen, and when there
I "switch" to a detailed WG that links to nodes very much defined as
action points—oven, stovetop, sink, refrigerator, countertop 1, countertop 2, pantry, dishwasher, and so forth, each with limited extent.
However (and here I refer to the kitchen in the home I share with
my wife), it also includes a spatially extended viewpoint, a place from
which I can admire the view of the back garden through the very large
picture window along the western wall. At an even finer level, when
retrieving or putting away cutlery, plates, and cooking utensils, I can
invoke knowledge of where and in what drawers and cupboards each
is to be stored.

These multiple scripts for how a space is to be used can provide competing claims on the spatial relationship of the places they invoke, places
initially determined by diverse considerations of form in relation to

aesthetics, function, and atmosphere. In designing the kitchen, the need for space to prepare and plate the meals for a dinner party provided one consideration for relating the positions of stovetop, oven, and countertops. Washing-up provided constraints for the relation between sink, dishwasher, and countertops—but also provided a secondary constraint of locating these in relation to a dividing wall in such a way that visitors in the dining room would not be subjected to a view of the dirty dishes as they piled up between courses. Our informal workflow analysis led us to trade off decisions about what went where as we (well, primarily my wife and son) designed a new and enlarged kitchen. This balancing act had to preserve a few prior features while developing new ones in relation to the available space: to incorporate transitions between the kitchen and the dining room/living room area, the hallway, and the back garden; and to preserve the unity of the exterior façade even as that new picture window transformed it dramatically.

Nonetheless, we do not live by the architect's scripts alone. The design meets a range of performance criteria but also offers a space in which we and our guests can share diverse experiences, whether primarily culinary or primarily social, or a blend of the two, to find new satisfactions.

With this background now in place, I invite the reader to proceed directly to Section 10.4, or to first read—or at least hum—one or both of the next two sections.

10.2. MULTIMODES AND THE ACTION–PERCEPTION CYCLE

A key lesson from VISIONS is that even *understanding* of a visual scene is a process of *mental construction*. It involves assembling schema instances, each associated with a particular region for which it provides the interpretation; downward paths associate each instance with attributes like location, form, depth, color, and texture. The scene is thus interpreted as an assemblage of objects in various spatial and other relationships. This exploits a loop between two levels of processing:

- *Segmentation/low-level vision*: Competition and cooperation
  at the level of local image features grows edges and regions to
  yield a first-pass subdivision of the image to ground semantic
  analysis; and
- *Recognition/high-level vision*: Schema instances compete and cooperate
  to interpret different regions with low-level and high-level processes
  communicating via the intermediate database.

The requisite knowledge for high-level vision is contained in a *network*
of perceptual schemas stored in long-term memory, but, crucially, the representation of the current scene is built up through the competition and
cooperation of schema *instances* in visual working memory:

- Schemas do not directly analyze the current scene. Crucially,
  this is accomplished by the activation of *schema instances* (both
  "bottom-up" by data extracted from the current scene, and "top-
  down" by cues based on the current task or from the activation of
  other schemas) attached to different regions of the scene, and these
  compete and cooperate. Thus, we may recognize the distinctive
  locations and appearances of two chairs in a scene—taking us
  beyond simply activating the chair schema as encoded in semantic
  memory.
- As certain regions are recognized (one schema instance "wins" over
  others), they, rather than the lower-level features that support them,
  become the units directing attention. In the Yarbus example (§3.2) of
  "remember the clothing of the people," the recognition of faces seemed
  to act as the anchor, with attention directed up and down beneath each
  face as the clothing was committed to memory.

Some relevant neuropsychology: Damage to the left inferior occipitotemporal junction (where the occipital lobe that contains primary visual
cortex meets the inferotemporal cortex that includes object recognition
processes) may result in *ventral simultagnosia*, in which patients cannot
visually recognize scenes even though they can recognize the individual

objects in the scenes one at a time. More specifically, such patients may recognize that several objects are present and thus navigate around them without recognizing them. (By contrast, bilateral lesions to the junction between the *parietal* and occipital lobes may yield *dorsal* simultanagnosia in which perception is limited to a single object without awareness of the presence of others.) In terms of VISIONS, it is as if a visual schema could be activated for each object as it is being attended to, but there is no visual working memory to accumulate schema instances over multiple fixations or to mediate the competition and cooperation involved in yielding a coherent, task-dependent, understanding of the scene.

Four comments now take us beyond the limits of the VISIONS model:

1. VISIONS seeks to classify what objects are present in the different regions of a scene and assess their spatial relation. However, our visual experience is not restricted to object recognition. One may, for example, simply appreciate a patch of color. Think of a garden where one enjoys the shapes and masses of color whether or not one refines that with a close-up view of details.

2. In general, experience is multimodal: the feel of a gravel path versus a springy lawn; birdsong and the hum of bees; the touch of spray on your cheeks blown from a sprinkler.

3. Activation of a visual schema instance may offer access to certain possibilities for action (affordances) and—through its linkage to lower level details—may even pass parameters to motor schemas that could control the action (recall the "what" and "how" pathways).

4. Our experience extends in time—episodes and not just scenes—as we act within the action–perception cycle, and as we recognize the actions of others, possibly as the basis for social interaction.

Addressing comment 1 simply involves extending the set of perceptual schemas to support conscious appreciation of patterns of color and tex-ture (as distinct from their subconscious role in low-level vision) as well as those engaged with the limbic system. We can recognize diverse forms for their aesthetic or emotional impact, irrespective of whether we can name what we observe. In particular, our discussion of the atmosphere of a building may relate to perceiving a unity (activating a general schema) in novel arrangements of diverse forms.

To address comment 2, I return to MULTIMODES (§3.6) as a *conceptual* extension of VISIONS. Here, processes of competition and cooperation of instances of perceptual schemas now exploit sensory cues from multiple modalities in developing a coherent understanding of dynamic episodes embedded within 3D space. All this is embedded within the inner and outer cycles of the action–perception cycle (Figure 1.4):

Actions in the *inner cycle* help us perceive more about the world. A sudden movement, an unexpected sound, a sting on the skin may attract our attention, or we may seek more context for what has been attended to. We may walk toward an object—either to get a closer look (inner cycle) or to act upon it, or interact with it, in some way (outer cycle). We may feel objects to learn more about them, or bring an object close to sniff it. Other mechanisms can direct a tongue to repeatedly find and probe a broken tooth.

Rather than having a single intermediate database restricted to vision, MULTIMODES has a separate intermediate database for each sensory modality, and these databases can be linked so that, for example, spatial layout cues can be coordinated between vision, audition, and touch—but they all contribute to the interpretation of the environment. Schemas in long-term memory now include schemas for recognizing actions as well as objects and agents and the relation between them. Working memory encompasses a range of schema instances that may be updated, added to, or removed according to the dynamics of both inner and outer cycles. Preprocessed data from the multiple modality-specific intermediate databases can interact to resolve ambiguities and discrepancies. Working memory will include a representation of recent actions, along with task and motivation information that can affect its dynamics. Schema instances may pass a critical threshold so that they and certain of their parameters may provide the perception of the episode that provides key data to direct or modulate ongoing action.

To begin to address comments 3 and 4, let's recall a functional magnetic resonance imaging (fMRI) experiment from §5.2 (Figure 5.6). The subject saw a video (no sound) of a person talking, a monkey making communicative orofacial movements, and a dog barking. The fMRI showed vigorous mirror system activity when the subject viewed the human, only modest activity when viewing the monkey, and none when viewing the dog. I inferred that *we don't need mirror neurons to recognize actions, but that mirror neurons can enrich perception of actions when they fall within our own repertoire.* Conversely, learning by imitation exploits a more general ability to recognize patterns of movement and in some cases relate them to goal-oriented behaviors. Only in certain cases will we come to map these performances onto our own body, master new actions, and develop related mirror neurons in the process.

There are intriguing neuroscience data that take us beyond Figure 10.2 and help us think about the diversity of neural pathways implicit in the previous paragraph. If you want a glimpse of these, read on. If not, jump to the next double lines.

Even if we restrict attention to vision, there are other dorsal and ventral streams beyond those sketched in Figure 10.2. Kravitz, Saleem, Baker, and Mishkin (2011) charted three dorsal visual pathways (Figure 10.3):

- The parieto-premotor pathway targets the premotor cortex and supports visually guided actions (this is the dorsal pathway in FARS).
- The parieto-prefrontal pathway targets the prefrontal cortex and supports spatial working memory and so may be a good candidate for at least part of the visual working memory as modeled in VISIONS.
- Bringing us to our concern with hippocampus, the parieto-medial temporal pathway targets the adjacent medial temporal lobe and supports navigation.

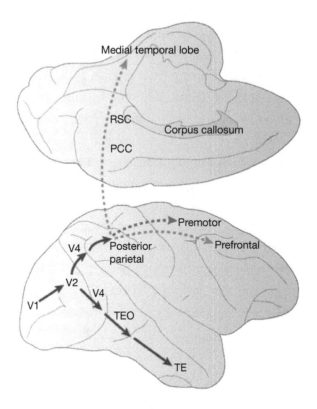

Figure 10.3 Three dorsal streams emanating from the posterior parietal cortex, as studied in the brains of macaque monkeys: the parieto-premotor pathway (*dashed red arrow*); the parieto-prefrontal pathway (*dashed green arrow*); and the parieto-medial temporal pathway (*dashed blue arrow*); see text for details. The diagram also shows the "classical" ventral "what" pathway from V2 to the inferotemporal cortex. PCC = posterior cingulate cortex; RSC = retrosplenial cortex; TE = rostral inferior temporal cortex; TEO = posterior inferior temporal cortex; V1= primary visual cortex. (Reprinted by permission of Springer Nature from Kravitz, D. J., Saleem, K. S., Baker, C. I., & Mishkin, M. © 2011. A new neural framework for visuospatial processing. *Nature Reviews Neuroscience*, 12, 217. doi:10.1038/nrn3008.)

Complementing this work (and going beyond the scope of the present discussion—but a good target for future A↔N conversation), Kravitz, Saleem, Baker, Ungerleider, and Mishkin (2013) went on to synthesize data from neuroanatomy and functional analysis to propose that the ventral pathway is best understood as a recurrent occipitotemporal network containing *at least six distinct cortical and subcortical systems*, with each system serving its own specialized behavioral, cognitive, or affective function.

A major neuroscience challenge is to understand how these pathways work together, and how they relate to memory and imagination in general. All this begins to structure the "spaghetti diagram" (Figure 3.9) of Felleman and Van Essen (1991). It diagrammed the many areas that are part of the visual system, and the multiplicity of connections between them, perhaps 30% of the possible total. In their diagram, the visual streams start at the retina at bottom, seem to converge within the dorsal prefrontal cortex where visually responsive neurons have access to both spatial and nonspatial information, and continue to hippocampus (HC) at top. But, of course, not all roads lead to Rome.

In extending MULTIMODES to IBSEN while taking the lessons of TAM-WGM into account, each of the three dorsal pathways (—for visually guided actions, spatial working memory, and navigation—must be augmented by multimodal input), and their reciprocal connections with ventral systems must be explored. Doing this may be important not only for the challenges to neuroscience thus provided but also as providing new ideas for the architecture-relevant dissection of phenomenology.

Varieties of learning in IBSEN

The conceptual design of IBSEN not only includes MULTIMODES (and thus VISIONS) but also has four new learning mechanisms:

1. Salient features of an episode can be extracted from the dynamics of this working memory to support *episodic memory.*
2. Procedural memory acquires skills that can reshape the body schema to better recognize affordances and pass the parameters to effectivities to support the graceful execution of a wide range of skills, with and without the involvement of tools.

3. *Working memory* patterns can be exploited, coupled with ongoing feedback or reinforcement from behavior, to update *semantic memory* (some open to conscious analysis, some not) for both the specifically sensory knowledge (the bottom-up cues that can evoke an instance of a schema) and the more general world knowledge (the lateral and top-down cues that can encode the knowledge that certain spatial relations between certain types of objects are more likely than others, and thus mediate the competition and cooperation of schema instances).

4. Moreover, *long-term working memory* that can link internal and external memory systems plays an essential role in the design process, providing priority access to (but not only to) memories that have proved relevant to the current design process. Some such memories may lose priority after they have served their role or been judged to be distractions, but the process of competitive computation may reactivate them in some circumstances.

IBSEN goes beyond the use of spatial context to provide memory structures that both exploit temporal context (given my assessment of what has happened in the past, how can I make sense of what I am seeing now?) and expectation (given my current assessment, what do I expect to happen next *and what actions might I perform next?*). Such expectation does not imply an exact prediction of what comes next—rather, we are in the domain of conditional probabilities, so that something turned the corner store.[5] Here, we see *scripts* as the temporal analog of "network schemas" like that in VISIONS that "if you see a region that may be a roof, then assess whether it is part of a house by checking the area beneath it for cues that the right type of wall is there."

---

5. Perhaps you noticed that the last clause ("we are in the domain of conditional probabilities, so that something turned the corner store") made little or no sense, but this was to illustrate the way in which expectations can accommodate a variety of possibilities, while rendering some so unlikely that they "set off alarm bells" (twice, in this example) that require a major reassessment of the situation.

IBSEN must not only capture the recognition of objects in spatial relationship but also capture the design of the spaces that support certain actions that link agents and objects, or two or more people, with each other in the building. On several occasions, we have suggested that architecture succeeds to the extent it satisfies the observer as a sculpture and also satisfies the user as to its functionality. Moreover, it has become clear that these are not either/or considerations—the skilled architect integrates diverse considerations. The environment (both of people and of buildings as well as natural landscape) can change our emotional state, and this in turn biases our likely courses of action. Thus, IBSEN must also incorporate the means to imagine ways in which buildings can create atmospheres that shape the moods and emotions of users.

10.3. LINKING MEMORY AND IMAGINATION: THE HIPPOCAMPUS AND MORE

When we consider how the architect's memories of past episodes may affect their designs, our concern is not with their accuracy as historical records but only with the ideas they may bring to mind, as in Utzon's experiences with Mayan and Chinese temples, or of sailing around Helsingør. This section introduces something of the neuroscience of the relation between memory and imagination. Here, our quest for relevant neuroscience leads us away from architecture, and so, at least on a first reading, many readers may prefer to omit this section, going directly to §10.4. Alternatively, you can get the highlights by initially skipping or humming the material between the pairs of double lines.

In "The Future of Memory: Remembering, Imagining, and the Brain," Schacter, Addis, Hassabis, Martin, Spreng, and Szpunar (2012) summarized studies showing that, while there are differences in brain activity between remembering and imagining, there is a shared network engaged in both. The key datum is that hippocampus is a core part of that overlap. Importantly, though, just as episodic memory is only one form of memory (§3.3), so is the hippocampus system only one route to imagination.

Linking episodic memory to autobiographical memory

An *episodic memory* captures something of an episode, grounded in (but not restricted to) who did what and to whom, and when. We may recall episodes in which we were actors, and others in which we served more as observers. In neither case is the accuracy of recall guaranteed. *Autobiographical memory* (something that may be unique to humans) is the basis on which we construct *narratives* for our lives, with the episodes situated in space and time—but in some very general sense of time to be explored shortly—and with some linked more tightly together than others. It should be noted that these memories are not fixed—a room we experienced as a child that seemed vast appears small when revisited; friends we remember from our youth may retain the qualities we remember when met years later, or may seem very different if (perhaps especially if) their personalities have not changed with the years. Moreover, memories are indeed multimodal, and may include the corporeal sensation of moving through a space as much as visual, auditory, or other exterosensory experience.

Some observations: The sense of "narrative" here is not limited to what can be expressed in words. Moreover, when we are in the domain of words, a "script" for a play or movie presents a narrative through words that specify a sequence of episodes in terms of what is spoken and what actions and interactions occur with and between these speeches. Note, however, that within our A↔N conversation, "script" refers not to a specific sequence of episodes but rather to set of general constraints or ground rules for how a certain class of behaviors might unfurl.

An episode may be as narrow as a single action or, more often, may embed a range of actions within a context that enriches their meaning. That context may itself be based on memories that were formed by earlier episodes. The first step from remembering episodes to autobiographical memory may thus be at the level of linking two episodes—the one that created the context and the one that exploited the context—in temporal relationship, but this will rarely involve "time by the clock." The "timeline" for self-episodes is highly flexible.

More generally, this linkage may be more one of "narrative coherence" than temporal contiguity. Recall of one episode may lead me to recall an earlier episode that led up to it, or something that followed from it,[6] perhaps even years later, as when I switch from recalling my time at high school to an episode that occurred at a class reunion 40 years after graduation. Clearly, there is no clock ticking in my brain that kept track of the passing minutes for 40 years. Rather, I have a general idea of my life's patterns, and a high school episode links to a specific few years of my life. By contrast, it was a distinctive feature of that class reunion that it occurred after 40 years. It then involves calendrical calculation, not a neurally ticking timeline, to determine the year that the reunion took place (note the use of spatial terminology to talk about time), and even then, I cannot recall the month, let alone the day, of its occurrence.

Autobiographical memory is relevant to the A↔N conversation in at least two ways:

1. Buildings are spaces where people make memories, and the architect must ponder in what ways the architecture may enrich those memories. What locations should become distinctive places and what associations, whether temporary or enduring, will they have for users of the building? Pondering what made a space memorable to them may enable the architect to develop new ideas. For example, a wooden staircase in a historical building may, after many years and

---

6. Of course, in the telling of a story (whether fictional or not), there will often be an underlying "timeline," but the order in which events are recalled in the narrative may be quite different from the order in which the corresponding episodes occurred. Indeed, a nonfictional narrative may start with a current event and then go back and forth in time in an attempt to explore its antecedents and suggest (and here imagination comes even more fully into play) its possible consequences. In designing a building, narratives are replaced by scripts that generalize across various ranges of behavior that may occur there.

possible renovations, still have a particular smell or creaky sound. What might this suggest in terms of enriching the multimodality of experience within a new building?

2. Understanding the linkage of episodes in autobiographical memories may enhance the architect's awareness of how to make each building a stage for the performance of scripts in our A↔N sense that yield the diverse narratives for those who visit, work, or dwell there. In *Body, Memory and Architecture*, Bloomer and Moore (1977) explore how body-image theory, aesthetics, and ballet extend our understanding of how bodily movement links to memories as they contribute to architecture. A very useful discussion contrasts aspects of buildings that support visual exploration (as in exploring the intricacies of the paintings on the interior of a dome) and those that invite locomotory exploration, engaging the whole body as we move around a space.

Implicating hippocampus in episodic memory and imagination

Diverse regions make their contributions to the dynamically shifting coalitions of brain circuits that underlie the *general* mechanisms of action, perception, memory, and imagination that find their *specialized* employment in the experience and design of architecture.[7]

Let's start with an fMRI study by Addis, Wong, and Schacter (2007). Participants were cued with a noun for 20 seconds and told to construct an account of a past (recalled) or future (imagined) event that occurred within a specified time period (week, year, 5–20 years). When participants had the event in mind, they pressed a button and for the remainder of the

---

7. There is a vast cognitive science and neuroscience literature related to memory and imagination, including diverse cognitive-level and neural-level models. I must confess that I have read only a small fraction of it. Thus, progress in this area will rest on sifting the current literature as well as designing new studies more attuned to the A↔N conversation.

scan elaborated on the event. Addis et al. call the first task "event construction" and the latter "event elaboration." Given this period of time, the subjects came up with a fairly extensive verbal narrative. Whatever the shortcoming of this terminology, note that, given the conditions of their study, their elaboration phase is in part converting fragments of memory that may be multisensory in their construction phase into a linguistic form that may discard some aspects of the earlier phase while elaborating others.

Here is a typical transcript of a participant's description of an imagined personally relevant future experience:

[Time scale: 5 years in future; cue: dress.] My sister will be finishing . . . her undergraduate education, I imagine some neat place, Ivy League private school . . . it would be a very nice spring day and my mom and my dad will be there, my dad with the camcorder as usual, and my mom with the camera as usual. My sister will be in the crowd and they'd be calling everyone's name . . . I can see her having a different hair style by then, maybe instead of straight, very curly with lots of volume. She would be wearing contacts by then and heels of course. And I can see myself sitting in some kind of sundress, like yellow, and under some trees . . . the reception either before or after and it would be really nice summer food, like salads and fruits, and maybe some sweets, and cold drinks that are chilled but have no ice. And my sister would be sitting off with her friends, you know, talking with them about graduating, and they'd probably get emotional.

This uses some autobiographical memory to suggest what might continue and what might change in family members. However, the passage of 5 years as such plays little role when used to establish that a college graduation will provide the frame.

Before reviewing the fMRI data, let's note how fertile the imagination of this typical subject is, not just the drumming up of diverse items—some essentially repurposed memories, others with variations, and some perhaps drawn from reading or viewing rather than experience—but also their ordering into some kind of coherence. If ideas can flow this freely, why does it take months or years to design a building? Or, if one can generate the previous imagined experience in 20 seconds, then why can't I write a 300-page book in a couple of days? Providing your own initial answer to these questions now may help you engage more fully in the later presentation of IBSEN.[8]

The separation of an (initial) construction period from an elaboration period in the Addis et al. fMRI study of episodic recall and imagination could in future research be applied to fMRI analysis of architects and others engaged in design tasks, seeking to distinguish brain activity during "bringing images to mind" to get a first pass on collecting "ingredients" for the design, from that involved in forming a coherent image of the newly imagined whole. Another architecture-centered fMRI study might involve comparing scans of architects asked (a) to recall a view of a familiar building (visually, rather than describing it in words) and (b) to imagine (again, without a verbal description) sketching a space with desired characteristics. Separate scans would request an emphasis on verbal description. Further data analysis might reveal that some architects make more use of verbal scaffolding of their visual recall and imagination than others.

The usual health warning: Don't let Figure 10.4 intimidate you. By all means, assess the details if you want to, but I want to single out just one aspect of these data. Yes, the figure gives a sense of the actual fMRI results, and contains data on many brain regions. However, all you need notice for now is not only how hippocampus is involved but also that *many other brain regions have significant activity in the construction or elaboration phase.*

In the *construction phase*, both past and future event construction engaged left hippocampus and posterior visuospatial regions.

---

8. A preliminary version of IBSEN, intended for computational neuroscientists, was published in the paper "From Spatial Navigation via Visual Construction to Episodic Memory and Imagination" (Arbib, 2020).

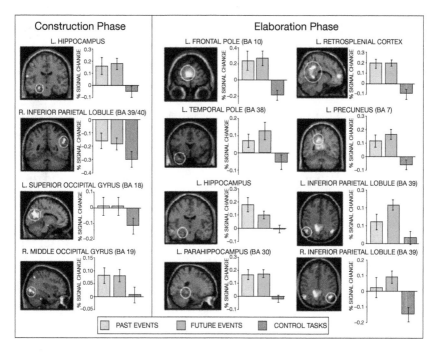

Figure 10.4 The key point of the figure for us is not the details, but rather how many regions are involved beyond the hippocampus. As in other fMRI experiments, it is necessary to have control tasks that, presumably, do not involve the mechanisms that are key to the processes under study. In this case, semantic memory and visual imagery trials were randomly interspersed through each scanning session, each with their own construction and elaboration phases. Neural regions shown are those commonly engaged during the (*left*) event (past + future) construction and/or (*right*) event elaboration relative to the control task. BA = Brodmann area. (Adapted from Addis, D. R., Wong, A. T., & Schacter, D. L. [2007]. Remembering the past and imagining the future: Common and distinct neural substrates during event construction and elaboration. *Neuropsychologia*, 45[7], 1363–1377, with permission from Elsevier.)

In the *elaboration phase*, left inferior parietal lobule was significantly more active for future events than past events, while other regions were notably more active in this case. Conversely, only left hippocampus was notably more active during past than future events.

Of course, if we were to more fully analyze these data in relation to hypotheses as to the contributions of the various brain regions, we would have to accept that there could be no strict separation between the construction phase and the elaboration phase, though we might (with second-by-second analysis of the fMRI) establish that certain processes are more important as the construction begins, while others become more active as elaboration proceeds. Further data of Addis et al. (2007) show brain areas with (a) significant increases in activity during the construction and elaboration of future events relative to that of past events; and (b) activations associated with the construction of past and future events relative to their elaboration and, conversely, elaboration of past and future events relative to their construction.

Addis et al. offer an interpretation of their data that is heavily theory-laden. By this I mean that if they see activation of a region and that region has been seen as significantly active in other papers for a particular process A > control, then they will comment that A may be involved in the phenomena studied here. They suggested that *future event construction* also recruited regions involved in *prospective thinking* while also implicating *right* hippocampus, *possibly as a response to the novelty of these events*. They attributed above-control activity of regions seen in elaboration to activity in the putative *autobiographical memory retrieval network, engaging elaboration, self-referential processing,* and *contextual and episodic imagery*.

In addition to their summary, it is worth pondering that they found a strong future > past effect during the elaboration phase in *left* BA 44/47 and *right* BA 45/46/47. *Left* BA 44/45 is traditionally seen as Broca's area, an area strongly involved in language production, whereas *right* BA 44/45 is not directly associated with language. Why might there be this greater involvement for future than past in both a language area and its right hemisphere analog? My speculation is that in recalling a past episode, language plays a secondary role to recalling the multimodal experience, whereas, in constructing a possible future event, a "language sketch" may precede any attempt to infuse that imagined event with fragments of multimodal sensation. However, in the elaboration phase, the difference may disappear because in each case this involves preparing the verbal description of the recalled or imagined event.

All this serves to remind us that, whatever progress is made on IBSEN in this chapter, it is only a beginning for understanding how diverse functional systems contribute to the design processes and much else besides, let alone being able to model how circuitry in various brain regions underlies these functions.

Eleanor Maguire's group has provided a steady stream of relevant papers, probing neural activity of hippocampus and the nearby parahippocampal gyrus region in relation to imagination and episodic memory. Hassabis and Maguire (2009; Hassabis, Kumaran, & Maguire, 2007) looked at healthy participants engaged in three tasks while in the scanner:

1. Vivid recall of recent real memories
2. Construction of new imaginary experiences in the scanner (but not linked to the subjects' future in some time period)
3. Vivid recall of previously created imaginary experiences (as in 2, but constructed outside the scanner)

Here is a typical transcript:

[Cue: Imagine standing by a small stream somewhere deep in a forest.] It's a pine forest. What I can see on the ground all around me are patches of pine needles and brown earth with nothing really growing. The tree trunks are quite narrow. Overhead are the spikes of the green pines and you can only just see the sky. There's a pine needle smell but down towards the stream there's a slightly rotting smell. It's quite a narrow stream with stones in it and dark water rushing round them causing little white water eddies. There's not much life around the stream and the banks are quite steep sloping down to the stream. It's peaceful and quiet.

As for the transcript from Addis et al., note how much detail is accumulated. A general issue, then, is what anchors each account and then what details get added via top-down and horizontal inferences (compare construction vs. elaboration in the sense of Addis et al.). What is engaged transiently but edited out of the articulated account?

Hassabis and Maguire demarcated the brain regions activated in common by the three tasks: hippocampus bilaterally, parahippocampal gyrus, retrosplenial and posterior parietal cortices, middle temporal cortices, and medial prefrontal cortex.[9] They claim that "this network is probably involved in scene or event construction, the primary process these three conditions have in common," and call it the *construction network*. Hassabis et al. (2007) further observe:

- The scan for episodic memory retrieval only adds right thalamus to the overlap.
- The scan for new fictitious experiences differs only in omitting left hippocampus.

The key point for us is the centrality of the hippocampus. Note, though, that different component processes may be differentially affected by hippocampal damage.

Mental construction in episodic memory and imagination

These two studies related to the recall of past episodes and the imagination of novel episodes support our claim that both of these are forms of *mental construction*. Recall of an episode is unlike retrieving a photograph; some aspects are recalled first, and then others are filled in, though not necessarily correctly, and many are not recalled at all.

9. While these "partners" of the hippocampus are of great interest to some neuroscientists, they lie outside the present scope (the parahippocampal gyrus will make a brief appearance in §10.4). Other relevant references (from a vast literature) include studies of "Discovering Event Structure in Continuous Narrative Perception and Memory" (Baldassano et al., 2017), and "Two Distinct Scene-Processing Networks Connecting Vision and Memory" (Baldassano, Esteva, Fei-Fei, & Beck, 2016).

The problem remains that the previous studies fail to address the key issue: What are the "pieces" that the construction process engaged in the fMRI studies assembles, and what is engaged in that construction? This is the task that IBSEN begins to address for architecture. Hassabis and Maguire assert that their construction network not only accounts for a large part of the episodic memory recall network but also bears a "striking resemblance" to networks activated by navigation, spatial and place tasks, but do not explain how this works. IBSEN will address this by building on the TAM-WGM in §10.4. But here we must extend our understanding of how hippocampus interacts with other brain systems.

Building on the *hippocampal memory indexing theory* (Teyler & Rudy, 2007), Moscovitch, Cabeza, Winocur, and Nadel (2016) developed a dynamic perspective on episodic memory and the hippocampus that runs from perception to language and from empathy to problem-solving. Their *component process model* holds that, when encoding episodes, hippocampus binds together into a memory trace or engram those neural elements in the medial temporal lobe and neocortex that give rise to the *perceptual, emotional, and conceptual experience,* together with a sense of *autonoetic consciousness* that engages the self in some form of reliving of the experience. They assert that the episodic memory trace binds activity in neocortical neurons with a sparsely coded hippocampal component that acts as "a pointer or index . . . to neocortical components that together represent the totality of the experience." Consequently, a partial cue that activated the index could activate the neocortical patterns and thus retrieve the memory of the episode.

This leaves open two complementary questions: (a) what binds together the different aspects of a memory, and (b) what would then permit "unbinding" so that fragments from different episodes could get activated, then interact, and possibly cohere into a new imagined episode?

Addis et al. (2007) showed that *right* hippocampus is more active for future events than past events during the construction phase (with no significant difference in left hippocampus), whereas left hippocampus is more active for past than future events during the elaboration phase. Alas, I have no insight into differences between left and right hippocampus. Five years after the 2007 study, Addis and Schacter (2012) ignore these differences and suggest that this hippocampal activation reflects recombining details into coherent scenarios—both encoding scenarios into memory as a combination of details and recombining details into novel but coherent scenarios.

However, if we use our analysis of VISIONS for guidance (as we did in §10.2), this fits what we might call a "naïve" construction view—assemble the pieces—but ignores the way in which one may recognize larger scale organization to provide the top-down cues for selecting what pieces to assemble and how to assemble them.

Perceiving an episode requires integration over some time interval in which dynamic changes in relationships can be observed, including "who did what and to whom (or which)" for persons and/or objects that attract the observer's attention (bottom-up), or to which the observer may direct attention (top-down) in pursuit of providing the perceptual base for a current task. At this point, though, recall that "top-down" in VISIONS refers to processes of interaction of schema instances that may be at the same level (e.g., seeing a hand makes one more likely to recognize a piece of fabric covering the wrist as a sleeve), and not just at the highest level. Note, too, that the overall organization that matches perceived details to a script is often highly flexible.

To the extent that a memory involves spatial and temporal relations between agents and objects, so too will these be more or less integral to the recall of the episode. Thus, the spatiotemporal framework for such recall will, I suggest, provide the "brain space" for the constructive recall and imagination of spatiotemporal episodes. A crucial challenge for further developing the model will be to also address the "experiential aspect" of an episode, and this includes the emotional shading present in that episode, whether this precedes or follows from the interpretive process. An episode you recall may be one in which you were actively involved, or one that you have observed. In recalling it, your autonoetic consciousness would engage the self in some form so that "reliving" the experience would include some sense of your role. Of course, nothing ensures that your memory is accurate—you may vividly recall your engagement in some activity for which, to the contrary, you were only a spectator.

In the §6.3 subsection on "The hippocampus in context," we looked at variation along the ventral-dorsal axis of the hippocampus (Figure 10.5) in relation to *spatial navigation*. Here we return to longitudinal variation in relation to *episodic memory*. Robin and Moscovitch (2017) suggest that the dorsal representation is finer than the ventral representation in relation to episodic memory, but offer a different view from that cited in §6.3:

- Ventral hippocampus may code information in terms of the general or global relations among entities, and is preferentially connected to anterior regions, such as
  - ventromedial prefrontal cortex (vmPFC), associated with *scripts* (though they call them schemas);
  - lateral temporal cortex, associated with *semantic information*; and
  - the temporal pole and the amygdala, associated with *social and emotional cues*.

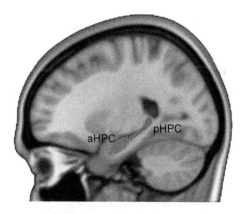

Figure 10.5 (A repeat of Figure 6.13). A cross section of the human brain, showing the lengthwise division of the hippocampus into the dorsal hippocampus (in primates, this is the posterior hippocampus [pHPC], both upper and to the rear) and the ventral hippocampus (in primates, this is the anterior hippocampus [aHPC], lower and toward the front). (From Li, X., Li, Q., Wang, X., Li, D., & Li, S. [2018]. Differential age-related changes in structural covariance networks of human anterior and posterior hippocampus. *Frontiers in Physiology*, 9[518]. doi:10.3389/fphys.2018.00518. Public access.)

- Dorsal hippocampus may code information in terms of precise positions within some continuous dimension, and is preferentially connected to perceptual regions in the posterior neocortex.

A *script-in-our-sense* is supported by a generic trace in long-term memory of what can be construed as a very high-level schema-in-our-sense that—unlike the purely spatial schemas of VISIONS—extends in time as well as space. *Semantic information* may correspond to the *schema instances* linked to the schemas in long-term memory that provide the knowledge base for VISIONS-like processes. These, along with emotional and social cues, might thus be the province of the ventral hippocampus. Indeed, Fanselow and Dong (2010) review relevant data to support the notion that dorsal hippocampus performs primarily cognitive functions, whereas ventral hippocampus relates to stress, emotion, and affect, a somewhat similar but nonetheless different division than that of Robin and Moscovitch.[10]

Turning to the dorsal hippocampus, we might relate its *highly specific representation* to the network of parameterized schema *instances* in working memory linked to the temporospatial regions within the episode. At a coarser grain, it might also include the *gist* as a collection of schema *instances* that provide the *context* for top-down influences on this highly specific representation (as in "my 10th birthday party").

Memory and imagination are not just episodic

The brain imaging studies described earlier link memory of episodes and imagination of narratives. But let's again "put hippocampus in its place," and then explore the notion that semantic memory and procedural

---

10. Fanselow and Dong (2010) also report that gene expression in the dorsal hippocampus correlates with cortical regions involved in information processing, while genes expressed in the ventral hippocampus correlate with regions involved in emotion and stress (amygdala and hypothalamus).

memory may be at least as important as episodic memory in architectural design.

Elward and Vargha-Khadem (2018, and Vargha-Khadem, personal communication) describe patients with *developmental amnesia*, resulting from oxygen deprivation during neonatal heart surgery. The lack of oxygen led to brain damage that included atrophy of hippocampus bilaterally (with greater atrophy of posterior hippocampus), but preservation of the nearby bilateral parahippocampal gyrus. Typically, they show *relatively preserved semantic memory and factual knowledge* about the natural world despite severe impairments in episodic memory. Children with developmental amnesia seem normal for 3 years or so, but at age 4 show amnesic symptoms: they forget belongings, repeat questions, and forget instructions. A parent will describe the child as "living in the moment, with flat affect"; a teacher will say the child is "friendly and polite, seems able but cannot deliver"; and the child will say, "I listened in class and understood everything, but a little later I forget everything." Although these subjects cannot remember events of their life, they have excellent fact memory *and recognition of what they have seen before*—they can encode and consolidate the scene and recognize it if they encounter it again, but cannot "bring it to mind" in their autonoetic consciousness. Compare recognizing an object as a potato peeler and knowing how to use it, but not being able to bring to mind an occasion on which you (or someone else) used it.

Recall that H. M. was amnesic because of surgery that removed hippocampus and adjacent temporal lobe bilaterally. He could understand visual scenes—he just could not commit them to episodic memory. Moreover, the evidence that he could get better at playing a game (procedural memory), even though he believed he had not seen it before, suggests that he lacks the developmental amnesics' ability to recognize that a scene had been seen before (and he certainly could not re-experience it as an episodic memory). To make sense of this, recall that H. M.'s surgery removed a massive amount of temporal cortex around the hippocampus, whereas the bilateral parahippocampal gyrus (adjacent to the hippocampus) was preserved in the developmental amnesics.

Combining these observations, we may formulate the following:

Hypothesis: Neocortical systems can support visual scene understanding (or episode perception generally) without involvement of
the hippocampus. Rather, the hippocampus provides a supplemen-
tal loop that evaluates episodes for "episodic memorability" and the
consequent strength with which an index (in the sense of Teyler
and others) is formed as a candidate for neocortical consolidation
and potential retrieval that involves autonoetic consciousness (i.e.,
the knowledge of the self's prior awareness during the episode).
The parahippocampal gyrus may be part of the system engaged
in encoding a scene into semantic memory, but without the hippocampus, that semantic memory cannot be linked into episodic
memory.

What, then, of the dorsal–ventral axis in hippocampus as assessed
by Robin and Moscovitch? The suggestion here is that this reflects the
differences in regions that provide input to these subdivisions of hippocampus, but these regions can function in the here and now without recourse to the "episodic memorability" system. Indeed, note that
VISIONS models visual scene understanding based solely on semantic memory and is enriched neither by linkage with prior episodes
nor through an ability to convert scene understanding into episodic
memory.

Memories do not sit in watertight compartments. Let's just consider
doors. There are procedural memories that allow you to use diverse doors
in diverse situations, even if you have not encountered them before. But
what about episodic memory? Suppose that you see a door and remember going through it before and finding yourself in a sweet-smelling garden. If so, that will tempt you to indeed go through that door and relive
the experience—though other motivations will compete to determine
whether or not you actually go through that door. However, such a memory may also take less episodic forms. If that particular door was visually distinctive and was associated with pleasing fragrances, then seeing

a similar door may tempt you to go through it, even if you do not recall any particular episode that contributed to these pleasurable associations.

Certainly, actions and emotions and the appreciation of visual form can all be part of a vivid episode in one's life, and can thus be integrated into episodic memory. Moreover, the hippocampus is part of the limbic system, which we have seen (§4.2) to be integral to the experience of emotion. And, yes, visual perception is integrated with the hippocampus in normal experience that can provide candidates for episodic memory. However, we have also seen that visual perception can proceed successfully in the absence of hippocampus. Recall, again, Teyler's index theory. The suggestion was not that the hippocampus provided the full memory of an episode, but that it provided an index to a multitude of cortical activations that between them would reconstitute the episode, while the hippocampus would link this to autonoetic consciousness. However, we saw that HM could still develop procedural memory, while the developmental amnesics could develop semantic memories of scenes even though they could not relive episodes that involved them.

Thus, while our demands on the architect's imagination do include imagination of episodes in the lives of future users of a building (framed but not exhausted by general scripts), they also include much more. They provide stimuli for experience in vision and other modalities; they imagine future actions for which affordances must be provided; and they imagine atmospheric and emotional impacts that are further parts of the package that must be integrated into the final design.

10.4. FROM SCRIPTS TO COGNITIVE MAPS TO BUILDINGS

The kitchen example of §10.1 introduced three key ideas:

1. Users of a building will develop multiple scripts for how they use it (which may incorporate social interaction and contemplation as well as practical behaviors).

2. These scripts may engage specific cognitive maps of relevant places.

3. The architect must not only imagine spaces that will support diverse scripts but must harmonize the places (and more) that ground the corresponding cognitive maps in the 3D realization of the building.

This section will more fully relate the first two issues to our earlier modeling of navigation, and sketch how IBSEN must support mechanisms that enable the designer to "invert" users' experience of the building as a stage for performing these various scripts. We will then address the third point: having developed initial ideas for how the building will support different script-related cognitive maps, the architect must then consider the extent to which certain places in the final building might serve as nodes in more than one map.

Revisiting TAM-WGM

TAM-WGM combined the taxon affordance model (TAM) and the world graph model (WGM) and was designed to address the differential engagement of multiple brain regions in two forms of wayfinding (§6.3), with hippocampus strongly engaged when exploiting a cognitive map (as modeled by WGM), but not when one simply follows responding to one affordance at a time (as modeled by TAM). Let's recall some of the phenomena captured by TAM and WGM before we consider how these ideas may factor into our sketch of IBSEN.

TAM captures the strategy of simply looking for affordances to meet our current needs within the sample of the environment that is currently within the range of vision or other senses. Affordances (registered in posterior parietal cortex) can be selected for action (as determined in premotor cortex). However, TAM also has a mechanism for evaluating the consequences of actions, reinforcing those actions that proved successful in a given situation. Crucially, TAM does not require a cognitive map, nor does it engage the hippocampus. Affordances for TAM may also include "signposts" (in some general sense) that point the way to the location of affordances for actions that meet our needs (e.g., seeing a sign pointing to a somewhat distant restaurant versus actually seeing the restaurant).

By contrast, WGM extends wayfinding beyond the proximate environment by implementing the formation and use of cognitive maps—modeled as WGs—of significant places. The model posited that prefrontal cortex could hold a variety of WGs, with one being invoked for the current navigation task. Navigation arenas could be quite diverse—around a house, or around a town—invoking some of the concepts architects gain from Lynch's *The Image of the City* (Lynch, 1960).

In each WG, nodes represented significant places, while a directed edge between two nodes encodes actions for getting from the first to the second. Nodes in a WG may serve simply as via points, such as places to turn off one road to another while driving, or they may satisfy basic needs like eating or drinking, or aesthetic needs such as offering a view of landscape or a painting. They may also serve social needs, as places to meet other people, or places that offer privacy. And there are also places that are fearsome in some sense, and so must be avoided.

Each node has features associated with knowing that you are approaching or at its place, as well as knowing the motivation-related properties that the place may address. Correspondingly, routes involve traversing from one node-place to another, and so each place must offer distinctive cues as to which direction from that place leads along a path corresponding to a particular edge in the cognitive map. Given some need or intention, WGM models how to plan a route to get from one's current location to a place where that need could be satisfied. Both exploration and reinforcement learning could update the map so that it could support discovery of new routes under varying conditions.

The abstract cognitive map of a WG is complemented by the *locometric map* encoded in hippocampus. When necessary to enforce the distinction, let's reserve the term *place* for a distinctive place that can ground a WG node. By contrast, a *location* is like a less distinctive "place" in the sense used in discussing the rat studies of hippocampus, where each "place cell" has a "place field" around some arbitrary location in the arena in which the animal is being studied. Let's recall, though, that the "place fields" of rat place cells change if the rat is transferred from one arena to the other. This led to the crucial metaphor of the "hippocampal chart table": different "charts" must be "installed" in hippocampus as the arena changes. WGM specifies (but does not model in detail) that the choice of current WG can drive installation of the appropriate hippocampal chart. Conversely, when hippocampus and WG are in register, the hippocampus can inform the WG about which node or edge best corresponds to the current location.[11]

Significant places

The forms and spaces of the building must establish affordances and atmosphere both to engage the users in scripts intended by the architect and to allow the users to create their own narratives and memories of experience in the building (episodic memory). We have all had the experience of driving repeatedly down certain streets where we have command of enough cues to navigate successfully, perhaps even anticipating certain sharp bends rather than responding to external affordances. But here's the rub. One day, when driving down a street after a prolonged absence, we recognize that there is a new house on our route—and yet, try hard as we may, we cannot remember what the previous house there looked like. However, there may be a house that provides a distinctive cue (it has been promoted to a WG node, one might say, as a "landmark"), such as "when

---

11. I have not pursued the mapping of components of WGM to specific brain regions, but it is worth noting that the *parahippocampal gyrus* is certainly relevant to future A↔N conversations. It surrounds the hippocampus and is part of the limbic system, and plays an important role in memory encoding and retrieval. Of particular interest is a subregion called the *parahippocampal place area* (PPA) that lies medially in the inferior temporo-occipital cortex. In fMRI studies, PPA becomes highly active when human subjects view stimuli for topographical scenes, such as images of landscapes, cityscapes, or rooms (Aguirre, Detre, Alsop, & D'Esposito, 1996; Epstein & Kanwisher, 1998)—thus the name "place area." Highlighting its relevance to us, Aguirre, Zarahn, and D'Esposito (1998) write about "An Area Within Human Ventral Cortex Sensitive to 'Building' Stimuli."

you get to that house, start looking for a right-hand turn that is hard to spot behind the trees." If that house is replaced, we will be able to recall it. The point? *The mechanisms that give a place enough salience to be promoted from the locometric map may be comparable to those that define a significant place within a building.* Accordingly, in a large building, significant choice points for navigation must be highlighted, whether by some memorable design feature or by useful signage (a less satisfying strategy, architecturally).

To consider this more fully, let's consider three kinds of places—*action points, viewpoints,* and *via points*—that might anchor scripts, and thus becomes nodes/significant places in a cognitive map/world graph. Some places may belong to multiple categories.

An *action point* is a place that offers affordances that inform the user that this is a place where certain actions may be performed. Such places must be defined for all the scripts that arise in developing the program for the building.

The next category is *viewpoints.* Utzon and Gehry both gave great importance (as, of course, do many other architects) not only to the overall distinctive form of their buildings in relation to their surroundings but also to how that form could be appreciated from different external viewpoints. Here, the "nodes" that define a building are not only places within the building itself but also related places that situate the building in relation to its environment. This builds on our deep ancestral assessment of landscapes. A viewpoint need not be a limited point in the locometric sense (move a meter and you are no longer there), but may have a considerable spatial extent. For example, the walkway on the east side of the Sydney Harbour Bridge serves as an extended viewpoint node for the Sydney Opera House. Nonetheless, this suggests how the position of a viewpoint provides constraints on the placement and design of what is to be viewed.

Now consider a doorway. It is primarily a *via point*, whether linking outside and inside, or one space within the building to another. As such, we might simply treat it as an edge in the WG for the building, connecting nodes for the spaces that the doorway connects. If there is a door to be opened or closed, then affordances must be provided for the necessary action, but these may belong to a more detailed WG focused on that doorway. Architecturally, though, the doorway may be more than a transition point or an action point—it can also be *two* viewpoints, one for each direction in which one passes through, opening to the view of the space beyond. I say "can be" because the architect has the choice of creating a sense of transition via a distinctive space (recall Le Corbusier's description of the Green Mosque in Asia Minor) or simply offering a way of getting from A to B, nothing more.

"Inverting" experiential processes

We have seen a sense in which an artist "inverts" vision. Let's recall from §4.4 (rearranging some of the material) what that means before extending this idea to suggest that the architect "inverts" experience.

> The task of the artist is in some sense to "invert" vision—creating an artificial object whose visual impact may achieve some intended effect or may, at least, offer some opportunity for contemplative visual exploration.

Where vision runs in one direction,

- real-world object (observed scene) → schema assemblage ("mental image")

drawing runs in the *inverse* direction:

- schema assemblage ("mental image") → real-world object (drawing).

This is the inverse (opposite) in effect, but requires different brain mechanisms for its success.

Certainly, viewing an artwork can be a dynamic experience but, even though we may at times "feel ourselves into" the work (§5.1), we remain observers. Our only actions are shifts of attention as we develop our own understanding and appreciation of the work. When viewing the external form of a building like the Sydney Opera House or Guggenheim Museum Bilbao, our cognitive processes are similar—and we may say that we are observing the result of the architect designing "in sculptor mode." However, we can also act and interact within and around a building. Thus, for the architect, the further challenge is to "invert the multimodal action–perception cycle," to create a new external environment for experience and behavior. In this spirit, we start by contrasting the WGs of users of the final building and the WGs that are embedded in the design process of the architect:

For the user of an extant building, a range of different WGs emerge that relate different places within the user's experience of the building. The nodes are abstracted from the user's ability to recognize and orient to significant places, as well as the actions that those places afford. The edges correspond to ways that the user has learned to get from one place to another.

For the architect, each WG may be a way of specifying places that the building must support, and the linkages that must be provided between them. Such a specification may be developed long before the details of the various places are elaborated, and their placement in 3D space, or linkage to locometric maps, has been worked out.

Note that the "final" WGs of the architect need not become WGs for users—both because each user may become familiar with only some aspects of the design of the building (as in the different cognitive maps that diners and staff may have for a restaurant) and because locations in the building may gain significance for a user that was not anticipated by the architect (perhaps the user finds a spot halfway down the stairs that is a good place to listen for what is happening below before proceeding further).

The experience ↔ design loop challenge now is to understand how the architect "inverts" the projected experiential processes of users as they act and interact within and around the planned building, exploiting and moving between different places in it. Thus, the forms and spaces of the building must, as stressed repeatedly, serve to establish affordances and atmosphere both to engage the user in scripts intended by the architect and to allow the user to create their own narratives and memories of experience in the building (episodic memory). In addition, the users abstract from those particular experiences (whether pre-scripted or not) various semantic and procedural memories they can deploy in their future behavior. Consider the experiencing of different operas at the Sydney Opera House, seeing it from the harbor, walking toward it from Circular Quay, or climbing the stairs to admire the view of the harbor from within the building. And then consider, for example, how the tentative exploration of how to enter the building, get to the right auditorium, and find one's seat coheres over repeated visits to an enduring cognitive map of the relevant parts of the building in relation to its immediate surroundings. Other long-term memories might capture how to behave during intermission, and where to stand for a favorite view of the harbor.

A mental image (visual or multimodal, action-oriented, and extended in time) may be very vague—for example, a general idea of a house, or the shape of a patch of color—or highly detailed as to form, size, and more. Compare paying less or more attention—from "I saw a cat over there" to "I saw a black cat with a ribbon around its neck sitting on the sofa and licking its paws." As the details of a drawing or painting emerge (recall Gehry's sketching, §9.3), such a process could invoke the internal processes of visual perception to assess how well the process of imagination was proceeding. But these processes would all involve competition and cooperation of image features and schema instances. In visual perception, schema instances compete and cooperate to match lower level features provided by the sensory input while being constrained, more or less (less so in the case of a Magritte painting—or when my wife and I observed a camel walking down a street in San Gimignano) by general knowledge of how different objects might relate to each other.

In VISIONS, the driver is the current sensory input, with top-down influences (e.g., mood, task) playing a secondary role in helping drive attention to potentially relevant aspects of the scene. In IBSEN, during the design process, the top-down images are determining what lower level schema details will satisfy the current burst of imagination. Multiple images at diverse levels of detail come to mind. Competition and cooperation determine which ones survive and how and where they are instantiated. Crucially, however, when imagination drives sketching (or model-making, or writing, or other physical construction), a new element comes into play. As design proceeds, imagination becomes externalized as markings or structures that provide an external memory of what imagination has wrought so far. Thereafter, the process of competition and cooperation bridges between the emerging "sketch" and the "very high level" schemas that constitute the extended internal working memory (possibly extending over days, months, or longer of the more viable ideas for a project) so that the sketches, the current ideas, and extended memory become dynamic interacting structures.

- In this way, the design begins to develop specifications for localized and extended sensory cues from multiple modalities that provide spatially distributed affordances for realizing diverse scripts that begin to cohere into an understanding of how dynamic episodes for the intended users will be embedded within a range of interconnected 3D physical spaces.

To close this section, then, let's adapt our initial quote on "inverting" vision to apply to the current situation: Experience starts with a static building (leaving aside for now the dynamics afforded by other people in the building, or as offered in neuromorphic architecture. However, rather than one viewing of a picture yielding the schema assemblage that captures our initial experience of it, we have that:

- Each exploration of a building → dynamic schema assemblages (mental images linking perception and action over some time period) that reveal affordances, certain of which are selected to guide behavior. The user may bring certain scripts to the use of the building, but repeated experience of it will develop a range of cognitive maps and, possibly, novel scripts, and these may change the way the building is experienced in future.

Design runs in the *inverse* direction, but the architect cannot anticipate the diverse specific experiences and episodes of users of the building. Instead, then, the design must not only be grounded in the program and site for the building but also must develop a set of scripts for the actions (practical and contemplative) of the user. So far, we have explored the first stage of the "inverse" process:

- Program and site → scripts → diverse WGs of significant places to support those scripts, only some of which are linked to actual locations in relation to the site.

Just as we have related WGs to locometric maps, so in the next subsection must we address how design completes the process:

- Diverse WGs → specific embedding of places within the 3D space defined by the site → the detailed specification of the building.

Harmonizing script-inspired world graphs

Recalling our earlier discussion of the interplay of desirability and executability, let's reflect further on the notion that "the effort of getting to the appropriate affordance can factor into the assessment of the executability of the action." Data for evaluating the effort of getting to the appropriate affordance may be contained in the WG of an individual user, but (beyond taking *types* of user into account, in most cases) the WG imagined by the architect will initially encode the properties of significant places and the key links between them.

Here's the turning point in the design: It is only the registration of the WG with the 3D space in and around the building site and this with a locometric map that spaces nodes according to the layout of the edges that makes the factoring of effort into executability possible. Moreover, the assessment of effort requires that the "locometric" map be extended to include metric relations relevant to spatially extended actions, and that the map include, where appropriate, 3D as well as 2D relations. In a kitchen, if two storage spaces for plates are equidistant from the dishwasher, getting to a space at waist height would be considered more executable/less effortful than getting to one on a top shelf or at floor level. A staircase included in an initial design may have to be reassessed if it will require undue effort of some people to use it.

This leads us to the crucial architectural challenge of *melding diverse scripts*. At early stages of design, there may be multiple scripts, with each script having its own separate preliminary WG with little or no locometric specification of where and how the nodes will be linked to locations in the 3D Euclidean space in which the various spaces of the building will be placed. The edges in the preliminary WG will simply mark transitions that will occur from one place to another in executing the corresponding script. As design proceeds, the WG's nodes must become anchored in the Euclidean space. This can include decisions to map certain nodes in distinct WGs to the same location, and this entails that the two WGs become merged into one as shared nodes inherit their properties and the edges of their progenitors. This in turn requires assessing whether features of one script do or do not block features of the other script as the new WG is refined to accommodate both scripts. For example, the scripts for cooking and for excreting in a home would normally require separation into different spaces; the scripts for food preparation and dishwashing in a home would normally involve using the same sink, whereas in a restaurant they might not. Culture can play a role, as in the Japanese use of futons removing the need for a separate bedroom. Thus, in a Western context, "go to bed" might require the action of locomotion to go to the bedroom, whereas the Japanese version might require that the action "go to the futon cupboard" precede "take the futon out of the cupboard," which in turn precedes setting up the bedding for use.

In basic WG theory, as we explore a terrain/building/town, we "grow" a cognitive map even as we use it. We might come upon an actual place under such different circumstances that we fail to recognize that the two psychologically different nodes correspond to the same place in the external world. If and when we have that "aha" moment when we realize that the two apparent places are one and the same, the merger of nodes in the WG may have far-reaching changes—as, for example, the discovery that a much shorter path opens up to meet certain conditions after one realizes this identity.

Where the user's navigation through existing spaces defines WGs "bottom-up," the architect may define a range of WGs "top-down"— whether dictated by scripts for a user's behavior, exploitation of the site, or atmosphere and other aesthetic considerations. However, the "node-merging" that occurs as the architect discovers that places dreamed up as part of two different scripts may be realized by the same place in the building may, but need not, be applied to a set of spaces previously defined in three dimensions (registration to which defines the expanded-sense locometric map for each WG) but may itself involve the reshaping of those spaces. The design of a building at the WG level constrains but does not determine the actual placement of "nodes" and "edges" in 3D space. The process of working this out may reflect back to modify the "what connects to what" of design at the WG level.

The following about the artist (from §4.4) adapts easily to the work of the architect:

This is the inverse (opposite) in effect, but requires different brain mechanisms for its success. . . . The work may develop through multiple sketches as the [architect] not only places (representations) of objects . . . but adjusts them and their relationships to achieve atmospheric as well as "semantic" effects—and, in the process, the original conception of the piece may change as the initial work reveals new possibilities and while, perhaps, some of the earlier ideas come to feel unsatisfactory.

Within the design process, scripts compete and cooperate. A given area may come to support multiple affordances (e.g., Utzon's provision of access to both the auditoriums and to the views of the Harbour), and ideas for the form of each begin to meld, or one reshapes the others. Similarly, the building may begin to morph as the spatial relationships between multiple scripts and the site are further developed. Each factor constrains the others, but the design process permits great flexibility even when site and program are specified: the top three designs in the Sydney Opera House competition offer very different ways to "solve" the same program.

After an architect (or team) has converged on an overall scheme for a building, attention can turn for a while to refining one of the subsystems or sub-subsystems, but with the understanding that each lower level decision may require changes in higher level decisions, and these effects may be contained or may propagate to modify or uproot higher level design decisions. All this is highly reminiscent of the dynamic interaction of bottom-up and top-down influences in activating *and parametrizing* diverse schemas that was exemplified in the VISIONS system.

Of course, real design is more complex than a direct transition from scripts to WGs to structures in 3D space. It involves not only matching the constraints of site and budget but also balancing diverse utilitarian and aesthetic demands. As design progresses, some parts of a design may seem sufficiently well worked out to provide "islands of reliability" that can anchor the ongoing design, at least for a while. But these may in turn be restructured as more satisfying islands of reliability emerge. In imagination and design, "part of the pattern" must remain stable long enough for other elements to fall into place in relation to it. This may yield a larger part of the pattern that itself becomes a new island of reliability—or the attempt to extend the initial island may prove unstable. Some subparts may survive for later use; others will be discarded, or greatly modified before they can re-enter the process. In particular, then, a certain embedding of parts of the building design in 3D space may provide the island of reliability for determining how best to merge certain WGs; conversely, attraction between WG nodes may place constraints on their 3D realization in the building. Such "islands" may vary from time to time and from one part of the building to another as design proceeds. As exemplified in our discussion of Frank Gehry's work, these processes within design are not "purely mental" in the way that visual perception is but involve the back and forth between the development and consideration of internal and external memories.

This perspective on scripts has implications for how architects develop the imaginative skills that will bolster the design process. Certain scripts are basic. How do you provide access to a building? How do you provide a kitchen that is well integrated with the dining room, and supports multiple functions? And so on. If one is not familiar with a range of designs that support these basic scripts, then one is perhaps unlikely to succeed in developing novel scripts that are likely to succeed both practically and aesthetically. But here is the point. Yes, one needs extensive experience of different buildings to master the design of buildings that support the basic scripts in varied ways. However, if all one knows are relatively routine examples of how to support a script, then one is probably doomed to provide relatively uninteresting buildings. Thus, the imagination needs to be fed by going through, or studying remotely, multiple buildings that use imaginative scripts or offer variations upon standard scripts in imaginative ways. This experience will build up a knowledge of diverse variations that can be made on scripts, and in combining building resources to support multiple scripts—and then these variations become available in developing imaginative scripts of one's own. The ability to deploy imagination in this way will depend not only on experience, but also on one's prior preparation, whether genetic or cultural, to learn from that experience.

10.5. AND SO WE COME TO THE END, WHICH IS
A BEGINNING

My aim has been to create a space for conversations that will engage both architects and neuroscientists (and, I hope, other readers as well), and frame future interactions between these communities. Our conversation has ranged over four different, but by no means independent, themes:

- Neuroscience of the experience of architecture
- Neuroscience of the design process
- Neuromorphic architecture
- The EvoDevoSocio perspective

While our focus in this chapter has been on design for architecture, IBSEN exploits capabilities rooted in the brain mechanisms that supported decisions made by protohumans and early humans, such as where to find materials to make stone tools, where to organize a fire for a campsite, where and how to dispose of the dead. The point is to again invoke our EvoDevoSocio framework. The biological underpinnings of IBSEN are deeply rooted in the biological evolution of *Homo sapiens*, but their exploitation by architects bears the marks of extended cultural evolution. Recall Mallgrave's (2009) analysis of how the architect's brain has changed over the centuries from the time of Alberti (himself inspired by Vitruvius) to the present day, and our observations on the diverse "languages" of architecture (§8.6). These changes are not biological, but rather reflect how developing in a particular environment shapes the human brain while leaving space for great variation in the imaginative abilities of different people. Perhaps more crucially, architecture does not evolve in isolation, but is both swept up in broader patterns of cultural evolution and, by transforming the built environment, can leave its mark on this flow, both literally and metaphorically. Indeed, it reflects a confluence of diverse strands of cultural evolution, including the development of language, sketching, and urbanism, as well as new materials and construction techniques.

These insights open up more questions than they answer. As we come to the end of the book, we are at the beginning of diverse new conversations both those (like this book) that seek to create a general framework and those that point the way to focused studies linking cog/neuro findings to specific problems in designing rooms, buildings, and larger environments that support human well-being. This final section first looks at some of the challenges opened up by the initial sketch of IBSEN, and then offers general observations on future A↔N conversations.

Beyond IBSEN

Although there has been some mention of contemplation and aesthetics, the focus of this chapter has been squarely on the design of a building to support affordances and the scripts that engage the user of a building in various action–perception cycles that exploit what the building has to offer. In this regard, IBSEN complements the ideas of Chapters 3, 4, and 5 on how the A↔N conversation may engage with issues like visual and motor aesthetics, balance of forms, atmosphere, and Einfühlung. Certainly, the visual impact of buildings was a dominant consideration in the case studies from Sydney and Bilbao in Chapter 9. However, IBSEN was designed to address what it is that distinguishes a successful building from a fine sculpture—that it provides a set of interconnected spaces in which people move, behave, and experience. Although this chapter touches on only a fraction of what goes through the architect's mind and brain during the design process, it does demonstrate the anchoring of a cognitive neuroscience of design in a set of key principles that have been developed in this volume:

- The approach to the experience of architecture via action-oriented perception can also inform the design of architecture, and bring its study within the ambit of cog/neuroscience.
- *Mental* construction holds the key to perception (and experience more generally), memory, and imagination and thus to the design process that develops the specifications for *physical* construction of buildings.
- Spaces are defined in great part by their spatial layout in relation to the affordances, both Gibsonian and non-Gibsonian, that they provide. Design in some measure inverts the processes of

action-oriented perception that will enable the user to exploit these relationships in the finished building.

- The design of a building involves the creation of multiple scripts for the intended use of the building, and these in turn support specification of cognitive maps/WGs whose nodes correspond to places (both inside and outside the building) that are significant in that they provide affordances for practical or contemplative actions.

- However, such places are not to be considered in isolation, but assessed for their relationship in diverse scripts for the expected use of the building. Design requires integration of the graphs for different scripts, and this may include the merging of nodes and their associated affordances and reconsideration of the adjacency relations between the nodes.

- Design must embed the resultant WGs in physical 3D space, and this may affect issues of executability that feed back into specification of WGs and even scripts.

- In many ways, the design process reiterates, on a larger scale and with great reliance on external memory, the processes of competition and cooperation that provides the framework for cooperative computation as the style of the brain.

In assessing a draft of this chapter, Mark Alan Hewitt (personal communication) argued that

there are "performance" criteria in all artifacts used by humans, but architects do not first assess their work according to these criteria. They have an intuitive, holistic appreciation for their task that, as Aalto says, allows them to "forget" all the functional, material and constructional requirements when they are in a creative groove, or "flow" state.

But must "flow" imply such "forgetting"? For Utzon, having two auditoriums side by side was an important constraint; for Gehry, the Guggenheim requirement for a long gallery provided a similar constraint. For Aalto himself, whatever the "flow" of aesthetic form-making that contributed to the design of his Paimio Sanatorium, his guiding concern remained to make the building a "medical instrument" to aid in the healing process for patients with tuberculosis. Chapter 9 gave a rich sample of the images that came to mind as Utzon and Gehry developed their designs, and the discussion of Gehry in particular gave a sense of the back and forth between the "flow" of semiautomatic sketching and the attention to programmatic demands.

In any case, we must distinguish the architects' introspection on their work, and the cog/neuroscientists' quest to understand the (in great part subconscious) cognitive and neural processes that make that work possible. A single chapter must, of course, be a simplification of the full design process, and my strategy has been to isolate some (not all) of what goes on in design within a conceptual model, in this case IBSEN, of cog/neuro processing that builds on the insights of the preceding chapters. Such insights provide a beginning, a basis for raising new challenges:

1. For much of the design process, the *details* of the physical construction, building the building, may be ignored, but at various stages they provide crucial constraints (cost, structural integrity, surface finish, and more) that will feed back to constrain various features of the design, in some cases forcing drastic changes in earlier design decisions, and in others simply filling in the details. The notion of "automatization" is relevant here— the architect may rely on a subconscious feel for what is feasible in the chosen medium of construction, and thus may come up with a design for which "filling in the details" is more feasible than would otherwise be the case. As construction details come into play, the shape of the forms may well have to be modified to meet the constraints of code and of physics. For example, the pronounced slope of the faces of the shells in Utzon's competition-winning entry is absent in the final building of the Sydney Opera House.

2. Mental construction in design is in great part separated from the physical process of constructing and using the building but may involve the discovery/invention of new "building blocks" and new forms of construction that may feed back into modifications of the design. Methods of construction of buildings are not restricted to joining assemblies into larger assemblies, but also involve the reshaping of components and may employ the forming of vast structures as units. Architecture as a design process may develop new building blocks (literally), changing the "lexicon" as when using new materials, or may even change the "grammar" when new construction methods are developed.

3. Many buildings are satisfying variations on a theme; others seek to offer something radically "new." Of course, novelty comes at a price—not just in economic terms but also (more cognitively) in terms of the reactions of viewers and users. There is a tradeoff between what people are prepared for in a new design, and what will require them to change some of their preconceptions to accept new forms or functionality. The latter may be affected both by social factors and by the rewards of the new functionality. Jerome Kagan's *discrepancy principle* (§3.2)—a preference for what is *slightly* different from what is familiar—leads to consideration of when a design should resemble other designs already adopted by a community, and when something truly new can become broadly admired. Here, the quest of certain individuals for novelty, the dissemination of opinions, and the simple familiarity that the years may bring may all serve to counter, yet welcome, *The Shock of the New* (Hughes, 1981). In §6.1, we speculated that the "joys" of exploration probably evolved as a survival strategy to support hunting and foraging, and the search for shelter— balanced by a primal fear of being lost or separated from "our group." Of course, this innate drive for exploration offers no guarantee that the place one finds is beneficial. Similarly, there is no guarantee that the architect's quest for novelty in place- making, and the consequent provision of enriching experience

and memories for a building's users, will be beneficial, or will—
though novel—prove to be the sort of kitsch that makes for bad
buildings and environments.[12]

4. Although for many buildings there may be one person who
    provides the guiding vision that shapes the work of others, there
    are other cases in which the final form emerges from interactions
    between multiple individuals. Understanding the final totality
    requires us to inquire who is responsible for what, and how
    the participants can communicate, so that, between them, they
    come up with the final coherent design. Chapter 9 showed how
    language, sketches, and models can each advance the interaction.
    A walk around the site together can provide a rich fund of shared
    images that may facilitate further interaction, developing ideas
    that may both compete and cooperate before an agreed-on (at
    least for a while!) part of the design may emerge. This raises
    challenges for *social* cognitive neuroscience as well as a reminder
    of our discussion of "external memory and the evolution of
    drawing" (§8.4), supporting the importance of sketches and
    architectural models in serving communication and innovation as
    well as memory.

Toward future A↔N conversations

Some might offer lessons from neuroscience, for which they would claim,
"Plug those in and that will help you do architecture," but my emphasis has
been, rather, to say to the architect, "Here are ways in which your understanding of the architectural experience and design may be enriched if
you understand how the brain is engaged in those processes." Another
aim, then, has been to encourage new studies by neuroscientists: "If you
think outside the box of the laboratory and look at people interacting with

---

12. In his Chapter 10, "Conceptual Architecture and the Digital Void," Hewitt (2020) places a
critique of novelty for novelty's sake in historical perspective.

each other and with buildings, you may come up with new challenges for your research." In some cases, these challenges may address very focused topics with immediate applications in architecture. In other cases, they may open up new avenues of basic research that only in the long run will feed back into the A↔N conversation.

All this leads me to declare, as we come to the end of the book, that we are at the beginning of a much richer interchange and collaboration between architecture and neuroscience, both broadly conceived. One hope I have for this chapter is that it will stimulate cog/neuroscientists to accumulate more data and systematize IBSEN in terms of explicitly modeled schemas and neuronal networks. Complementing this, my hope for the architect and the general reader is that, in thinking about buildings in their own experience, they will reinforce their understanding of the principles they have gleaned from this book, and that this understanding will equip many architects to more fully engage in the A↔N conversation.

Some architects have worried that neuroscience is going to provide algorithms that say "humans are like this; therefore you must build like that" and that this will remove all opportunity for spontaneity in architectural design. This will not happen, but perhaps there is some danger that certain findings from neuroscience might become overrated, so that many architects will design according to the same general observation about human response, and ignore the fact that humans vary greatly. However, complementing the neuroscience of design, recall (§1.3) John Eberhard's concern with understanding that the brains of different types of people vary greatly, and that this should be factored into the design of different typologies of buildings. Of course, most architects know that it is not helpful to design a building without understanding something of the experience of the client and factoring this into the design, but the notion here is that this can be enriched by more general insights from cog/neuroscience. Knowing something about the differences between the brain of a young child, a teenager, a mature adult, and someone suffering from dementia may help one understand what cues are needed to support wayfinding in the different populations.

Very often, an architect imagines that the neuroscientist is not so much to be engaged in conversation but to be a consultant who will be presented with a highly specific problem and provide a cost-efficient solution—in the same way that one engages a structural engineer without any interest in talking about engineering research. Perhaps, in future, there will be professionals devoted to such consultation. Even then, the consultant who can help with how ceiling heights combine with color are different from those with expertise on choice of materials in relation to acoustics. However, for myself, the emphasis is on conversations in which the architect really wants to understand what it is that neuroscientists think about, and neuroscientists really want to think about how their lessons from focused experiments in their lab can be merged with the work of many others to develop the built environment in such a way that it will be both useful and enjoyable for those who experience it.

This book has placed neuroscience in a larger context with psychology and other human sciences on the one side and artificial intelligence on the other, disciplines that shelter under the broad umbrella of *cybernetics*. A crucial reminder is that we need to complement phenomenology with rational analysis not only of how people interact with buildings (or vice versa!) but also of social interactions. Through conversations with this range of disciplines, architects will enrich their understanding of human action, perception, and social interaction, and this will inform the way they think about the design of buildings and the larger systems of which they are part. Complementing this, some neuroscientists and other scientists may become more familiar with the translational science of moving from lab studies to real-world situations, which include how people react to the built environment. These two efforts will combine to constitute a conversation in which questions can be raised about how different buildings affect different people, and how buildings and larger environments can be better adapted to the needs of diverse kinds of people—not only the better-off people whom one normally thinks of as hiring architects but also people who are disadvantaged. Perhaps the needs of the latter will best be met by some form of social housing, whether by explicit design by architects and urban planners or by providing support for the self-organization demonstrated with varying degrees of success in the favelas and shanty-towns of the world.

Since this is not a "how-to" book, I have not emphasized prior collaborations between architects and neuroscientists, nor do I offer explicit guidance for future collaborations. However, here are some examples that help point the way for further such collaborations:

Perhaps the most famous study linking cognitive science and architecture is Roger Ulrich's (1984) "View Through a Window May Influence Recovery," that may be seen as adding a new script, or rather a family of scripts, to architecture, based on assessment of the power of biophilia:

> Records on recovery after [gall bladder surgery] of patients in a suburban Pennsylvania hospital between 1972 and 1981 were examined to determine whether assignment to a room with a window view of a natural setting might have restorative influences. Twenty-three surgical patients assigned to rooms with windows looking out on a natural scene had shorter postoperative hospital stays, received fewer negative evaluative comments in nurses' notes, and took fewer potent analgesics than 23 matched patients in similar rooms with windows facing a brick building wall.

An important control was that patients were assigned to rooms as they became vacant, ruling out the possibility that richer (and thus possibly healthier) patients could afford rooms with the external view. On the other hand, this study does not determine what aspects of the view made it beneficial. Would indoor potted plants or a large TV screen projecting a similar image serve as well, or could architectural tweaks or changes in room layout have similar benefits? Again, more studies are required to assess whether benefits for surgical recovery would also be benefits for other hospital patients, let alone for different uses and users of different types of buildings.

In noting all this, in no way do I belittle the importance of Ulrich's study—I simply note that it is too big a leap from this focused study to general claims for the general benefits of biophilic architectural designs.

Indeed, some experiences of nature can be downright horrifying. Follow-up studies already exist, but in each case the architect must assess whether the special conditions involved do or do not make the findings relevant to a current design project. Here, let me note that Grant Hildebrand's (1999) *Origins of Architectural Pleasure* involves no neuroscience in the strict sense—but provides analyses of various buildings that are highly relevant for future work studying variations in neural correlates of mood and emotion with experience of different architected spaces. Complementing the assessment of architectural features that augment human well-being, there are studies of the effects of poor environments, or what might be called environmental deprivation. The challenge is to transfer insights from such studies into programs to provide housing for the poor that enriches their lives, rather than creating new high-rise slums. A chronic problem, and a challenge that takes us beyond the neuroscience of the experience of architecture to the need to devise new studies linking brain, body, and environment with *politico-architecture* as a branch of environmental studies, in raising political momentum for the support of public housing that is affordable, beneficial, and enjoyable.

We examined (§4.5) an exploratory fMRI study of "contemplative" spaces by Bermudez et al. (2017) to note the challenges of designing such studies. How meaningful was the restriction of subjects to be architects to conclusions about design for other users of buildings? And was the study really looking at response to contemplative versus noncontemplative spaces, or to "famous" versus "ordinary" buildings? We showed how such questions point the way to future studies. Later, in §5.7, "Neuroaesthetics revisited, and more," we sampled a range of A↔N efforts. And, of course, when we focus on different specific aspects of building design, we can discover a range of studies of human experience that can factor back into parametric information that can modulate the design process. To offer just one example, Amber Dance (2017) begins her review of "Science and Culture: The Brain Within Buildings" by discussing the collaboration of neuroscientist Satchinananda Panda, an expert on circadian rhythms, and architect Frederick Marks (Academy of Neuroscience for Architecture [ANFA] President, 2019–2020) to characterize how lighting affects people in the built environment. Many further examples can be found on the Conference pages of the ANFA website.

Such studies gain a new dimension as we bring neuroscience to play on the development of smart architecture (dynamic buildings, responsive computational infrastructure) in general, and *neuromorphic architecture* in particular. Here, we must assess human behavioral, cognitive, and neural responses to assess which interaction patterns prove most attractive or productive for people in different typologies, whether in utilitarian or aesthetic terms, and then factor this into new ideas for design practice. In the latter case, the design of the sensors, effectors, and "brain" (interaction infrastructure) of the building will be enriched by studies in neuroethology, looking at the evolved differences in body, brain, and behavior that fit animals to their specific ecological niche. As we saw in Chapter 7, a crucial ethical challenge for the linkage of architecture with cybernetics comes from the increasing use of artificial intelligence in the home. Already, devices supplied by Amazon, Google, and other providers are gathering immense amounts of data about individuals, not to mention the increasing use of surveillance cameras in public spaces. A great debate is already underway on privacy, and this will continue with respect to broader concerns about the nature of a just society that will spill over into issues that concern architects specifically.

All this is complemented by our development (especially in Chapter 8) of the EvoDevoSocio framework in which we seek to understand the dynamics of niche construction whereby cultural evolution has reshaped human brains and human environments across tens of thousands of millennia. What does this mean when rapid changes occur on a time scale of decades or less, rather than centuries or millennia?

If it succeeds, this book will encourage detailed case studies of how different types of people experience specific aspects of different buildings, as well as historical case studies like those of Chapter 9 in which the aim is to enrich our understanding of the mental and neural processes that underlie the design practices of diverse architects. Chapter 9 made no pretence to reveal neural particularities that distinguish the brains of Utzon or Gehry from those of other architects. Rather, it helped us probe more deeply how architects learn from experience—their experience within buildings, and their experience designing buildings—and are shaped by and can reshape the world around them.

The conversation between architecture and neuroscience that has *begun* here may thus reflect back into the education of architects who, by thinking more explicitly about their cognitive processes and the action–perception cycles of those who experience buildings, can get a new handle on what goes on in the experience and then design of buildings. The further hope is to stimulate neuroscientists and cognitive scientists to find new challenges for their own research. I also hope to have engaged many others who share an interest in both brains and buildings.

Let's be candid. Very few neuroscientists will become architects, and very few architects will become neuroscientists, but that does not deny the power of partnerships. More broadly, the aim of the conversations in this book has been to build enough of a shared vocabulary and range of examples to enable the neuroscientist to think more richly about the experience of the built environment, and the architect to embrace the idea that understanding key ideas about cognitive and neural processes can enrich, rather than inhibit, a creative approach to design. Hundreds of architects and a lesser number of neuroscientists engage in the activities of the Academy of Neuroscience for Architecture (anfarch.org), or engage in related meetings hosted by other organizations. Yet I have found that too few neuroscientists have gone much beyond proclaiming the importance of their specialized studies to explore their relevance to architecture, and few architects currently know enough about brains to sustain a deep conversation. My hope is that the conversations synthesized in this book will indeed encourage many architects and neuroscientists (in the broadest sense) to learn more about each other's work and concepts—whether to engage in lively conversations or even to develop active partnerships.

With the understanding of both what we have achieved and the many focused issues in the experience and design of (possibly neuromorphic) architecture that remain, it is clear that, as we come to the end of this book, we are only at the beginning of many, and highly varied, A↔N conversations as architects and cog/neuroscientists work together to address focused challenges in better linking future rooms, buildings, and towns to the needs and capabilities of their human users. Of course, architects must engage in a number of vital conversations complementing those charted in this volume. Perhaps the most important conversations in the coming decades will be those in which humanity either faces or fails to face how human habitation, work, and play can adapt to meet the challenges of climate change and inequality. In this connection, the use of remote work will play an important role as a way to decrease pollution, and not just to avoid pandemic contact. More generally, the transition to renewable energy sources will complement development of new materials and techniques for "green" buildings. At the same time, the plight of essential workers during the pandemic reminds us that there is a crisis of inequality that cannot be solved by architects alone, but that requires architects to work with city planners, developers, and, yes, even politicians to provide low-cost housing of high quality for workers that places them within easy commuting distance of their work.

REFERENCES

Addis, D. R., & Schacter, D. (2012). The hippocampus and imagining the future: Where do we stand? *Frontiers in Human Neuroscience*, 5(173). doi:10.3389/fnhum.2011.00173

Addis, D. R., Wong, A. T., & Schacter, D. L. (2007). Remembering the past and imagining the future: Common and distinct neural substrates during event construction and elaboration. *Neuropsychologia*, 45(7), 1363–1377. doi:10.1016/j.neuropsychologia.2006.10.016

Aguirre, G. K., Detre, J. A., Alsop, D. C., & D'Esposito, M. (1996). The parahippocampus subserves topographical learning in man. *Cerebral Cortex*, 6(6), 823–829. doi:10.1093/cercor/6.6.823

Aguirre, G. K., Zarahn, E., & D'Esposito, M. (1998). An area within human ventral cortex sensitive to "building" stimuli: Evidence and implications. *Neuron*, 21(2), 373–383. doi:10.1016/S0896-6273(00)80546-2

Amado Lorenzo, A. (2012). Kahn and Barragán: Convergence in the Salk Institute plaza. *EGA-Revista de Expresion Grafica Arquitectonica*, 19, 126–135.

Arbib, M. A. (2020). From spatial navigation via visual construction to episodic memory and imagination. *Biological Cybernetics*, 114, 139–167. doi:10.1007/s00422-020-00829-7

Arbib, M. A., Érdi, P., & Szentágothai, J. (1998). *Neural organization: Structure, function, and dynamics*. Cambridge, MA: MIT Press.

Baldassano, C., Chen, J., Zadbood, A., Pillow, J. W., Hasson, U., & Norman, K. A. (2017). Discovering event structure in continuous narrative perception and memory. *Neuron*, 95(3), 709–721.e705. doi:10.1016/j.neuron.2017.06.041

Baldassano, C., Esteva, A., Fei-Fei, L., & Beck, D. M. (2016). Two Distinct Scene-Processing Networks Connecting Vision and Memory. *eNeuro*, 3(5), ENEURO.0178–0116.2016. doi:10.1523/ENEURO.0178-16.2016

Bermudez, J., Krizaj, D., Lipschitz, D. L., Bueler, C. E., Rogowska, J., Yurgelun-Todd, D., & Nakamura, Y. (2017). Externally-induced meditative states: an exploratory fMRI study of architects' responses to contemplative architecture. *Frontiers of Architectural Research*, 6(2), 123–136. doi:10.1016/j.foar.2017.02.002

Bloomer, K. C., & Moore, C. W. (1977). *Body, memory, and architecture*. New Haven and London: Yale University Press.

Caligiore, D., Arbib, M. A., Miall, R. C., & Baldassarre, G. (2019). The super-learning hypothesis: Integrating learning processes across cortex, cerebellum and basal ganglia. *Neuroscience and Biobehavioral Reviews*, 100, 19–34. doi:10.1016/j.neubiorev.2019.02.008

Dance, A. (2017). Science and culture: The brain within buildings. *Proceedings of the National Academy of Sciences*, 114(5), 785–787. doi:10.1073/pnas.1620658114

Elward, R. L., & Vargha-Khadem, F. (2018). Semantic memory in developmental amnesia. *Neuroscience Letters*, 680, 23–30. doi:10.1016/j.neulet.2018.04.040

Epstein, R., & Kanwisher, N. (1998). A cortical representation of the local visual environment. *Nature*, 392(6676), 598–601. doi:10.1038/33402

Ericsson, K. A., & Kintsch, W. (1995). Long-term working memory. *Psychological Review*, 102, 211–245.

Fanselow, M. S., & Dong, H.-W. (2010). Are the dorsal and ventral hippocampus functionally distinct structures? *Neuron*, 65(1), 7–19. doi:10.1016/j.neuron.2009.11.031

Felleman, D. J., & Van Essen, D. C. (1991). Distributed hierarchical processing in the primate cerebral cortex. *Cerebral Cortex*, 1, 1–47.

Hassabis, D., Kumaran, D., & Maguire, E. A. (2007). Using imagination to understand the neural basis of episodic memory. *Journal of Neuroscience*, 27(52), 14365–14374. doi:10.1523/jneurosci.4549-07.2007

Hassabis, D., & Maguire, E. A. (2009). The construction system of the brain. *Philosophical Transactions of the Royal Society B: Biological Sciences*, 364(1521), 1263–1271. doi:10.1098/rstb.2008.0296

Hewitt, M. A. (2020). *Draw in order to see: A cognitive history of architectural design*. San Francisco: ORO Editions.

Hildebrand, G. (1999). *Origins of architectural pleasure*. Berkeley, CA: University of California Press.

Hughes, R. (1981). *The shock of the new: The hundred-year history of modern art its rise, its dazzling achievement, it's fall*. New York: Knopf.

Kandel, E. R., Schwartz, J. H., Jessell, T. M., Siegelbaum, S. A., & Hudspeth, A. J. (2013). *Principles of neural science* (5th ed.). New York: McGraw-Hill, Health Professions Division.

Kravitz, D. J., Saleem, K. S., Baker, C. I., & Mishkin, M. (2011). A new neural framework for visuospatial processing. *Nature Reviews Neuroscience*, 12, 217. doi:10.1038/nrn3008

Kravitz, D. J., Saleem, K. S., Baker, C. I., Ungerleider, L. G., & Mishkin, M. (2013). The ventral visual pathway: An expanded neural framework for the processing of object quality. *TRENDS in Cognitive Sciences*, 17(1), 26–49. doi:10.1016/j.tics.2012.10.011

Lynch, K. (1960). *The image of the city*. Cambridge, MA: MIT Press.

Mallgrave, H. F. (2009). *The architect's brain: Neuroscience, creativity, and architecture*. New York: Wiley-Blackwell.

Moscovitch, M., Cabeza, R., Winocur, G., & Nadel, L. (2016). Episodic memory and beyond: The hippocampus and neocortex in transformation. *Annual Review of Psychology*, 67, 105–134.

Rauschecker, J. P., & Tian, B. (2000). Mechanisms and streams for processing of "what" and "where" in auditory cortex. *Proceedings of the National Academy of Sciences*, 97(22), 11800–11806. doi:10.1073/pnas.97.22.11800

Robin, J., & Moscovitch, M. (2017). Details, gist and schema: Hippocampal–neocortical interactions underlying recent and remote episodic and spatial memory. *Current Opinion in Behavioral Sciences*, 17, 114–123. doi:10.1016/j.cobeha.2017.07.016

Romanski, L. M., Tian, B., Fritz, J., Mishkin, M., Goldman-Rakic, P. S., & Rauschecker, J. P. (1999). Dual streams of auditory afferents target multiple domains in the primate prefrontal cortex. *Nature Neuroscience*, 2(12), 1131–1136.

Schacter, D. L., Addis, D. R., Hassabis, D., Martin, V. C., Spreng, R. N., & Szpunar, K. K. (2012). The future of memory: remembering, imagining, and the brain. *Neuron*, 76(4), 677–694.

Teyler, T. J., & Rudy, J. W. (2007). The hippocampal indexing theory and episodic memory: Updating the index. *Hippocampus*, 17(12), 1158–1169. doi:10.1002/hipo.20350

Ulrich, R. (1984). View through a window may influence recovery. *Science*, 224(4647), 224–225.

For the benefit of digital users, indexed terms that span two pages (e.g., 52–53) may, on occasion, appear on only one of those pages.

Figures are indicated by *f* following the page numbers. Notes are indicated by n.

Printed in the USA
CPSIA information can be obtained
at www.ICGtesting.com
CBHW050807230424
7300CB00010B/35